P9-CKX-717

Methods in Cell Biology

VOLUME 51
Methods in Avian Embryology

Series Editors

Leslie Wilson
Department of Biological Sciences
University of California, Santa Barbara
Santa Barbara, California

Paul Matsudaira
Whitehead Institute for Biomedical Research and
Department of Biology
Massachusetts Institute of Technology
Cambridge, Massachusetts

Methods in Cell Biology

Prepared under the Auspices of the American Society for Cell Biology

VOLUME 51
Methods in Avian Embryology

Edited by

Marianne Bronner-Fraser

Developmental Biology Center
University of California
Irvine, California

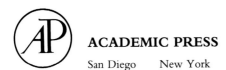

ACADEMIC PRESS

San Diego   New York   Boston   London   Sydney   Tokyo   Toronto

Cover photograph (paperback edition only): Section through the trunk
region of a stage 18 HH chick embryo. From Chapter 16, Fig. 6 by Sechrist
and Marcelle. For details see color insert.

This book is printed on acid-free paper. ∞

Copyright © 1996 by ACADEMIC PRESS, INC.

All Rights Reserved.
No part of this publication may be reproduced or transmitted in any form or by any
means, electronic or mechanical, including photocopy, recording, or any information
storage and retrieval system, without permission in writing from the publisher.

Academic Press, Inc.
A Division of Harcourt Brace & Company
525 B Street, Suite 1900, San Diego, California 92101-4495

United Kingdom Edition published by
Academic Press Limited
24-28 Oval Road, London NW1 7DX

International Standard Serial Number: 0091-679X

International Standard Book Number: 0-12-564153-2 (Hardcover)

International Standard Book Number: 0-12-135275-7 (Paperback)

PRINTED IN THE UNITED STATES OF AMERICA
96 97 98 99 00 01 EB 9 8 7 6 5 4 3 2 1

CONTENTS

Contributors   xi

Preface   xiii

1. Culture and Microsurgical Manipulation of the Early Avian Embryo

Mark A. J. Selleck

    I. General Introduction   1
    II. Culture of the Avian Embryo   2
    III. Tools for Microsurgery   13
    IV. Microsurgical Approaches to the Young Embryo   14
    References   19

2. Quail-Chick Transplantations

Nicole Le Douarin, Françoise Dieterlen-Lièvre, and Marie-Aimée Teillet

    I. Introduction   24
    II. Differential Diagnosis of Quail and Chick Cells   27
    III. Material and Equipment   29
    IV. Preparation and Sealing of Eggs   35
    V. Neural Tissue Transplantations   35
    VI. Early Transplantations in Blastodiscs   40
    VII. Hemopoietic Organ Rudiment Transplantations   44
    VIII. Results, Discussion, and Perspectives   51
    References   54

3. Manipulations of Neural Crest Cells or Their Migratory Pathways

Marianne Bronner-Fraser

    I. Introduction   61
    II. Preparation of Avian Neural Crest Cultures   62
    III. Microinjection of Cells and Antibodies into Embryos   70
    IV. Labeling of Neural Crest Cells *in Vivo* with Vital Dyes   72
    V. Grafting Techniques   74
    VI. Conclusions   78
    References   78

4. Manipulation of the Avian Segmental Plate *in Vivo*

Brian A. Williams and Charles P. Ordahl

    I. Introduction   81
    II. Materials   82

 III. Methods 84
 IV. Critical Aspects of the Procedure 90
  V. Results and Discussion 91
 VI. Conclusions and Perspectives 91
   References 92

5. Somite Strips: An Embryo Fillet Preparation

Kathryn W. Tosney, Robert A. Oakley, Mia Champion, Lisa Bodley, Rebecca Sexton, and Kevin B. Hotary

  I. Introduction 94
  II. Fillet Preparation 94
 III. Critical Aspects 101
 IV. Analyzing Neurites to Assess Guidance Interactions 104
  V. Conclusions and Perspectives 104
   References 107

6. Embryo Slices

Kevin B. Hotary, Lynn T. Landmesser, and Kathryn W. Tosney

  I. Introduction 109
  II. Cutting and Culturing Embryo Slices 110
 III. Embryo Slice Characteristics 116
 IV. Experimental Results Using Embryo Slices 117
  V. Conclusions and Perspectives 122
   References 123

7. Operations on Limb Buds of Avian Embryos

John W. Saunders, Jr.

  I. Introduction 125
  II. Preparing to Operate 126
 III. Extraembryonic Membranes 131
 IV. Making Various Kinds of Grafts 133
  V. Manipulations Involving the Apical Ectodermal Ridge 139
 VI. Grafts to Test Polarizing Activity 141
 VII. Enzymatic Dissociation and Recombination of Limb Tissues 142
   References 144

8. Iontophoretic Dye Labeling of Embryonic Cells

Scott E. Fraser

  I. Introduction 147
  II. Iontophoretic Microinjection of Lineage Tracers 149
 III. Iontophoretic Application of DiI 158
 IV. Relative Advantages of Dextran and DiI 159
   References 160

9. Gene Transfer Using Replication-Defective Retroviral and
Adenoviral Vectors

Steven M. Leber, Masahito Yamagata, and Joshua R. Sanes

I.	Introduction	162
II.	Retroviral Vectors	162
III.	Adenoviral Vectors	168
IV.	Injection of Virus into Chick Embryos	173
V.	Histology and Histochemistry	174
VI.	Uses of Viral Vectors	177
	References	181

10. Manipulating Gene Expression with Replication-Competent
Retroviruses

Bruce A. Morgan and Donna M. Fekete

I.	Introduction	186
II.	Materials	195
III.	Methods	196
IV.	Results and Discussion	214
V.	Conclusions and Perspectives	216
	References	217

11. *In Situ* Hybridization Analysis of Chick Embryos in Whole Mount and
Tissue Sections

M. Angela Nieto, Ketan Patel, and David G. Wilkinson

I.	Introduction	220
II.	When to Hybridize to Sections or Whole Mounts	221
III.	Solutions	221
IV.	Whole Mount *in Situ* Hybridization	222
V.	Double Detection of Two RNAs	228
VI.	Double Detection of RNA and Protein	229
VII.	Combined DiI Labeling and *in Situ* Hybridization	230
VIII.	*In Situ* Hybridization to Tissue Sections	230
IX.	Troubleshooting Guide	233
	References	235

12. Micromass Cultures of Limb and Other Mesenchyme

Karla Daniels, Rebecca Reiter, and Michael Solursh

I.	Introduction	237
II.	Micromass Culture Technique	238
III.	Use of Micromass Cultures in Teratology	245
IV.	Discussion and Perspectives	246
	References	246

13. Autonomic and Sensory Neuron Cultures

Rae Nishi

    I. Introduction   249
    II. Materials   251
    III. Methods   252
    IV. Critical Aspects of the Procedures   259
    V. Results and Discussion   261
    VI. Summary and Conclusions   262
    References   262

14. Retinal Cultures

Deborah Finlay, George Wilkinson, Robert Kypta, Ivan de Curtis, and Louis Reichardt

    I. Introduction   265
    II. Obtaining Primary Cells   266
    III. Cell Culture   275
    IV. Neuronal Cell Assays   278
    V. Concluding Remarks   282
    References   282

15. Migration and Adhesion Assays

Thomas Lallier

    I. Introduction   285
    II. Materials   285
    III. Assay Methods   287
    IV. Conclusions   299
    References   299

16. Cell Division and Differentiation in Avian Embryos: Techniques for Study of Early Neurogenesis and Myogenesis

John Sechrist and Christophe Marcelle

    I. Cell Cycle and Cell Specialization   301
    II. Cell Division and Neural Differentiation   303
    III. Cell Division and Somite Differentiation   307
    IV. Primary Methods Selected to Detect Dividing Cells   309
    V. Selected Histological Procedures   316
    References   327

17. Time-Lapse Cinephotomicrography, Videography, and Videomicrography of the Avian Blastoderm

H. Bortier, M. Callebaut, and L. C. A. Vakaet

    I. Introduction   331
    II. General Methods   332

III. Time-Lapse Cinephotomatography, Videography, and
       Videomicrography Installation   341
  IV. Critical Aspects of Time-Lapse Video Registration   343
   V. Results and Discussion   343
  VI. Conclusions and Perspectives   353
       References   353

Index   355
Volumes in Series   365

CONTRIBUTORS

Numbers in parentheses indicate the pages on which the authors' contributions begin.

Lisa Bodley (93), Department of Biology, The University of Michigan, Ann Arbor, Michigan 48109

H. Bortier (331), Laboratory of Human Anatomy and Embryology, University Centre Antwerpen (RUCA), 2020 Antwerpen, Belgium

Marianne Bronner-Fraser (61), Developmental Biology Center, University of California, Irvine, California 92717

M. Callebaut (331), Laboratory of Human Anatomy and Embryology, University Centre Antwerpen (RUCA), 2020 Antwerpen, Belgium

Mia Champion (93), Department of Biology, The University of Michigan, Ann Arbor, Michigan 48109

Karla Daniels (237), Department of Biological Sciences, University of Iowa, Iowa City, Iowa 52242

Ivan de Curtis[1] (265), Howard Hughes Medical Institute and Department of Physiology, University of California, San Francisco, California 94143

Françoise Dieterlen-Lièvre (23), Institut d'Embryologie Cellulaire et Moléculaire du CNRS et du Collège de France, 94736 Nogent-sur-Marne, France

Donna M. Fekete (185), Department of Biology, Boston College, Chestnut Hill, Massachusetts 02167

Deborah Finlay (265), Howard Hughes Medical Institute and Department of Physiology, University of California, San Francisco, California 94143

Scott E. Fraser (147), Division of Biology, Beckman Institute, California Institute of Technology, Pasadena, California 91125

Kevin B. Hotary (93, 109), Department of Internal Medicine and Comprehensive Cancer Center, The University of Michigan Medical School, Ann Arbor, Michigan 48109

Robert Kypta (265), Howard Hughes Medical Institute and Department of Physiology, University of California, San Francisco, California 94143

Thomas Lallier (285), Department of Cell Biology, University of Virginia, Charlottesville, Virginia 22908

Lynn T. Landmesser (109), Department of Neuroscience, Case Western Reserve University School of Medicine, Cleveland, Ohio 44106

Nicole Le Douarin (23), Institut d'Embryologie Cellulaire et Moléculaire du CNRS et du Collège de France, 94736 Nogent-sur-Marne, France

Steven M. Leber (161), Division of Pediatric Neurology, University of Michigan Medical Center, Ann Arbor, Michigan 48109

[1] Present address: Department of Biology and Technology, San Raffaele Hospital, 20132 Milano, Italy.

Christophe Marcelle (301), Developmental Biology Center, University of California, Irvine, California 92717

Bruce A. Morgan (185), Cutaneous Biology Research Center, Harvard Medical School and Massachusetts General Hospital, Charlestown, Massachusetts 02129

M. Angela Nieto (219), Instituto Cajal, 28002 Madrid, Spain

Rae Nishi (249), Department of Cell and Developmental Biology, Oregon Health Sciences University, Portland, Oregon 97201

Robert A. Oakley (93), Department of Biology, The University of Michigan, Ann Arbor, Michigan 48109

Charles P. Ordahl (81), Department of Anatomy and Cardiovascular Research Institute, University of California, San Francisco, California 94143

Ketan Patel (219), Laboratory of Developmental Neurobiology, National Institute for Medical Research, London NW7 1AA, United Kingdom

Louis Reichardt (265), Howard Hughes Medical Institute and Department of Physiology, University of California, San Francisco, California 94143

Rebecca Reiter (237), Department of Biological Sciences, University of Iowa, Iowa City, Iowa 52242

Joshua R. Sanes (161), Department of Anatomy and Neurobiology, Washington University School of Medicine, St. Louis, Missouri 63110

John W. Saunders, Jr. (125), Department of Biological Sciences, State University of New York, Albany, New York 12222

John Sechrist (301), Developmental Biology Center, University of California, Irvine, California 92717

Mark A. J. Selleck (1), Department of Developmental and Cell Biology and Developmental Biology Center, University of California, Irvine, California 92717

Rebecca Sexton (93), Department of Biology, The University of Michigan, Ann Arbor, Michigan 48109

Michael Solursh[2](237), Department of Biological Sciences, University of Iowa, Iowa City, Iowa 52242

Marie-Aimée Teillet (23), Institut d'Embryologie Cellulaire et Moléculaire du CNRS et du Collèege de France, 94736 Nogent-sur-Marne, France

Kathryn W. Tosney (93, 109), Department of Biology, The University of Michigan, Ann Arbor, Michigan 48109

L. C. A. Vakaet (331), Laboratory of Experimental Cancerology, University Hospital, 9000 Gent, Belgium

David G. Wilkinson (219), Laboratory of Developmental Neurobiology, National Institute for Medical Research, London NW7 1AA, United Kingdom

George Wilkinson (265), Howard Hughes Medical Institute and Department of Physiology, University of California, San Francisco, California 94143

Brian A. Williams (81), Department of Anatomy and Cardiovascular Research Institute, University of California, San Francisco, California 94143

Masahito Yamagata (161), Division of Molecular Neurobiology, National Institute for Basic Biology, Okazaki, Aichi, Japan

[2] Deceased.

PREFACE

For over a century, embryologists have been intrigued with the central question in developmental biology: How does a complex organism develop from a single cell? In the past decade, the application of modern techniques in molecular biology to the study of this longstanding embryological question has led to a resurgence of interest in this fascinating field.

The questions in embryology are wide-ranging and include how cells proliferate, migrate, and differentiate. A number of different developing tissues have proved extremely valuable in studying these issues. These include the nervous system, somites, neural crest, limb, and many other organ systems.

For studies of vertebrate develoment, a number of organisms, each with its relative merits and weaknesses, have proved readily accessible to analysis. Bird and frog embryos are easily accessible to transplantation and experimental manipulations, whereas mouse and zebrafish embryos are ideally suited to genetic manipulation. However, no individual organism can serve to answer all embryological questions. In fact, it is becoming increasingly common to take a multiorganismal and evolutionary approach to studying complex developmental questions.

The avian embryo represents an important model system for developmental and cell biological studies because of its ease of manipulation and its similarity to mammalian development. This book is a compilation of diverse techniques that are used to study a number of questions in avian development. The methodologies range from classical embryological approaches to modern molecular biological and image analysis techniques. Chapters include descriptions of embryonic transplantations, cell culture, organ culture, *in situ* hybridization, dye labeling techniques, classical histological techniques, and retrovirally mediated gene transfer. The unique feature of this book is that it is specifically devoted to providing detailed approaches with adaptations that work optimally for avian embryos.

The authors have attempted to include detailed methodologies that describe both the potentials and the pitfalls of various embryological and cell biological approaches. The goal was to allow direct implementation of these techniques in the reader's laboratory.

I thank all of the authors for their thoughtful and thorough contributions and particularly for their attention to detail. I also take this opportunity to thank the excellent staff of Academic Press, particularly Jasna Markovac, for helping bring this volume to fruition.

Marianne Bronner-Fraser

CHAPTER 1

Culture and Microsurgical Manipulation of the Early Avian Embryo

Mark A. J. Selleck

Department of Developmental and Cell Biology and
Developmental Biology Center
University of California
Irvine, California 92717

I. General Introduction
II. Culture of the Avian Embryo
    A. Introduction
    B. Accessing the Avian Embryo *in Ovo*
    C. New Culture
    D. Alternative Culture Methods
III. Tools for Microsurgery
IV. Microsurgical Approaches to the Young Embryo
    A. Explantation of Donor Embryos
    B. Enzymes for Dissection
    C. Culture of Young Embryos: Tips and Special Considerations
    References

I. General Introduction

The early stages of chick embryo development are arguably the most appealing for study. Within the first 48 hr of incubation, the embryo changes from a relatively patternless disc of cells to a trilaminar embryo with a discernible rostrocaudal axis and with nearly all major organ systems under construction. Unfortunately, the early embryo is also the most challenging to the developmental biologist in terms of its culture and manipulation. The embryos are incredibly small, fragile, and sensitive to many substances that are harmless to older embryos. Much to our advantage, the innovative and pioneering work of the experimental embryologists in the first half of this century has provided us with the

Copyright © 1996 by Academic Press, Inc. All rights of reproduction in any form reserved.

means to overcome these difficulties. A brief foray into any of the classic papers and books of that time will reveal that many of the techniques employed are practically identical to those in use currently. Moreover, many of the older approaches to embryo culture that have since lost favor with developmental biologists should be seriously reconsidered for use in today's laboratory.

The culture of chick embryos and microsurgical techniques have received attention from many authors. Some excellent books that contain detailed descriptions include those by Hamburger (1960), New (1966), and Stern and Holland (1993). This chapter briefly reviews methods that have been used to culture avian embryos at all stages of development and discusses in more detail those techniques commonly used for culturing young chick embryos. Useful variations in the basic techniques are considered, followed by a discussion of microsurgical procedures as they relate to young avian embryos.

II. Culture of the Avian Embryo

A. Introduction

The problem of how to gain access to the avian embryo while allowing it to grow normally has been the subject of many studies. Essentially four different approaches have been used for the cultivation of avian embryos:

1. culture of the embryo in the shell (Hamburger, 1960; New, 1966; Barnett, 1982; Callebaut, 1983; Iyengar, 1983; Perry, 1988; Naito and Perry, 1989; Naito *et al.,* 1990; Stern, 1993b; Ono *et al.,* 1994),
2. culture of the embryo after removal of the shell ("shell-less culture") (Romanoff, 1943; Corner and Richter, 1973; Auerbach *et al.,* 1974; Dunn, 1974; Palén and Thörneby, 1976; Ono and Wakasugi, 1983),
3. culture of the embryo on its vitelline membrane after explantation from the yolk (New, 1955, 1966; Flamme, 1987; Kucera and Burnand, 1987; Flamme *et al.,* 1991; Stern, 1993a), and
4. culture of the embryo on a plasma or agar clot (Waddington, 1932; Spratt, 1947a,b; Mitrani and Shimoni, 1990; Bortier and Vakaet, 1992; Eyal-Giladi *et al.,* 1994; Schoenwolf, 1995) or on the chorioallantoic membrane of a host embryo (Willier, 1926).

The choice of culture method depends on a number of variables, including the age of the embryo at the start of the experiment, the length of time the embryo must be cultured, and the nature of the intervention (ranging from no perturbation of the embryo to extensive incisions and fragmentation). Figure 1 illustrates the times during which various culture techniques may be used. For young embryos, culture of the embryo in the shell (so-called "*in ovo* culture") and culture of the embryo on its vitelline membrane are most widely used. A consensus approach to each of these culture methods is described next, followed by a brief discussion of modifications and alternative culture methods.

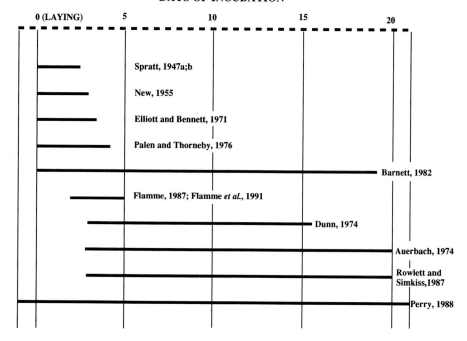

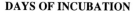

Fig. 1 A range of methods have been developed for culturing avian embryos. This chart indicates the period during avian development for which a technique is particularly useful. A representative sample of published culture methods has been selected for inclusion.

B. Accessing the Avian Embryo *in Ovo*

Two approaches to the long-term cultivation of avian embryos have been taken: (i) culture of embryos in the shell, and (ii) shell-less culture. Embryos cultured in shell-less conditions are easily visible and accessible to both mild manipulations (such as chorioallantoic grafting) and to test chemicals for teratological studies. But despite quite extensive growth of avian embryos in shell-less culture systems (Fig. 1) (Romanoff, 1943; Corner and Richter, 1973; Dunn, 1974; Auerbach *et al.,* 1974; Palén and Thörneby, 1976; Ono and Wakasugi, 1983), the birds will not reach hatching, unlike those left in their shells. Furthermore, most shell-less culture systems use eggs preincubated for 72 hr as their starting point. In some cases, unincubated eggs can be grown in shell-less systems, but only for a much shorter duration (a mean of 3–4 days) (Elliott and Bennett, 1971; Palén and Thörneby, 1976).

The cultivation of embryos in the shell offers many advantages over culture of the explanted embryo. The egg's supporting structures such as shell, shell membranes, albumen, and chalazae are vital for maintaining optimal physicochemical conditions, providing protection, and supporting the extraembryonic tissues (Hamilton, 1952; Wittmann *et al.*, 1987; Deeming *et al.*, 1987; Tullett and Burton, 1987). In addition, the shell is an important source of calcium for building skeletal elements. By taking a few precautions, embryos cultured in this way can reach hatching. While in-shell culture systems offer many advantages, shell-less culture has been effective in the culture of fertilized ova obtained prematurely from hens. The subsequent transfer to surrogate shells (Callebaut, 1983; Rowlett and Simkiss, 1987) permits the embryos to grow to hatching (Perry, 1988; Naito and Perry, 1989; Naito *et al.*, 1990). This approach has been used successfully to generate transgenic birds (Ono *et al.*, 1994).

Two methods are described below by which embryos may be accessed and cultured in their shells. While the techniques work well for embryos at 1–2 days of incubation, the same technique might be applied to older embryos, provided that precautions are taken to prevent disruption of the extensive network of extraembryonic tissues present in older eggs (Callebaut, 1981).

1. Materials

Egg holder (made from modeling clay or something similar)
3-ml syringe
1-ml syringe
18G1.5-gauge needle
25G5/8-gauge hypodermic needle
Scotch Magic Tape, Type 810 (3M)
Small scissors, one pair
Fine-tipped watchmakers' forceps, two pairs

For the alternative method:

Scalpel (No. 3) and blade (No. 10)
Petroleum jelly (Vaseline) or silicone grease
Grease gun: this is constructed from a 20-ml syringe and a yellow pipetter tip
Scotch Super 33+ electrical tape (3M)

2. Solutions

70% ethanol
Tyrode's saline (Tyrode, 1910; New, 1966; Stern, 1993a)
    80 g NaCl
    2 g KCl
    2.71 g $CaCl_2 \cdot 2H_2O$
    0.5 g $NaH_2PO_4 \cdot 2H_2O$
    2 g $MgCl_2 \cdot 6H_2O$

10 g glucose

Distilled water to 1 liter

This 10× stock solution can be autoclaved and diluted with sterile distilled water prior to use. Bicarbonate is used as a buffer in the original recipe (1 g $NaHCO_3$ per liter), but solutions to which it has been added cannot then be autoclaved.

Chick Ringer's saline (New, 1966)

9.0 g NaCl

0.42 g KCl

0.24 g $CaCl_2$

Distilled water to 1 liter

Ink solution

Before use, mix one part of Pelikan Fount India ink with nine parts of saline.

3. Easy Method

The following procedure is well suited for many simple experiments (see Tickle, 1993). The technique is illustrated in Fig. 2.

1. Place the egg on its side in the egg holder and swab with 70% ethanol. Allow to air dry.

2. Using a 3-ml syringe with a 18G1.5-gauge hypodermic needle, penetrate the blunt end of the egg, slightly below the equator of the shell, and gently withdraw about 1.5–2.5 ml of thin albumen. To avoid damage to the yolk, ensure that the needle points downward, almost vertically, as it is passed into the shell (Fig. 2A).

3. Take two 6-cm strips of scotch tape and apply them to the uppermost surface of the shell so that they overlap lengthwise. Ensure that as much of the tape adheres to the underlying shell as possible.

4. Using one tip of a scissors, penetrate the tape-covered shell and cut a 2-cm-diameter circle of shell from the egg. The embryo should be visible through the window (Fig. 2B).

5. Carefully drip a little saline (Tyrode's or chick Ringer's) onto the blastoderm to keep it moist.

6. India ink diluted in saline can be injected beneath the blastoderm to render it clearly visible. Use a 1-ml syringe fitted with a 25G5/8-gauge needle, ensuring that no air bubbles are present in the ink solution. Rotate the shell until the edge of the blastoderm appears in the shell window. Penetrate the vitelline membrane outside the *area opaca* and advance the needle such that its tip comes to lie about 1 mm beneath the center of blastoderm, with the axis of the needle lying parallel with the blastoderm. Gently inject ink until the entire embryo is

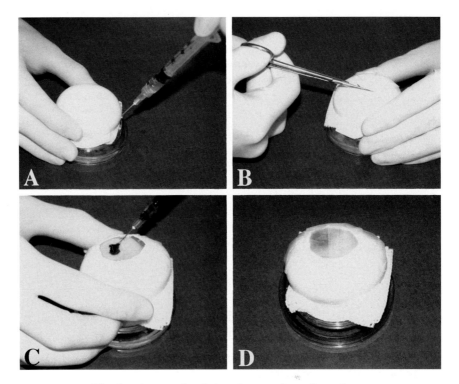

Fig. 2 The "easy" technique for accessing embryos *in ovo*.

visible above the ink background. By rotating the shell in this way to inject ink at the margin of the blastoderm, any ink that spills from the hole in the vitelline membrane tends to sink downward in the egg and does not float above the embryo to obscure it from view (Fig. 2C)

7. The egg can then be mounted on the stage of a dissecting microscope, illuminated, and operations performed.

8. After surgery, moisten the embryo with a little saline and carefully cover the window with two strips of Scotch tape (Fig. 2D). Place the egg into a humidified incubator at 38°C.

4. Alternative Method

For some operations, accessing the embryo by the method just described is not suitable because there is insufficient saline above the embryo during the surgery. As a consequence, surface tension effects can make grafting difficult and some illumination techniques, which require a bubble of saline over the embryo, cannot be used (see below). Slight modifications to the easy method can overcome this problem (Fig. 3) (Stern and Keynes, 1987; Selleck and Stern, 1991; Stern, 1993b):

1. Swab the egg with 70% ethanol and drain albumen from the blunt end of the egg as described earlier (Fig. 3A).

2. Using a scalpel, carefully score a 1-cm square on the uppermost shell of the egg. Applying gentle pressure and using small strokes, continue to score around the shell until it can be lifted free from the underlying shell membrane (Fig. 3B). WARNING! The scalpel can easily slip on the shell, so care should be taken to position fingers out of the way of the blade! Some workers prefer to use a dental drill to score the egg shell. A Dremel Moto-Tool (Model 395) fitted with a small bit works well.

3. Moisten the shell membrane with a little saline and remove sufficient membrane to generate a window to the embryo beneath (Fig. 3C).

4. Apply a 1-mm ribbon of high vacuum silicon grease or Vaseline to the edge of the window. A simple grease gun makes the procedure easier: use a 10/20-ml syringe fitted with a simple nozzle made from a cut-off yellow pipetter tip (Fig. 3D).

5. Drip enough saline into the egg to cause the yolk to float, bringing the embryo into the window. Continue to drip saline onto the embryo so that it is covered by a bubble which is contained by the ribbon of grease. If ink is to be used, it can be injected beneath the embryo as described earlier (Fig. 3E).

6. After the surgical manipulation, drain about 2 ml of saline/albumen from the blunt end of the egg using the syringe. This causes the embryo to drop into the egg away from the window.

7. Scrape away the grease from the edge of the window and swab with 70% ethanol, ensuring that none makes contact with the inside of the egg. Dry the area (Fig. 3F).

8. Seal the window with electrical tape: cut a 5- to 6-cm length of tape and, holding it taut, apply it to the surface of the shell (Fig. 3G). Make sure that the window is completely covered and that the tape is firmly applied to the shell surface. Place the egg into a humidified incubator at 38°C.

C. New Culture

With the advent of tissue culture at the start of this century, many experimental embryologists attempted to apply such culture techniques to the embryo (reviewed by Rawles, 1952). In early experiments, embryos or embryo fragments were grown on clots of plasma or agar (see below), but embryos grown by such methods failed to develop normally because they lacked the vitelline membrane on which they expand. New culture, named after Dennis New who published the method in 1955, is a yolkless cultivation technique in which the blastoderm can be successfully grown on a vitelline membrane supported by a glass ring

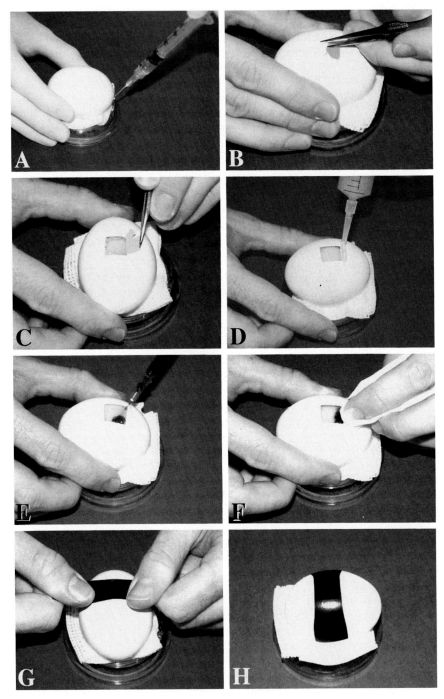

Fig. 3 An alternative technique for accessing the embryo *in ovo*. By cutting a small window in the shell and applying a ribbon of grease around the margins of the window, the embryo can be floated to the top of the egg.

over a pool of thin albumen. It can be used for growing young embryos at preincubation to early neurula stages, to about the 19 somite-pair stage (stage 13).

This method has many advantages over the culture of gastrula and neurula stage embryos *in ovo*. First, young embryos in New culture can easily be studied using either transmitted or incident light. Second, both dorsal and ventral aspects of the embryo are accessible to manipulation in New culture. Third, full-thickness incisions, i.e., those penetrating all three germ layers, can be made into New-cultured blastoderms. Similar operations performed *in ovo* result in yolk erupting through the hole and death of the embryo. New culture is particularly useful for teratological studies because the embryo is fully accessible to applied substances.

New culture also has significant drawbacks. The technique permits expansion of the blastoderm on the vitelline membrane and the subsequent formation of a healthy area vasculosa. However, once the margins of the blastoderm reach the inner aspect of the ring, further expansion of the blastoderm is prevented, development ceases, and the embryo dies. This means that embryos can be cultured only briefly, typically 24–36 hr after explantation of a stage 4 embryo. Furthermore, embryos with more than a few somite pairs cannot be placed into New culture because the blastoderm is already as large as the culture rings. A number of researchers have attempted to circumvent these problems by employing modifications discussed later in this chapter.

1. Materials

Clear glass baking tray, approximately 5 cm deep; dishes about 28 cm long and 18 cm wide are of optimal size

Concave watch glasses; one or two

Glass or plexiglass rings (about 22 mm outer diameter, 19 mm inner diameter, 5 mm thick); one ring required per culture

Pasteur pipettes

Pasteur pipette with smooth tip; a smooth tip can be created by repeatedly passing a regular Pasteur pipette through a Bunsen flame until no rough edges remain

Small beaker to hold the thin albumen

Tissue culture dishes (35 mm diameter, 10 mm depth, with lid); one per culture

Scissors, fine forceps, blunt-ended forceps

Dissecting microscope

2. Solutions

70% ethanol

Pannett and Compton saline (Pannett and Compton, 1924; New, 1966; Stern, 1993a)

Stock solution A:

121 g NaCl

15.5 g KCl

10.42 g CaCl$_2$ · 2H$_2$O

12.7 g MgCl$_2$ · 6H$_2$O

Distilled water to 1 liter; autoclave prior to storage

Stock solution B:

2.365 g Na$_2$HPO$_4$ · 2H$_2$O

0.188 g NaH$_2$PO$_2$ · 2H$_2$O

Distilled water to 1 liter; autoclave prior to storage

Immediately prior to use, mix solutions A, B, and distilled water in the ratio of 4:6:90. Avoid mixing A and B directly since insoluble precipitates form. Make sufficient saline to fill the baking tray.

3. Method

The method described next differs in a few ways from New's original technique (New, 1955, 1966) and is based on the modifications of Stern and Ireland (1981; see also Stern, 1993a). The glass rings used by New were circular in cross section, while those used in the method described next are cut from glass tubing and are rectangular in cross section. This modification permits the ring/membrane/blastoderm preparation to be transferred from the watch glass (in which New cultured his embryos) to a flat-bottomed plastic dish for culture. The technique is illustrated in Fig. 4.

1. Make fresh Pannett and Compton saline and pour into the baking tray.

2. Swab the egg shell with 70% ethanol and allow to air dry.

3. Holding the egg with the blunt end uppermost, gently break the uppermost shell with large forceps and pare away the shell and shell membranes.

4. After removing about one-quarter of the shell, gently tip the egg to drain the albumen from it. Thin albumen will easily pour from the egg and should be retained for later use. In contrast, thick albumen is somewhat more difficult to remove and can be separated from the yolk by tilting the egg and using forceps to tease it from the yolk. Take particular care to ensure that the vitelline membrane surrounding the yolk is not punctured.

5. Continue to pare away the shell and drain the albumen until almost all the albumen surrounding the yolk has been removed and the yolk lies in a shallow bowl of egg shell. The more thick albumen that is removed at this stage, the easier subsequent steps will be!

6. Submerge the egg in the Pannett and Compton saline and tilt the shell to pour the yolk into the baking tray. Discard the remaining shell and remove any albumen remaining on the yolk.

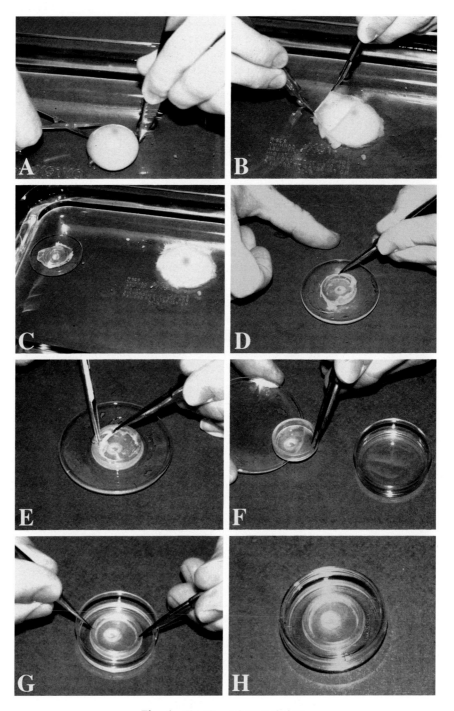

Fig. 4　The New culture technique.

7. Using the smooth sides of the forceps, rotate the yolk until the embryo lies uppermost. At this stage the yolk surface should be inspected to ensure that no yolk is leaking from small holes in the vitelline membrane. Any holes in the membrane above the equator will likely prevent the embryo from developing in culture.

8. With scissors, puncture the vitelline membrane at the yolk equator, or slightly below. Gently rotate the yolk with the smooth edge of the forceps and, at the same time, cut the vitelline membrane around the yolk equator until the uppermost membrane is completely separate from that below the equator (Fig. 4A).

9. Submerge a watch glass and a glass ring in the saline, close to the yolk.

10. With fine forceps, grasp the cut edge of the vitelline membrane bearing the embryo at two points, about 15 mm apart. Gently reflect the vitelline membrane and pull the grasped edge toward the opposite side of the yolk mass to peel the membrane from the yolk (Fig. 4B). Once free, the embryo lies on top of the membrane, ventral side uppermost.

11. Float the vitelline membrane onto the submerged watch glass and place the glass ring onto the center of the vitelline membrane, around the embryo (Fig. 4C).

12. Lift the watch glass from the saline and concomitantly drain a little saline from outside the ring. Place the watch glass on the stage of a dissecting microscope.

13. Using fine-tipped forceps, pull the free edge of the vitelline membrane over the side of the glass ring. Work around the ring so that the membrane at its center is pulled taut (Fig. 4D). At this time, it often helps to trim away any excess vitelline membrane (Fig. 4E). The culture is now at a suitable point for experimentation. Keep the embryo covered with saline during the microsurgical operations.

14. Using the fire-polished Pasteur pipette, drain all the saline from inside the glass ring.

15. Pour a little thin albumen into the bottom of a plastic culture dish and moisten the lid of the dish with a little albumen.

16. Firmly grasping the edge of the glass ring with forceps, slide the culture from the watch glass (Fig. 4F) and place it into the center of the culture dish. With forceps, fix the ring onto the bottom of the dish (Fig. 4G), replace the culture dish lid, and place the completed New culture into a humidified incubator at 38°C for further development (Fig. 4H).

D. Alternative Culture Methods

A number of less common embryo culture methods have been devised that may prove useful for some applications.

1. Variations on the New Culture Method

Conventional New cultures have been placed into dishes containing a 1-mm-deep agar substratum instead of thin albumen (DeHaan, 1963). The agar clot contains equal parts of thin albumen and saline, with 1% agar and 1% glucose. Bortier and Vakaet (1992) make their substrate with 25 ml of thin albumen mixed with 150 mg Bacto agar (Difco) in 25 ml Ringer's saline.The advantage of using a solid substratum is that holes in the vitelline membrane do not prove disastrous to development and less care needs to be taken in preparing the cultures.

In an attempt to extend the New technique to the culture of older embryos, a number of modifications have been developed (Flamme, 1987; Kucera and Burnand, 1987; Flamme *et al.,* 1991; Stern, 1993a). Typically, stage 13 embryos can be grown to 4–5 days (stages 20–25) using these new methods.

2. Agar and Plasma Clots

One easy method used to culture young chick blastoderms to the 20/30 somite stage is to explant them directly onto a solid nutrient "clot" made from blood plasma or agar. Waddington (1932) used plasma clots made from three parts chicken plasma and one part chick embryo extract for his culture experiments. Agar clots (Spratt, 1947a,b; New, 1966) have superseded plasma as a culture substrate and many workers currently use them for culturing young gastrula and neurula stage embryos (Mitrani and Shimoni, 1990; Eyal-Giladi *et al.,* 1994). An excellent description of the protocol can be found in Schoenwolf (1995). Briefly, 200 mg of low melting point agarose is dissolved in 3 ml of water and autoclaved. While cooling, 8 ml of Rosewell Park Memorial Institute (RPMI) saline is mixed with the agarose, along with 10 μl of penicillin and 100 μl glutamine. The medium is poured into 35-mm petri dishes and allowed to gel. Blastoderms are grown on this medium at 37°C, 100% humidity, and with 5% CO_2.

Blastoderms are cultured endoderm-side down on the clot. For culturing preincubation stage blastoderms, Spratt and Haas (1960) recommend placing them ectoderm-side down on the medium. The major drawback of this method is that the blastoderm does not expand on the culture substrate in the way that it will on the vitelline membrane. Furthermore, some reports indicate that the morphogenetic movements of embryos cultured in this way are abnormal. One possible solution is to leave the blastoderm attached to the vitelline membrane which is spread over the agar (as described earlier).

III. Tools for Microsurgery

Most experiments performed on young embryos may be conducted using standard dissection instruments and simple tools that can be made by the experimenter. A dissection kit containing coarse forceps, a few pairs of fine-tipped watchmakers' forceps (No. 4 or 5), and a pair of small scissors is required for preparing the chick embryo cultures. For microsurgery and manipulations, some workers like to use specialized, commercially available microsurgical instruments such as iridectomy knives and microscissors. These instruments can sometimes prove useful but their cost is considerable and it may not be cost-effective to purchase them unless they are used on a regular basis. Excellent alternatives can be made easily; a superb description of microinstrument construction can be found in Hamburger (1960).

Small incisions in the embryo are made using entomology pins or sharpened needles constructed from tungsten wire or capillary glass. Glass needles can be made by pulling capillary glass in a conventional microelectrode puller. Typically, aluminosilicate glass (Kimble Products) is used, with the following dimensions: an internal diameter of 0.8 mm, an outer diameter of 1.1 mm, and a length of 100 mm. Care should be taken to ensure that the puller settings are such that the shank of the microelectrode is short and sturdy. Long, wispy shanks are harder to control and may prove difficult to use. Microsurgical needles can also be made from small lengths of tungsten wire, approximately 0.3 mm in diameter. One end of the wire is sharpened for use in delicate dissections. Sharpening is best achieved electrolytically by connecting the tungsten wire to a 10- to 12-V dc power source and immersing both the indifferent electrode and the tip of the wire into a 10 N NaOH solution. Glass and tungsten needles can be mounted in commercially available needle holders or glued into the tip of Pasteur pipettes for added control.

Many surgical procedures involve the transfer of small fragments of tissue from one culture dish to another. The control that one has over conventional Pasteur pipettes and bulbs is inadequate for moving most small grafts, but these pipettes can be specially adapted for the purpose. Directions for making one of these "Spemann micropipettes" is given in Hamburger (1960). Briefly, a hole is made into the neck of a Pasteur pipette (i.e., where the body of the pipette starts to taper) and is sealed with a strip of rubber (Fig. 5A). Alternatively, the tapered portion of the pipette may be separated from the body and the two joined with a short length of rubber tubing (Fig. 5B). With a conventional pipette bulb in place, small inward and outward movements of solution and tissue fragments can be produced by applying slight pressure to the rubber strip. An alternative solution is to use a standard laboratory pipetter set to 3–5 μl. If the grafts stick to either the glass or the plastic surfaces, the transfer pipettes or pipetter "yellow tips" can be precoated with a siliconizing liquid.

IV. Microsurgical Approaches to the Young Embryo

A. Explantation of Donor Embryos

Graft tissue can be dissected from embryos maintained *in ovo* or cultured by the technique of New, but unless the donor embryo is to be cultured further,

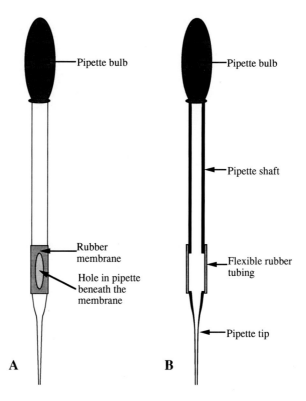

Fig. 5 Spemann pipettes can be used to transfer tissue fragments in small quantities of fluid. (A) An opening is made at the neck of a Pasteur pipette and is covered with a rubber membrane. Alternatively (B), the shaft of a Pasteur pipette is joined to a Pasteur pipette tip with a length of rubber tubing. Squeezing and releasing the rubber tubing cause small inward and outward movements of fluid that are sufficient to suck up and release the tissue.

preparing the embryos in this way wastes time. It is far easier to explant the embryos from the egg into saline prior to dissection. Proceed as follows:

1. Swab the egg with 70% ethanol and allow to air dry.

2. Holding the blunt end of the egg uppermost, crack the shell with large, blunt-ended forceps and carefully remove the shell and shell membranes. Drain albumen from the egg as described earlier for the New culture.

3. With the side of the forceps, stroke the yolk until the embryo lies uppermost in the center of the yolk mass.

4. With small scissors, make four cuts in the shape of a square through the vitelline membrane around the blastoderm. Ensure that the cuts meet so that the vitelline square with the attached blastoderm is freed from the surrounding membrane (Fig. 6A).

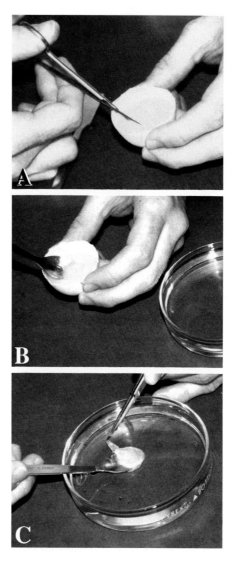

Fig. 6 A method for explanting young avian embryos that uses a shallow spoon to scoop the blastoderm from the underlying yolk.

    5. For embryos older than stage 8: Grasp a corner of the vitelline membrane and blastoderm with fine-tipped forceps and lift the embryo from the yolk and transfer it to a dish containing saline (Tyrode's or chick Ringer; see earlier discussion).

    For embryos younger than stage 8: Younger embryos tear if they are lifted from the yolk directly. Use a small shallow spoon or a spatula with concavity to scoop the embryo from the yolk. Moisten the spoon and insert it beneath the blastoderm (Fig. 6B). Lift the embryo from the yolk and submerge it completely in a dish containing saline. With the spoon beneath the embryo, grasp one corner of the vitelline membrane with fine-tipped forceps and gently peel the membrane with the attached embryo from the surface of the yolk (Fig. 6C). The yolk and spoon can then be lifted from the saline.

Sorokin's filter paper method: Both young and old embryos can be explanted from the yolk using a simple method attributed to Sorokin (see Menkes *et al.,* 1961; Flamme, 1987). After draining albumen from the egg, an annulus of filter paper is laid onto the vitelline membrane with the embryo lying at its center. Scissors are used to cut through the vitelline membrane around the filter paper. Because the vitelline membrane and blastoderm adhere to the filter paper, the annulus can then be lifted from the yolk by means of forceps, with the embryo lying taut across the center.

6. After transferring the embryo to saline, remove the vitelline membrane from the blastoderm. In the case of older embryos, the blastoderm will fall off with gentle agitation or can be removed with forceps. In contrast, the peripheral cells of younger blastoderms tend to adhere to the vitelline membrane. In this case, hold one corner of the membrane with forceps and work around the edge of the blastoderm with a sharpened dissection needle to separate the embryo and the membrane.

7. Transfer the blastoderm to a dissection dish using a wide-mouth Pasteur pipette, the end of which has been fire-polished.

8. For many intricate dissections it helps to pin the embryo out flat. To provide a suitable surface for pinning, the bottom of the dish can be coated with paraffin wax (black wax is especially useful) or with Sylgard 184 (Dow Corning), a silicone rubber made by mixing two liquid components (see Stern and Holland, 1993). The pins can be made from sharpened tungsten wire or commercially available entomology pins can be used. Four to five pins per dish are sufficient.

B. Enzymes for Dissection

The tissues of older embryos tend to stick tightly to one other and do not easily dissociate in normal Tyrode's or chick Ringer's salines. In some cases, Tyrode's saline (see Section II,B,2) lacking the calcium and magnesium salts (Tyrode's–CMF) is sufficient to separate some tissues. Stern (1993a) recommends using double-strength calcium- and magnesium-free saline at 30°C. In other instances, enzymes must be added to the saline to assist in the dissection, but special considerations should be given to the possible deleterious effects of using enzymes in such experiments. Trypsin (0.1% in saline; Selleck and Bronner-Fraser, 1995) or collagenase (1 mg/ml in Howard Ringer's saline; Pettway *et al.,* 1990; Selleck and Bronner-Fraser, 1995) is typically used. After dissection, tissues may be allowed to recover in a culture medium containing serum prior to grafting.

C. Culture of Young Embryos: Tips and Special Considerations

While shell-less and in-shell cultures permit the long-term growth of embryos, there are significant drawbacks to their use for early avian embryos. Primarily, embryos at these young stages are exquisitely sensitive to the ink injection. While not all embryos die, the survival rate is low and they are often abnormal. A number of alternatives eliminate the need to inject ink beneath the blastoderm. New (1966) describes the use of Nile blue- or neutral red-containing agar blocks to lightly stain the embryo. Alternatively, he recommends illuminating the embryo with an oblique blue or green light source. Schoenwolf (1995) describes a method in which a carbon powder and agar mixture is injected beneath the blastoderm. A technique originally reported by Hara (1970, 1971) has proved especially effective. Light is focused onto a large saline bubble overlying the embryo so that its rays travel parallel to the surface of the blastoderm. The light is reflected onto the blastoderm in such a way that its structures become clearly visible. In a similar way, a fine fiber optic cable, the tip of which rests inside the bubble, has been used to successfully illuminate a definitive streak stage embryo. It follows that the "alternative method" of *in ovo* culture must be used since only by this technique is a bubble of saline generated above the embryo.

Another major problem relates to the thinness of 1- to 2-day-old embryos. It is very easy at these stages to inadvertently make a full-thickness hole through all three germ layers of the embryo. When this occurs *in ovo,* yolk spills from the hole and the embryo (which is under tension) frequently tears. Provided the vitelline membrane is not punctured, this is not a problem for embryos grown in New culture. In fact, full-thickness holes can be made through New-cultured embryos in the course of a microsurgical procedure, and the embryo will heal and grow if simple precautions are taken. Those cells at the periphery of the blastoderm are the ones that attach to the vitelline membrane and "crawl" along it to generate expansion of the blastoderm (New, 1959; Spratt, 1963). Therefore, if a hole is made through all three germ layers of a cultured embryo, this expansion can widen the hole and ultimately split the embryo. To prevent this, the edge of the area opaca can be trimmed away, allowing the hole enough time to heal before the blastoderm reattaches to the vitelline membrane (Bellairs, 1963; Selleck and Stern, 1992). Healing is also accelerated by removing as much saline as possible from the hole. On occasion, it is advantageous to remove a New-cultured embryo from the vitelline membrane in order to operate on it in a Sylgard-coated dissection dish. After returning the embryo to the New culture, the blastoderm will reattach to the vitelline membrane and development will proceed as normal.

Acknowledgments

This work is dedicated to the memory of Michael Solursh. I am grateful to Marianne Bronner-Fraser for her advice and support and to Claudio Stern for having taught me many of the techniques presented in this chapter. Thanks also go to Mouner N. Salem for help with photography and to

Drs. Meyer Barembaum, Cathy Krull, Seth Ruffins, and Jack Sechrist for helpful comments on the manuscript. M.A.J.S. is funded by NIH Grant HD-25138.

References

Auerbach, R., Kubai, L., Knighton, D., and Folkman, J. (1974). A simple procedure for the long-term cultivation of chicken embryos. *Dev. Biol.* **41,** 391–394.

Barnett, S. B. (1982). A method for the observation of long term development in chick embryos. *Poul. Sci.* **61,** 172–174.

Bellairs, R. (1963). The development of somites in the chick embryo. *J. Embryol. Exp. Morphol.* **11,** 697–714.

Bortier, H., and Vakaet, L. C. A. (1992). Fate mapping the neural plate and the intraembryonic mesoblast in the upper layer of the chicken blastoderm with xenografting and time-lapse videography. *Development (Cambridge, UK), Suppl.,* pp. 93–97.

Callebaut, M. (1981). A new method for making an artificial air space on top of fertilized avian eggs. *Poult. Sci.* **60,** 723–725.

Callebaut, M. (1983). Autoradiographic demonstration of the penetration of albumen-derived material through the vitelline membrane into the egg yolk, exterior to the avian blastoderm. *Poult. Sci.* **62,** 1657–1659.

Corner, M. A., and Richter, A. P. J. (1973). Extended survival of the chick embryo in vitro. *Experientia* **29,** 467–468.

Deeming, D. C., Rowlett, K., and Simkiss, K. (1987). Physical influences on embryo development. *J. Exp. Zool., Suppl.* **1,** 341–345.

DeHaan, R. L. (1963). Organization of the cardiogenic plate in the early chick embryo. *Acta Embryol. Morphol Exp.* **6,** 26–37.

Dunn, B. E. (1974). Technique of shell-less culture of the 72-hour avian embryo. *Poult. Sci.* **53,** 409–412.

Elliott, J. H., and Bennett, J. (1971). Growth of chick embryos in polyethylene bags. *Poult. Sci.* **50,** 974–975.

Eyal-Giladi, H., Lotan, T., Levin, T., Avner, O., and Hochman, J. (1994). Avian marginal zone cells function as primitive streak inducers only after their migration into the hypoblast. *Development (Cambridge, UK)* **120,** 2501–2509.

Flamme, I. (1987). Prolonged and simplified in vitro culture of explanted chick embryos. *Anat. Embryol.* **176,** 45–52.

Flamme, I., Albach, K., Muller, S., Christ, B., and Jacob, H. J. (1991). Two-phase in vitro culture of explanted chick embryos. *Anat. Rec.* **229,** 427–433.

Hamburger, V. (1960). "A Manual of Experimental Embryology." Univ. of Chicago Press, Chicago.

Hamilton, H. L. (1952). Sensitive periods during development. *Ann. N.Y. Acad. Sci.* **55,** 177–187.

Hara, K. (1970). "Dark-field" illumination for micro-surgical operations on chick blastoderms in vitro. *Mikroskopie* **26,** 61–63.

Hara, K. (1971). Micro-surgical operations on the chick embryo in ovo without vital staining. *Mikroskopie* **27,** 267–270.

Iyengar, B. (1983). A new in situ organ culture technique using the early chick blastoderm. *Chemotherapy* **29,** 68–70.

Kucera, P., and Burnand, M.-B. (1987). Routine teratogenicity test that uses chick embryo in vitro. *Teratogen. Carcinog. Mutagen.* **7,** 427–447.

Menkes, B., Miclea, C., Elias, St., and Deleanu, M. (1961). Researches on the formation of axial organs. I. Studies on the differentiation of the somites. *Acad. Repub. Pop. Rom., Baza Cercet. Stiint., Timisoara, Stud. Cercet. Stiint. Med.* **8,** 7–34.

Mitrani, E., and Shimoni, Y. (1990). Induction by soluble factors of organized axial structures in chick epiblasts. *Science* **247,** 1092–1094.

Naito, M., and Perry, M. M. (1989). Development in culture of the chick embryo from cleavage to hatch. *Br. Poult. Sci.* **30,** 251–256.

Naito, M., Nirasawa, K., and Oishi, T. (1990). Development in culture of the chick embryo from fertilized ovum to hatching. *J. Exp. Zool.* **254,** 322–326.

New, D. A. T. (1955). A new technique for the cultivation of the chick embryo in vitro. *J. Embryol. Exp. Morphol.* **3,** 320–331.

New, D. A. T. (1959). The adhesive properties and expansion of the chick blastoderm. *J. Embryol. Exp. Morphol.* **7,** 146–164.

New, D. A. T. (1966). "The Culture of Vertebrate Embryos." Logos Press, London.

Ono, T., and Wakasugi, N. (1983). Development of cultured quail embryos. *Poult. Sci.* **62,** 532–536.

Ono, T., Murakami, T., Mochii, M., Agata, K., Kino, K., Otsuka, K., Ohta, M., Mizutani, M., Yoshida, M., and Eguchi, G. (1994). A complete culture system for avian transgenesis, supporting quail embryos from the single-cell stage to hatching. *Dev. Biol.* **161,** 126–130.

Palén, K., and Thörneby, L. (1976). A simple method for cultivating the early chick embryo in vitro. *Experientia* **32,** 267–268.

Pannett, C. A., and Compton, A. (1924). The cultivation of tissues in saline embryonic juice. *Lancet* **205,** 381–384.

Perry, M. M. (1988). A complete culture system for the chick embryo. *Nature (London)* **331,** 70–72.

Pettway, Z., Guillory, G., and Bronner-Fraser, M. (1990). Absence of neural crest cells from the region surrounding implanted notochords in situ. *Dev. Biol.* **142,** 335–345.

Rawles, M. (1952). Transplantation of normal embryonic tissues. *Ann. N.Y. Acad. Sci.* **55,** 302–312.

Romanoff, A. (1943). Cultivation of the early chick embryo in vitro. *Anat. Rec.* **87,** 365–369.

Rowlett, K., and Simkiss, K. (1987). Explanted embryo culture: In vitro and in ovo techniques for domestic fowl. *Br. Poult. Sci.* **28,** 91–101.

Schoenwolf, G. C. (1995). "Laboratory Studies of Vertebrate and Invertebrate Embryos: Guide and Atlas of Descriptive and Experimental Development." Prentice-Hall, Englewood Cliffs, NJ.

Selleck, M. A. J., and Bronner-Fraser, M. (1995). Origins of the avian neural crest: The role of neural plate-epidermal interactions. *Development (Cambridge, UK)* **121,** 525–538.

Selleck, M. A. J., and Stern, C. D. (1991). Fate mapping and cell lineage analysis of Hensen's node in the chick embryo. *Development (Cambridge, UK)* **112,** 615–626.

Selleck, M. A. J., and Stern, C. D. (1992). Commitment of mesoderm cells in Hensen's node of the chick embryo to notochord and somite. *Development (Cambridge, UK)* **114,** 403–415.

Spratt, N. T., Jr. (1947a). A simple method for explanting and cultivating early chick embryos in vitro. *Science* **106,** 452.

Spratt, N. T., Jr. (1947b). Development in vitro of the early chick blastoderm explanted on yolk and albumen extract saline-agar substrata. *J. Exp. Zool.* **106,** 345–365.

Spratt, N. T., Jr. (1963). Role of the substratum, supracellular continuity, and differential growth in morphogenetic cell movements. *Dev. Biol.* **7,** 51–63.

Spratt, N. T., Jr., and Haas, H. (1960). Morphogenetic movements in the lower surface of the unincubated and early chick blastoderm. *J. Exp. Zool.* **144,** 139–157.

Stern, C. D. (1993a). Avian embryos. *In* "Essential Developmental Biology: A Practical Approach" (C. D. Stern and P. W. H. Holland, eds.), pp. 45–54. Oxford Univ. Press, Oxford.

Stern, C. D. (1993b). Transplantation in avian embryos. *In* "Essential Developmental Biology: A Practical Approach" (C. D. Stern and P. W. H. Holland, eds.), pp. 111–117. Oxford Univ. Press, Oxford.

Stern, C. D., and Holland, P., eds. (1993). "Essential Developmental Biology: A Practical Approach." Oxford Univ. Press, Oxford.

Stern, C. D., and Ireland, G. W. (1981). An integrated experimental study of endoderm formation in avian embryos. *Anat. Embryol.* **163,** 245–263.

Stern, C. D., and Keynes, R. J. (1987). Interactions between somite cells: The formation and maintenance of segment boundaries in the chick embryo. *Development (Cambridge, UK)* **99,** 261–272.

Tickle, C. (1993). Chick limb buds. *In* "Essential Developmental Biology: A Practical Approach" (C. D. Stern and P. W. H. Holland, eds.), pp. 119–125. Oxford Univ. Press, Oxford.

Tullett, S. G., and Burton, F. G. (1987). Effect of two gas mixtures on growth of the domestic fowl embryo from days 14 through 17 of incubation. *J. Exp. Zool., Suppl.* **1,** 347–350.

Tyrode, M. V. (1910). The mode of action of some purgative salts. *Arch. Int. Pharmacodyn.* **20,** 205–223.

Waddington, C. H. (1932). Experiments on the development of chick and duck embryo, cultivated in vitro. *Philos. Trans. R. Soc. London, Ser. B* **221,** 179–230.

Willier, B. H. (1926). The development of implanted chick embryos following the removal of the primordial germ cells. *Anat. Rec.* **34,** 158.

Wittmann, J., Kugler, W., and Kaltner, H. (1987). Cultivation of the early quail embryo: Induction of embryogenesis under in vitro conditions. *J. Exp. Zool., Suppl.* **1,** 325–328.

CHAPTER 2

Quail–Chick Transplantations

Nicole Le Douarin, Françoise Dieterlen-Lièvre, and Marie-Aimée Teillet

Institut d'Embryologie Cellulaire et Moléculaire du CNRS
et du Collège de France
94736 Nogent-sur-Marne, France

I. Introduction
II. Differential Diagnosis of Quail and Chick Cells
    A. Nucleolar Marker
    B. Species-Specific Antibodies
    C. Species-Specific Nucleic Probes
III. Material and Equipment
    A. High Quality Fertilized Eggs
    B. Incubators
    C. Egg Holders
    D. Optical Equipment
    E. Microsurgery Instruments
    F. Other Equipment
    G. Feulgen–Rossenbeck Staining
IV. Preparation and Sealing of Eggs
V. Neural Tissue Transplantations
    A. Neural Tube Transplantations
    B. Transplantations of Anterior Neural Folds and Neural Plate at Early Neurula Stage
    C. Transplantations of Brain Vesicles
VI. Early Transplantations in Blastodiscs
    A. Blastodermal Chimeras
    B. Germ Layer Combinations
    C. Transplantation of Epiblast or Primitive Streak Fragments
VII. Hemopoietic Organ Rudiment Transplantations
    A. Grafts on Chorioallantoic Membrane and Injections into Chorioallantoic Vessels
    B. Grafts in Somatopleure
    C. Grafts in Dorsal Mesentery

METHODS IN CELL BIOLOGY, VOL. 51
Copyright © 1996 by Academic Press, Inc. All rights of reproduction in any form reserved.

      D. Parabiosis
      E. Orthotopic Transplantations of Thymus and Bursa of Fabricius
      F. Yolk Sac Chimeras
VIII. Results, Discussion, and Perspectives
      References

I. Introduction

Easily accessible to experimentation as it is, the avian embryo has long been a popular object of study for embryologists. The association of cells or rudiments from two avian species (quail, *Coturnix coturnix japonica,* and chick, *Gallus gallus*), advocated as a means to identify cells that migrate during embryogenesis (Le Douarin, 1973a), was rapidly recognized in this context as a useful tool for the study of many developmental biology problems. The rationale underscoring of the use of quail–chick associations is the need to label certain cells selectively in order to follow their migrations and interactions during the prolonged period of time encompassing morphogenesis and organogenesis.

The method is based on the observation (Le Douarin, 1969) that the constitutive heterochromatin in all embryonic and adult cells of the quail is condensed in one (sometimes two or three) large mass(es) in the center of the nucleus and is associated with the nucleolus, making this organelle strongly stained with the Feulgen–Rossenbeck reaction (1924). When combined with chick cells, quail cells can readily be recognized by the structure of their nucleus which thus provides a permanent genetic marker without any need for particular premanipulation of the cells (Fig. 1).

The main purpose in constructing quail–chick chimeras was to follow the fate of definite embryonic territories. Not only was their ultimate fate in the mature bird the point of interest but so were the intermediate states undergone by the embryonic cells to achieve their fate. The investigations carried out on the neural crest provide a good example of the possible use of the quail–chick chimera system as they have disclosed the nature of the tissues and organs derived from this structure while showing the migratory pathways taken by crest cells to reach their destination (Le Douarin, 1982). Another example concerns the mapping of the neural primordium which has been, and still is, under scrutiny in our laboratory (Le Douarin, 1993). The transformation from the early neural ectoderm to the mature brain involves an enormous level of complexity, built up through differential growth of the various regions of the neuroepithelium, cell migrations, and assembly of the very complicated wiring taking place between the neurones of the central nervous system (CNS). As will be shown in this chapter, quail–chick chimeras provide a means to unveil some of these mechanisms.

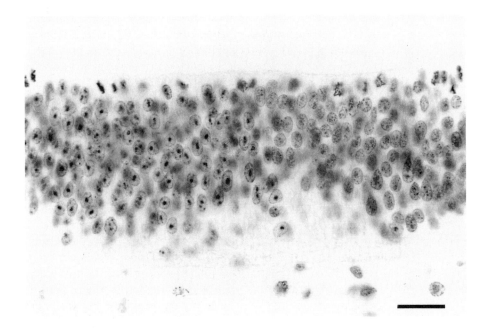

Fig. 1 Chimeric neuroepithelium at 4 days of incubation. A quail hemimesencephalon was grafted orthotopically, 2 days earlier, in a 2-day-old chick embryo. Quail cell nuclei (to the left) show the typical quail nucleolus with a large heterochromatin clump, whereas chick cells (to the right) display dispersed heterochromatin. The section is 5 μm thick; Feulgen–Rossenbeck staining with counterstain. Scale bar: 20 μm.

The purpose of this type of study implies that the developmental processes unfold in the chimeras as they do in the normal embryo. To achieve this, transplantations of quail tissues into chick embryo (or vice versa) do not consist of adding a graft to an otherwise normal embryo but rather in removing a given territory in the recipient and replacing it as precisely as possible by the equivalent region of the donor that is at the same developmental stage.

Quail and chick are closely related in taxonomy, although they differ by their size at birth (the quail weight is about 10 g and the chick is 30 g) and by the duration of their incubation period (17 days for the quail and 21 days for the chick). However, during the first week of incubation, when most of the important events take place in embryogenesis, the size of the embryos and the chronology of their development differ only slightly. When the dynamics of development of a given organ is to be studied by the quail–chick substitution method, the exact chronology of development of this organ in each species must first be established. This is necessary in order to choose the exact stage of donor and host embryos at operation time and to interpret the results later on. An example of this requirement can be found in the study that was performed on the origin of the calcitonin-producing cells that develop in the ultimobranchial body and of the enteric nervous system (see Le Douarin, 1982, and references therein).

In order to rule out possible differences in developmental mechanisms in the two species, it is beneficial to carry out the grafts not only from quail to chick (the most often performed because it is easier to recognize one isolated quail cell within chick tissues than the other way around) but also to perform some control experiments from chick to quail.

The isochronic–isotopic substitution method is not the only one that can be used. Certain developmental processes can be studied by performing a graft onto an otherwise normal embryo, i.e., without previous extirpation of the corresponding territory. This was instrumental in demonstrating the colonization of the primary lymphoid organ rudiments (thymus and bursa of Fabricius) by hemopoietic cells and in showing that this process occurs according to a cyclic periodicity (Le Douarin *et al.*, 1984, and references therein).

Because the quail–chick chimeras resulting from the isotopic–isochronic substitution of embryonic territories seemed to develop normally, the chimeras were subjected to a functional test for normality: that of hatching and postnatal survival. This was done in a variety of experimental designs: neural chimeras in which parts of the CNS (including the brain) or the peripheral nervous system of chick were replaced by their quail counterpart (Kinutani *et al.*, 1986; Le Douarin, 1993, and references therein) or by immunological chimeras in which the thymus rudiment of the chick was replaced by that of the quail (Ohki *et al.*, 1987). Neural chimeras are able to hatch and exhibit an apparently normal sensory motor behavior even when their brain is chimeric. Quail and chick are endowed with species-specific behavioral characters. The problem is thus raised as to whether a particular character is linked to a determinant located within a special area of the neuroepithelium. This type of problem is amenable to a precise analysis as demonstrated for certain species-specific traits of the song in quail and chick (Balaban *et al.*, 1988).

However, the analysis of quail–chick chimeras after birth is limited in time. Although no immune reaction against the graft takes place during embryogenesis when the immune system is building up, the transplant triggers its own rejection which occurs at various times after birth. For neural grafts, a long delay is observed between the onset of immune maturity and rejection. This is due to the relative isolation of the CNS from the circulating lymphocytes by the blood–brain barrier and to the low immunogenicity of the neural cells that do not (or at a very low rate) express molecules of the major histocompatibility complex (MHC). This delay, which may be more than a month, allows behavioral studies to be carried out in early postnatal life.

The immune rejection of the implant, albeit present in the chimera during immune system maturation, raised a series of interesting problems concerning the mechanisms of self–nonself discrimination and this system turned out to be instrumental in showing an unexpected role of the epithelial component of the thymus in tolerance to self (Belo *et al.* 1989; Martin, 1990; Ohki *et al.*, 1987, 1988).

In a number of instances the immune reaction of the host toward the graft could be studied not only in xenogeneic (quail–chick) associations but also in allogeneic (chick–chick) associations. It was found that embryonic neural grafts between MHC-mismatched individuals of the chick species did not trigger an immune response (or only a very mild one) from the host. This was at the origin of a new avenue of investigations in which the brain areas responsible for an autosomic form of genetic epilepsy were identified (Teillet *et al.,* 1991; Guy *et al.,* 1992, 1993; Fadlallah *et al.,* 1995).

For many years the analysis of the chimeras relied on the differential staining of the nucleus by either the Feulgen–Rossenbeck reaction or any other method revealing specifically the DNA profiles such as acridine orange or bizbenzimide (Hoechst 33258, Serva, Heidelberg) which could be combined with immunocyto-chemistry (see, for example, Fontaine-Perus *et al.,* 1985; Nataf *et al.,* 1993). Later on, significant progress was accomplished when species-specific antibodies recognizing either quail or chick cells were prepared. Now, not only species but also cell type-specific reagents are available either as monoclonal antibodies (Mabs) or as nuclear probes which distinguish, at the single cell scale, whether a cell produces a particular product and if it belongs to the host or the donor.

The next section reviews the technical aspects and requirements of the experiments performed to study the previously mentioned problems.

II. Differential Diagnosis of Quail and Chick Cells

A. Nucleolar Marker

The interphase nucleus of quail cells has an immediately apparent feature even when stained with a common nuclear dye like hematoxylin. The nucleus contains a very large, deeply stained inclusion, the so-called "quail nucleolus," even in cells where the nucleolar ribonucleoproteins are not abundant. DNA-specific techniques like the Feulgen–Rossenbeck reaction or the use of acridine-orange or bizbenzimide and electronic microscopy have revealed that this inclusion is essentially composed of heterochromatin associated with the nucleolus (Le Douarin, 1973b; also see Fig. 2). This is in contrast with the nucleoli of most species which contain only minute amounts of chromatin, usually below the limit of detectability in the light microscope. The quail type of nucleolus has been found in several other bird species, belonging to different groups (Le Douarin, 1971).

Some variations in the morphology of the quail nucleolar DNA are observed depending on the cell type (Le Douarin, 1973b; also Fig. 3). In early embryonic cells, e.g., in young blastoderms, the centronuclear chromatin mass is very large, but is not stained very deeply, with irregular outlines and a reticulated structure. A similar aspect is characteristic of early hemopoietic precursors. In most later embryonic cells and differentiated cells, the nucleus contains one or two centronu-clear chromatin clumps, which are compact, brightly stained, and precisely out-lined, e.g., in kidney, lung, thyroid, suprarenal gland, neural tube, and neural

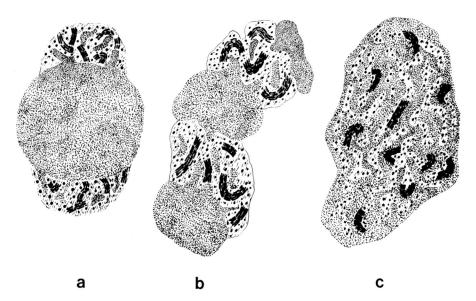

a   b   c

Fig. 2 The quail nucleolus: schematic drawings of the ultrastructural organization of quail nucleoli. (a) Type 1 nucleolus of quail cells; a large chromatin condensation is flanked by lateral clumps of nucleolar material (granular and fibrillar containing structures and amorphous matrix) inside which chromatid strands are located; (b) type 2 nucleolus of quail cells observed in hepatocytes; several DNA condensations are linked by nucleolar RNA; and (c) type 3 nucleolus of quail cells; RNA granules and fibrils are localized inside the large centronuclear DNA condensation. Reprinted with permission from Le Douarin (1973b).

derivatives. In hepatocytes there may be two to four heterochromatin masses, some attached to the nuclear membrane. In lymphocytes, many chromocenters are dispersed in the nucleus and smaller ones are located against the nuclear membrane. In muscular fibers, three to five masses line up along the axis of the elongated nuclei.

In the chick (see Fig. 3), the chromatin network is made up of inconspicuous chromocenters, homogeneously distributed in the nucleoplasm. Variations in this pattern are usually small from one cell type to another. In hepatocytes where the nucleolus is large, the nucleolus-associated DNA appears as a thin ring around the nucleolar RNA. In thymocytes, numerous tiny chromocenters are scattered in the whole nucleus.

As a rule, the differences between nuclei of corresponding cell types from the two species are obvious and can be used as markers to distinguish the origin of cells in combinations at all times of an experiment. Before diagnosis, it is important to compare the relevant cells or tissues in each species and to establish diagnostic criteria and the possible variations from the standard aspect.

B. Species-Specific Antibodies

Antibodies have been prepared which recognize virtually all cell types of the quail and nothing in the chick. Such is the case for the chick anti-quail serum raised by Lance-Jones and Langernaur (1987) and for the Mab QCPN prepared by Carlson and Carlson, which is available at the hybridoma bank (Department of Biology, University of Iowa, Iowa City, IA). The QCPN Mab is particularly instrumental in studying the derivatives of any quail graft in the young embryo and its use can be easily combined with that of other antibodies (Fig. 4, see color insert). Other Mabs are not only species-specific but also cell type specific; such is the case of the MB1 and QH1 Mabs (Péault *et al.*, 1983; Pardanaud *et al.*, 1987) which recognize a glycosylated epitope carried by surface proteins expressed in quail leucocytes and endothelial cells at the exclusion of any cell type of the chick (Péault and Labastie, 1990). These antibodies are very useful in studying the development of the vascular and hemopoietic systems in quail and chimeric embryos (Pardanaud *et al.*, 1989; Pardanaud and Dieterlen-Lièvre, 1993, 1995).

A series of reagents are available to study the development of the immune function. They concern MHC molecules such as TAC1 and TAP1 which identify a public determinant of quail and chick class II MHC, respectively (Le Douarin *et al.*, 1983), and a number of T-cell markers that are strictly specific for the chick (see Table I) and have been widely used in the study of the maturation of the immune function in quail–chick chimeras (Bucy *et al.*, 1989; Coltey *et al.*, 1989).

Finally, the analysis of neural chimeras is greatly facilitated by the availability of Mabs which recognize either neuronal cell bodies or neurites of one or the other species (Tanaka *et al.*, 1990; also see Table I).

C. Species-Specific Nucleic Probes

Species-specific cDNA probes have been used to analyze quail–chick chimeras. Such is the case of the chick probe for the homeobox gene *goosecoid* which has been used to demonstrate induction of this gene in a chick host by grafting quail goosecoid-producing tissues (Izpisùa-Belmonte *et al.*, 1993). The quail-specific Schwann cell myelin protein probe (Dulac *et al.*, 1992) is currently used in quail–chick neural chimeras to distinguish quail and chick oligodendrocytes (Cameron-Curry and Le Douarin, 1996). Chick *Wnt1* and quail *Wnt1* probes have been combined to demonstrate ectopic *Wnt* expression in heterotopic quail–chick chimeras (Bally-Cuif and Wassef, 1994).

III. Material and Equipment

A. High Quality Fertilized Eggs

Freshly laid eggs from vigorous strains of chick and quail should be selected. The eggs should be stored no more than 1 week at 15°C. The choice of a rapidly

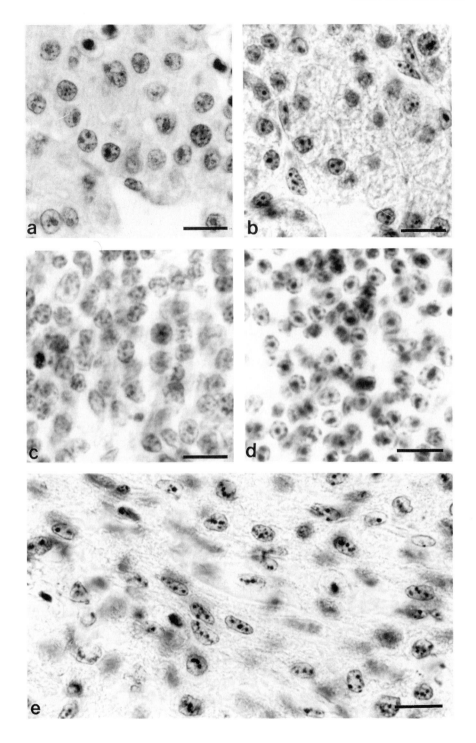

growing strain of chickens is judicious because early stages of development will proceed at the same speed in donor and recipient embryos. Such is the case for the JA57 strain (I. S. A. Lyon, France), which is particularly resistant and normally shows a high rate of hatching. Other features may guide the choice of the host strain, e.g., feather pigmentation may serve as an additional marker when grafts of neural crest cells are involved. Usually the chick host is obtained from a nonpigmented strain as the quail wild-type phenotype is heavily pigmented.

B. Incubators

Incubators must be equipped with temperature (38+/−1°C) and humidity regulators [45% up to embryonic day 17 (E17) for the chick, 75% thereafter, up to hatching time]. Automatic rocking is required in certain cases. A timed programmer is also useful in order to ensure precise stages, especially for operations performed at the early phases of development. The developmental tables of Hamburger and Hamilton (HH) (1951), Eyal-Giladi and Kochav (1976), and Zacchei (Z) (1961) are used to stage chick and quail embryos.

C. Egg Holders

There are several kinds of egg holders with different uses. Multiple wire tongs are used to hold series of chick eggs in a horizontal position and to manipulate them prior to operations. Wooden circles of appropriate sizes serve to hold eggs during operations. After the operation, eggs are stocked horizontally in the incubator on hollowed out wooden slats.

D. Optical Equipment

Microsurgery is performed under a stereomicroscope allowing a continuously progressive magnification (Zoom), e.g., from ×6 to ×50. The possibility of adding photographic or video equipment without losing stereoscopic vision is appreciated. Illumination is usually obtained from optic fibers. Formerly used conventional light bulbs with a condensor tend to radiate heat and cause traumatic drying to the embryos during surgery.

Fig. 3 Appearance of nuclei in different types of chick and quail cells. (a) Hepatocytes in a 15-day-old chick embryo. Very fine heterochromatin dots and an occasional pale staining nucleolus are shown. (b) Hepatocytes of a 15-day-old quail embryo. Chromatin condensations are larger and more deeply stained. (c) Chick thymic cell nuclei display several fine, dispersed chromocenters. (d) Quail thymic cells present one large heterochromatin mass and several smaller ones against the nuclear membrane. (e) Myocardal cells of a quail 10 days after birth. As in skeletal muscle quail cell nuclei, several chromatin condensations are present. Feulgen–Rossenbeck staining. Scale bars: 10 μm.

Table I

Cell type	Quail	Chick
All	Chick anti-quail serum (Lance-Jones and Lagenaur, 1987) QCPN (B. M. Carlson and J. A. Carlson, personal communication, 1993) (Hybridoma Bank)	
Neurones	QN (neurites) (Tanaka *et al.*, 1990)	37F5 (neuronal cell bodies), 39B11 (neurites) (Takagi *et al.*, 1989), CN (neurites) (Tanaka *et al.*, 1990)
Hemangioblastic lineage	MB1/QH1 (Péault *et al.*, 1983; Pardanaud *et al.*, 1987)	
MHC	TAC1 (Cl II) (Le Douarin *et al.*, 1983)	TAP1 (Cl II) (Le Douarin *et al.*, 1983)
T-cell markers		αTCR1 (γδ) (Chen *et al.*, 1988) αTCR2 (αβ) (Cihak *et al.*, 1988) αCT3 (Chen *et al.*, 1986) αCT4 (Chan *et al.*, 1988) αCT8 (Chan *et al.*, 1988)

E. Microsurgery Instruments

Microscalpels adapted to each type of operation are needed. Microscalpels manufactured by stropping and honing steel needles on an Arkansas oil stone are the most convenient for excising fragments of the neural tube or brain vesicles because they can be both extremely thin and resistant (Fig. 5a). Prepared with a smooth tip, they are used for dissociating tissues after enzymatic treatment. Tungsten microscalpels (Conrad *et al.*, 1993) or microscalpels made from entomology needles are quicker to prepare but are more fragile. They are useful for dissecting very small pieces of tissues precisely. Other instruments (Fig. 5b) involve curved and straight small scissors, iridectomy scissors (Pascheff-Wolff, Moria-Instruments, Paris), thin forceps, a transplantation spoon, microscalpel holders, and black glass needles.

F. Other Equipment

Glass micropipettes are hand drawn from Pasteur pipettes, curved, and calibrated according to use, injections of liquid, or transfer of pieces of tissues (see Fig. 5b). Calibration of the micropipette according to the size of the rudiment to be transplanted (for instance, neural tube versus brain) is an important requirement. The pipettes are equipped with plastic tubes for mouth use. Indian ink diluted with a physiological solution containing antibiotics can be usefully injected under the embryo to create a dark background against which young embryos

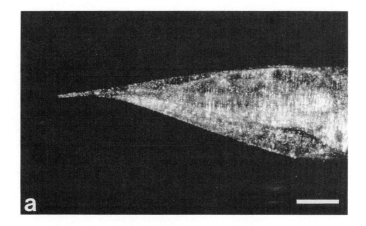

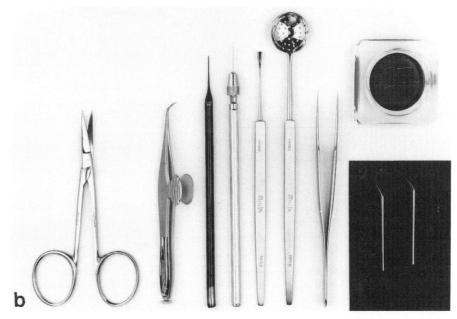

Fig. 5 (a) Microscalpel made from a steel needle. Only the extreme tip is used for microsurgery. Scale bar: 200 μm. (b) Microsurgery instruments: from left to right, curved scissors; Pascheff–Wolff iridectomy scissors; black glass needle; microscalpel in a holder; transplantation spoon and skimmer; and No. 5 Dumont forceps. Top right: glass dish with black rhodorsil base and entomology needles. Bottom: Micropipettes.

become easily visualized (Fig. 6). Phosphate-buffered saline (PBS) or Tyrode solution devised for avian cells may be indifferently used for dissections and treatments of the embryos. They are currently supplemented with antibiotics, penicillin, and streptomycin. Enzymes for tissue dissociation, trypsin, pancreatin,

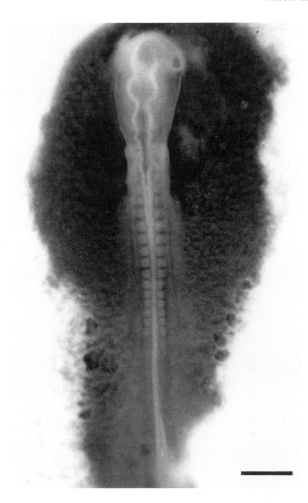

Fig. 6 Chick embryo with 15 pairs of somites prepared for *in ovo* surgery against a black background. A few drops of diluted Indian ink (1 vol/1 vol PBS) have been injected beneath the blastoderm using a curved glass micropipette inserted through the extraembryonic area. Scale bar: 200 μm.

or collagenase are used to dissociate the epithelia from the mesenchyme. The concentration of the enzyme diluted in normal or Ca^{2+}, Mg^{2+}-free Tyrode solution and the application time have to be determined for each rudiment since the purpose is to partly degrade the basement membrane without interfering with cell-to-cell adhesion in order to separate cleanly a still coherent epithelial sheet from the mesenchyme. A dish with a black resilient base and entomology needles are needed to contain and immobilize the donor embryo for dissection. A rhodorsil base (Rhône-Poulenc) is now preferred to paraffin. Animal carbon is added to the commercial transparent preparation in order to obtain a black suspension which is poured in a dish of adequate size and shape and polymerized by UV illumination (according to provided directions). Disposable syringes (1 or 2 ml) and needles (0.8 mm) are used to remove albumin from host eggs. Transparent scotch tape (5 cm in width) serves to seal the shell of operated eggs.

G. Feulgen–Rossenbeck Staining

Zenker's or Carnoy's fluids are used to prepare the tissues adequately for the Feulgen–Rossenbeck reaction (1924). Carnoy's fluid is particularly appreciated because it allows the application of both the Feulgen–Rossenbeck technique and various antibodies or nuclear probes on alternate paraffin sections. Feulgen–Rossenbeck staining is carried out according to the directions recorded in Gabe (1968). This staining is performed on 5-μm paraffin sections.

IV. Preparation and Sealing of Eggs

Eggs are incubated with their long axis horizontal for operations before E4 and their long axis vertical (air chamber up) for operations from E4 onward. The blastoderm normally develops on the upper surface of the yolk and is located against the shell membrane. If the egg was incubated horizontally, the blastoderm would be injured when a window is cut in the shell; thus, usually, a small quantity of albumin (about 1 to 3 ml) is removed before the window is opened, using a 1- or 2-ml syringe equipped with a 0.8-mm needle inserted at the pointed pole of the egg. The hole is then closed with a drop of paraffin or a small piece of tape. A more practical way to open the shell without injuring the E2 or E3 embryos is to perforate the air chamber and turn the egg upside down. The blastoderm comes back to the top immediately and lies away from the shell. If the eggs are incubated air chamber up, from E4 onward a window can be cut through the upper part of the shell (i.e., in contact with the air chamber) without any other premanipulation.

After Indian ink injection, if necessary, the vitelline membrane is torn open with a microscalpel at the site chosen for the graft. When the grafting operation has been performed, the window is sealed with a piece of tape and the egg is reincubated in the same orientation. Daily gentle manual rocking of the operated eggs enhances embryo survival.

V. Neural Tissue Transplantations

Different types of neural tissue transplantations have been classified according to the purpose of the experiments.

A. Neural Tube Transplantations

1. Orthotopic Grafting

This operation (Fig. 7) has allowed the detection of crest cell migration pathways and the construction of a neural crest fate map (Le Douarin and Teillet, 1973; Le Lièvre and Le Douarin, 1975; Le Douarin, 1982).

Neural crest cells leave the dorsal aspect of the neural tube progressively from rostral (5–6 somite stage at the dimesencephalic level; Le Lièvre and Le Douarin, 1975) to caudal levels (E4.5 and E5 in quail and chick embryos, respectively) (M. Catala, unpublished data). The interspecific graft is performed at a level where the crest cells are still inside the apex of the neural anlage, i.e., in the neural folds (see next paragraph) of the cephalic area and at the level of the last formed somites for the cervical and dorsal regions. Quail and chick embryos are stage matched (the most precise way to determine the stage at E2 is to rely on the number of somites formed); the stage is selected according to the rostrocaudal level of the neural tube that is to be transplanted since neural crest migration starts at the level of a given somite only a few hours after it is formed.

a. Excision of Host Neural Tube

The selected neural tube fragment is excised from the host embryo by microsurgery *in ovo* (Fig. 8a). A longitudinal slit through the ectoderm and between the

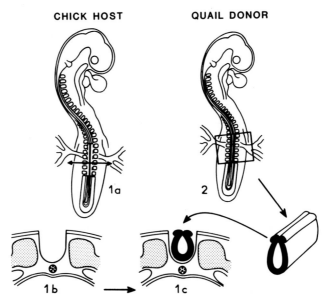

Fig. 7 Scheme of neural tube orthotopic transplantation. A fragment of the neural tube is microsurgically removed *in ovo* from the chick host at the level of the last segmented somites (1a, 1b). The corresponding level of a quail embryo at the same stage is submitted to enzymatic digestion (2) and is dissociated. The neural anlage free from surrounding tissues is inserted in the chick host (1c).

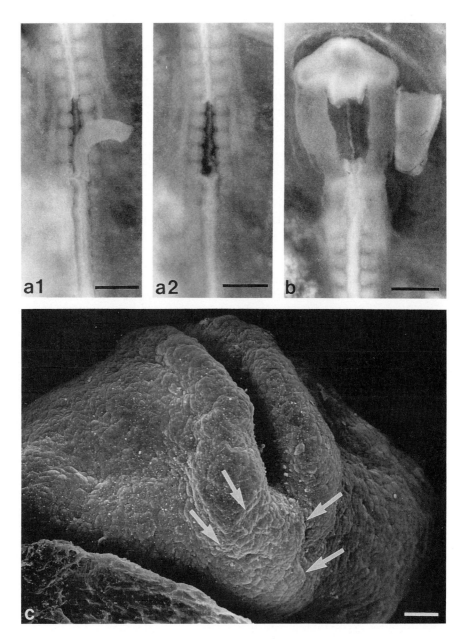

Fig. 8 Neural tissue microsurgery photographed at different steps of the procedure. (a) Ablation of a fragment of the neural tube at the level of the last segmented somites in a 18 somite stage embryo *in ovo*. Scale bars: 100 μm. (a1) The neural tube is partially removed. (a2) The notochord is visible at the level from which the neural tube has been completely removed. (b) The mesencephalic and metencephalic vesicles have been microsurgically excised from a 12 somite stage chick embryo *in ovo*. The equivalent quail vesicles that are to be grafted in the free space are positioned next to the host encephalon. Scale bar: 100 μm. (c) Scanning electron micrograph of a rostral neural fold graft (arrows) in a 5 somite stage chick embryo, 2 hr after the operation. The neural fold has been replaced at the 3 somite stage by an equivalent fragment excised from a quail embryo. This region of the neural fold gives rise to the adenohypophysis (Couly and Le Douarin, 1985). Note the perfect incorporation of the quail grafted tissue (courtesy of G. Couly and P. Coltey). Scale bar: 25 μm.

tube and the adjacent paraxial mesoderm is made bilaterally along the chosen part of the neural tube. The latter is then gently separated from the neighboring somites and is cut out transversally, rostrally, and caudally. Using a microscalpel, it is then progressively severed from the underlying notochord and is finally sucked out with a glass micropipette.

b. Preparation of Graft

The transverse region of the donor embryo comprising the equivalent fragment of the neural tube plus surrounding tissues (ectoderm, endoderm, notochord, and somites) is retrieved with iridectomy scissors, is subjected *in vitro* to enzymatic digestion (pancreatin 1:3 in PBS or Tyrode) for 5 to 10 min on ice or at room temperature according to the age of the embryo, and is then rinsed with PBS or Tyrode. The addition of calf serum accelerates the elimination of the proteo-lytic enzymes.

c. Grafting Procedure

The donor neural tube is transplanted to the host embryo using a calibrated micropipette and is placed in the groove produced by the excision in the normal rostrocaudal and dorsoventral orientations.

Labeling of neural crest cells by orthotopic grafting of a fragment of quail neural anlage into a chick embryo (or vice versa) can be made theoretically at any rostrocaudal level. However, the lumbosacral and caudal neural tube arising from the tail bud develops late (at E3–E4), when this type of microsurgery becomes virtually impossible because of the curvature of the tail. For this reason, operations bearing on the region caudal to somite 25 have to be made on presumptive territories during E2 and checked for accuracy on the following days using the newly segmented somites as landmarks (Catala *et al.,* 1995).

2. Heterotopic Grafting

This type of grafting of fragments of the neural tube is instrumental in studying whether the fate of neural crest cells is specified when the operation is carried out. The graft is taken from the donor at a more rostral or more caudal level than the acceptor level (see Le Douarin and Teillet, 1974). Depending on the latter, the donor embryo will be older or younger than the recipient (see Le Douarin, 1982, and references therein).

3. Grafting of a Neural Tube Compartment

A unilateral compartment of the neural tube can be selectively exchanged in order to disclose contralateral crest cell migrations.

B. Transplantations of Anterior Neural Folds and Neural Plate at Early Neurula Stage

Fate maps of the early rostral neural primordium have been established. They involved substitution of neuroepithelial territories at the neurula stage when zero to five somites are formed (Couly and Le Douarin, 1985, 1987, 1988; Couly *et al.*, 1993).

Very thin, sharp microscalpels (made up from tungsten fibers or entomology needles) are used to excise precise fragments of the folds. The grafts are not subjected to enzymatic treatment since no mesoderm is present in the neural folds at that stage. An ocular or objective micrometer is used to measure the pieces of tissue that are to be removed and grafted. Pieces of neural folds are grafted orthotopically (Fig. 8c) for studying the normal development of the cells composing this structure or heterotopically to discover the level of autonomy of the grafted territory (Grapin-Botton *et al.*, 1995).

C. Transplantations of Brain Vesicles

This operation has been devised to label defined regions of the brain and to study cell migration within the neuroepithelium itself (Alvarado-Mallart and Sotelo, 1984; Martinez and Alvarado-Mallart, 1989; Hallonet *et al.*, 1990; Tan and Le Douarin, 1991) or to transfer a genetic behavioral or functional trait from host to recipient in either xenogeneic or isogeneic combinations (Balaban *et al.*, 1988; Teillet *et al.*, 1991; Le Douarin, 1993, and references therein). For these different purposes, either the entire encephalon or fragments of encephalic vesicles can be exchanged between chick and quail or between normal and mutant chick embryos.

Donor and recipient embryos are chosen around somite stage 12, which is particularly appropriate for the following reasons: (i) brain vesicles, still uncovered by the amnion, are clearly demarcated by constrictions in the absence of brain curvature; (ii) the neural tissue does not adhere strongly to the notochord; and (iii) the neuroepithelium is not yet vascularized. At younger stages, landmarks are lacking and precise measures have to be taken to know exactly what part of the brain has to be dissected and grafted (see Couly and Le Douarin, 1985). Moreover, separation of the neural tissue from the underlying notochord is much more difficult (see Grapin-Botton *et al.*, 1995).

Equivalent brain vesicles or parts of them are excised microsurgically in the stage-matched donor and recipient (Fig. 8b). The dorsal ectoderm is slit precisely at the limit between the neural tissue and the cephalic mesenchyme on each side of the selected part of the brain. The neural epithelium is then separated from the cephalic mesenchyme, cut out transversally (and longitudinally) at the chosen levels, and finally severed from the notochord if necessary. Heterotopic grafts can be made to study specific problems (Nakamura, 1990; Martinez and Alvarado-Mallart, 1990; Grapin-Botton *et al.*, 1995; Martinez *et al.*, 1991; Le Douarin, 1993, and references therein).

In order to study the extent of the territory that yields the cerebellar cortex, very refined experiments have been performed (Hallonet and Le Douarin, 1993). Fragments of the alar plate extending from 20° to 120° from the sagittal plan were exchanged between chick and quail embryos at the level of the mesencephalon and metencephalon (Fig. 9). This allowed the pathways of cell migrations, taking place within the neural epithelium in this area, and a precise insight into the nature and extent of the morphogenetic movements affecting this region of the brain to be perceived.

Interestingly, when the graft is successfully incorporated into the host encephalon, the chimeric brains develop with a gross anatomy very close to normal (Fig. 10). Brain chimeras can hatch and show apparently normal behavior (Fig. 11). Histologically, one can see that the grafted cells are perfectly integrated into the host tissues. Cell migrations are so abundant in the brain that small- and medium-sized grafts become entirely chimeric due to the penetration of host cells. Similarly, the host neural structures are invaded by donor cells. It is remarkable that the pattern of these migrations is highly reproducible for each type of graft. Therefore it can be assumed that these migrations reflect normal cell movements in the neuroepithelium. Notably, the cells of the ependymal epithelium do not mix, which means that the quail–chick limit at this level indicates in fact the initial limits of the graft. This allows evaluation of the extent of migration of the host cells into the graft and vice versa (Fig. 12).

VI. Early Transplantations in Blastodiscs

A. Blastodermal Chimeras

These chimeras can be made for investigating immunological tolerance or with the aim of producing transgenic birds (Watanabe *et al.*, 1992). Area pellucida of stages XI–XIII (Eyal-Giladi and Kochav, 1976) quail blastoderms are dissected out and cleaned free of yolk in Tyrode's solution, then cells are dissociated with or without enzymatic treatment. Seven hundred to 2000 cells suspended in 1.3 ml of Tyrode are injected into the subgerminal cavity of Stage XI to two (HH) chick embryos with a 70- to 100-μm tip diameter siliconized glass pipette using a micromanipulator. Injections are made in different locations of the blastodisc (central or posterior) according to the stage of development of the chick host. Chick–chick chimeras have been constructed according to the same pattern and were able to hatch (Petitte *et al.*, 1990).

B. Germ Layer Combinations

Such chimeras have been constructed and cultured *in vitro* and have been used to study gastrulation (Vakaet, 1974; Fontaine and Le Douarin, 1977). Blastoderms incubated for 5 to 8 hr are dissociated mechanically into a hypoblast and an epiblast. The layers are then exchanged between quail and chick, and the recombinants are cultured, epiblast side down, for 24 to 50 hr according to New's (1955) culture technique. At slightly later stages [head process to head fold (stages 5–6 of Hamburger and Hamilton, HH)], pieces of the area pellucida are

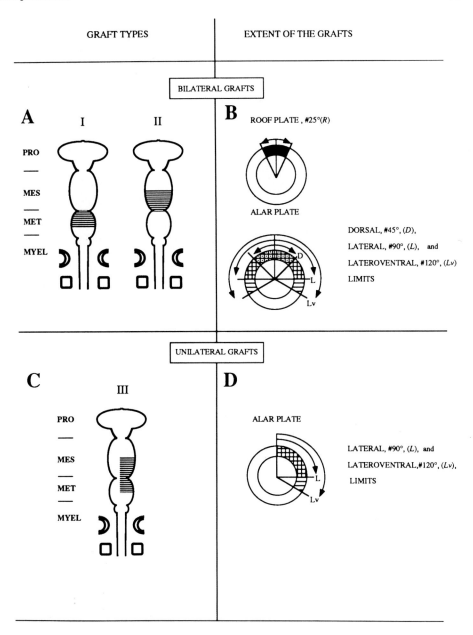

Fig. 9 Different types of isotopic and isochronic reciprocal changes made between chick and quail embryos in order to study cerebellum origin and development. These grafts are bilateral (A and B) or unilateral (C and D) and cover different dorsoventral sectors of the alar plate (B and D). Reprinted with permission from Hallonet and Le Douarin (1993).

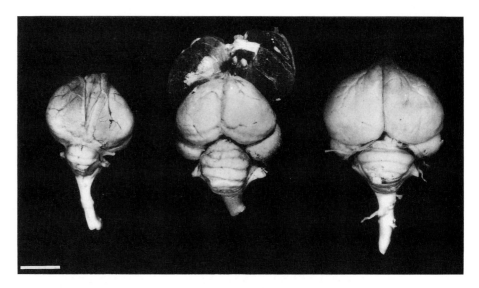

Fig. 10 The brain of a chimera (center) 7 days after hatching between the brains of normal quail (left) and chick (right) of the same age. The chimera was constructed by replacing the prosencephalon of a chick embryo with that of a quail. The grafted quail hemispheres are narrower than the optic tecta of chick origin. The eyes have been left in place in the chimera. Scale bar: 5 mm.

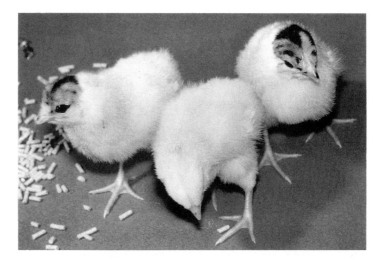

Fig. 11 Two quail–chick brain chimeras and a control chick 4 days after hatching. In the chimeras, a quail dorsal prosencephalon was grafted *in ovo* at the 12 somite stage. Quail melanocytes of a neural crest origin decorate the head feathers of the chimeras at the level of the graft.

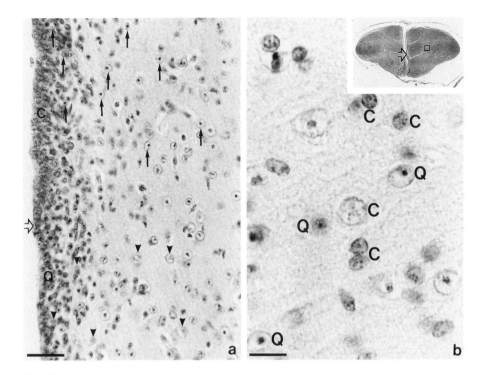

Fig. 12 A Feulgen-stained section through the cerebral hemispheres of a brain chimera in which the dorsal part of a quail prosencephalon has been orthotopically grafted at the 12 somite stage. (a) At the level of the ventricular epithelium, quail (Q) and chick (C) cells are clearly segregated (open arrow). A mixing of quail (arrows) and chick (arrowheads) cells in the subventricular zone indicates tangential cell movements during development; this produces chimeric brain regions, one of which framed in the insert is enlarged in b, where quail and chick neuronal and glial cells are mixed. The large open arrow indicates the ventricular boundary of the graft. Scale bars: a, 30 μm; b, 10 μm. Reprinted with permission from Balaban *et al.,* (1988).

dissociated by trypsin treatment (0.1% in Tyrode solution minus calcium and magnesium) into ectoderm on the one hand and endomesoderm on the other hand. Recombined layers are cultivated for 12 hr on a semisolid medium to ensure their association and are then grafted onto the chorioallantoic membrane (CAM) of chick hosts (Fig. 13).

C. Transplantation of Epiblast or Primitive Streak Fragments

These transplantations, bearing on small segments of the selected structures, are used to map territories in the young blastodisc and to disclose the cell movements which occur during gastrulation and early neurulation (Schoenwolf *et al.,* 1989, 1992). Isotopic and isochronic grafts of a plug of epiblast or of short segments of the primitive streak are made *in vitro* from quail to chick or

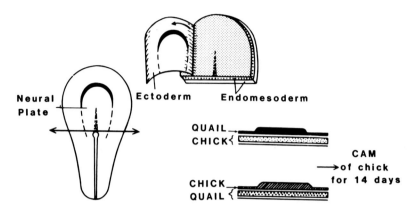

Fig. 13 Germ layer recombination.

conversely. Host blastoderms are cultured ventral side up according to New's technique for an additional 24 hr. Similar experiments can also be performed *in ovo* (Catala *et al.*, 1996).

VII. Hemopoietic Organ Rudiment Transplantations

Similar to the cells of the neural primordium, migrations of cells are an in-built feature of hemopoietic cells. However, these migrations are more extensive in the hemopoietic system than in the nervous system since they continue past the period of ontogenesis, they may affect cells at different times of their maturation process, they can be resumed after a period of arrest, they do not need to follow defined pathways, and they respond to physiopathological cues. Cell labeling has revolutionized the long-held classical view of the ontogeny of the hemopoietic system by revealing one of its essential features: that stromal cells of hemopoietic organs do not yield hemopoietic cells. This developmental dissociation was first hypothesized from chicken combinations where the sex chromosomes were used as markers (Moore and Owen, 1965, 1967) and could be definitively and precisely established by means of quail/chick transplantations (for a review see Le Douarin *et al.*, 1984).

A. Grafts on Chorioallantoic Membrane and Injections into Chorioallantoic Vessels

The CAM of the chick embryo is an excellent culture environment for many viruses, microorganisms, and normal or tumoral tissues. When avian hemopoietic organ rudiments are grafted onto it, they are colonized by blood-borne extrinsic stem cells and thus become chimeric. The advantages of this technique are ease and rapidity. Indeed, it suffices to deposit the tissue or rudiment in an area devoid of large vessels on the CAM of 6- to 10-day embryos for the tissues to become vascularized. If the stromal frame of a rudiment is grafted, hemopoietic cells provided by the host colonize it even across species barriers between various avian species (e.g., quail and chick) or across vertebrate class barriers in the case of reptiles and birds (e.g., quail and turtle; Vasse and Beaupain, 1981) but not between birds and mammals. Thus a mouse thymic rudiment grafted onto the quail or chick CAM remains uncolonized (Moore and Owen, 1967). Blood vessels of the rudiment may connect with those of the CAM. If the rudiment is not yet vascularized, blood vessels from the CAM invade it.

Alternatively, it is possible to inject these cells into a vein of the CAM at 13 days of incubation. To that end, the egg is candled and branching vessels are identified and marked on the shell. Using a circular saw, a triangle is cut from the shell around the branching, making sure that the shell membrane remains undamaged. A drop of paraffin oil is applied to the window, making it transparent, so that the vessels become visible. The vessels remain adherent to the shell membrane, and the needle may be inserted tangentially into the direction of the branching. This procedure is mainly used to study the influence of adult lymphoid cells on the avian embryo and to analyze the process known as the graft versus host reaction (reviewed in Simonsen, 1985; Fedecka-Bruner *et al.*, 1991).

B. Grafts in Somatopleure

When the host has reached a stage of about 30 pairs of somites (around 52 hr of incubation), the vitelline membrane is torn apart using watchmaker's forceps, and the amnion is split away. The graft, marked with a few particles of carbon black, is deposited near the grafting site. The somatopleura, i.e., the body wall constituted by ectoderm and mesoderm, is split and the graft is inserted into the cleft in such a way that it remains wedged into the opening. The size of the cleft has to be adapted to that of the graft. Somatopleural grafting (Fig. 14) has been extensively used by Le Douarin's group to investigate the colonization schedule of the thymus and bursa of Fabricius (Le Douarin and Jotereau, 1975; Le Douarin *et al.*, 1975, 1984).

C. Grafts in Dorsal Mesentery

Purely mesenchymal tissues, introduced through a deep cleft made along the ventral aspect of the aorta, embed within the dorsal mesentery of the host, which provides a hemopoietic microenvironment (Fig. 15). The wall of the dorsal aorta, grafted in this location, gives rise to hemopoietic foci (Dieterlen-Lièvre, 1984).

D. Parabiosis

Parabiosis between two chicken embryos is a classical technique (see Metcalf and Moore, 1971). A simple method has been developed to achieve parabiosis between two quail embryos (Le Douarin *et al.*, 1984). The contents of two quail

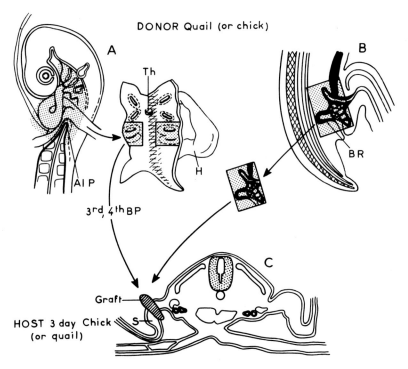

Fig. 14 Somatopleural grafting in the case of the thymus or bursa of Fabricius. AIP, anterior intestinal portal; BP, branchial pouch; H, heart; S, somatopleura; Th, thyroid. (A) A 3-day donor for the floor of the pharynx, (B) a 6-day donor for the bursa rudiment (BR), and (C) a transverse section in the trunk of a 2-day recipient showing the position of the graft.

eggs are poured into an emptied chick shell that serves as a culture dish. Vascular anastomoses form when the two embryos develop. The transfer of the two eggs to the empty shell can be accomplished until day 2 of incubation. This system has been used to demonstrate the physiological nature of the cyclic periodicity of thymus colonization by hemopoietic precursors in intact embryos (Le Douarin *et al.*, 1984).

E. Orthotopic Transplantations of Thymus and Bursa of Fabricius

The heterotopic transplantation of the thymus and bursal rudiments into the somatopleure of an E3 host has been instrumental in demonstrating the hemopoietic origin of the T and B lymphocytes, the colonization schedule of the primary lymphoid organs, and the emergence of T-cell subpopulations within the thymus (see Dieterlen-Lièvre and Le Douarin, 1993, and references therein). More refined techniques have been devised (Martin, 1983; Belo *et al.*, 1985) to substitute *in ovo* the thymic and bursal epitheliomesenchymal rudiments of the chick by their quail counterpart prior to their colonization.

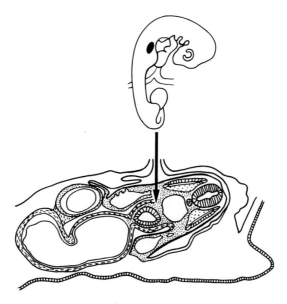

Fig. 15 Grafting into the dorsal mesentery. The graft is inserted through a cleft in the body wall at the wing level just ventral to the aorta (black dot in the schematized embryo). The arrow indicates the location of the graft, ventral to the aorta in a section.

1. Microsurgery of Thymus

a. Extirpation of Thymus

Extirpation is carried out when the chick embryo is at stage 25–26 of HH (E5). The shell is opened above the air chamber, and the shell membrane is removed. Using forceps, a window is carefully opened in the chorion and the amnion. The tegument of the neck is then incised with a microscalpel above the vagus nerve, which can be seen transparently through the skin. The two thymic primordia that derive from the third and the fourth branchial pouches appear as white masses between aortic arches III–IV and IV–V, respectively. They are dissected and sucked out with a micropipette that has an internal tip diameter of 0.1 mm. The proximity of the aortic arches and jugular veins makes the operation quite delicate. If these vessels are injured, the embryos most often die within 24 hr. The glossopharyngeal nerves are present near the posterior thymic primordia and make their complete ablation uneasy. For bilateral thymectomy, the embryo that usually lies right side upwards is first operated on the right side and is then rotated inside the amniotic cavity.

b. Grafting

The quail thymuses that are to be grafted are taken either from 5-day-old embryos, therefore still uncolonized by lymphoid precursor cells, or from 6- to 8-day embryos, then already seeded. Each thymic rudiment, which includes a minimum of surrounding mesenchyme, is inserted into the space made by the extirpation of the host thymic primordium.

2. Microsurgery of Bursa of Fabricius

The bursa develops much better when it is grafted in an orthotopic position instead of a heterotopic site. This experimental model has been used to study the immunological status of birds in which B-cell progenitors develop in a foreign microenvironment (Belo *et al.*, 1985; Corbel *et al.*, 1987). As in the case of the thymus, surgery involves two steps: bursectomy followed by *in situ* implantation of a foreign bursal rudiment (Fig. 16). The method, described next, which permits precise replacement of the recipient bursa by a foreign rudiment, is well tolerated so that animals hatch and survive until adulthood. This method has replaced a former operation in which the rump of the embryos was cut out at 72 hr of incubation (Fitzsimmons *et al.*, 1973). This resulted not only in the absence of the bursa but also of the caudal gut and was not compatible with prolonged postnatal survival.

a. Bursectomy

Bursectomy is performed in the E5 chick embryo. After opening the shell and the shell membrane, a window is made in the chorion and the amnion, above the posterior part of the embryo. The right hind limb of the embryo is maintained in deflection by means of a humidified cotton thread, the ends of which are

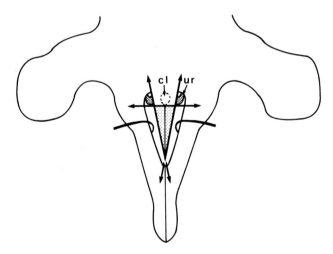

Fig. 16 The posterior part of a chick embryo at 5 days of incubation after a superficial section over the cloacal area. Arrows indicate the transverse and lateral cuts that will liberate the bursal region (represented as a dotted area), which will be removed. Ur, arrival of the uretera in the cloaca; cl, view of the cloacal cavity across the superficial ectoderm.

applied to the egg shell where they adhere. The tail is extended with curved forceps, thus providing access to the cloacal region. The bursal rudiment is isolated by a transversal cut in the anal plate just behind the ureters and is then removed by two lateral cuts.

b. Isotopic and Isochronic Transplantation of Quail Bursal Rudiment

The quail bursal primordium to be grafted is taken from quail embryos at E5, and the graft is inserted at the exact site of chick bursa removal. The superficial sheets of mesenchymal cells are peeled off from the quail bursal rudiment in order to avoid contaminating the graft by peribursal blood vessels and donor blood cells. The quail bursa, slightly smaller than its chick counterpart, is deposited in the space made by the extirpation of host bursal rudiment; care should be taken to position the graft with the proper anteroposterior and dorsoventral orientation. The leg and the tail of the recipient embryo are then placed back in their normal positions. The amnion is sealed by joining and cutting together the edges of the opening. The shell membrane is pushed back into its initial position, covering the embryo, and the shell is sealed with adhesive tape.

F. Yolk Sac Chimeras

This microsurgical technique (Martin, 1972) consists of suturing the quail embryonic body onto the chick extraembryonic area (Fig. 17). The operation is

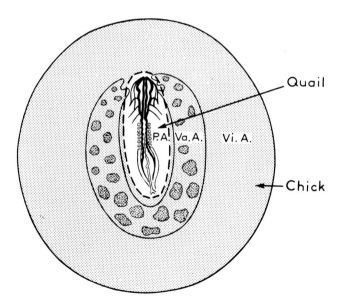

Fig. 17 Construction of a yolk sac chimera. The stippled line indicates the suture between the two components. P.A., pellucid area; Va.A., vascular area; Vi.A., Vitelline area.

performed during the second day of incubation on embryos ranging from 8 to 22 pairs of somites. The blastodiscs providing the two components of the association are matched for stage. White Leghorn chick eggs are incubated 6 hr earlier than the quail to achieve synchrony. The quail blastoderms, donors of the embryonic area, are taken out in Tyrode's solution and the vitelline membrane is removed. The central area of the blastoderm is trimmed, but a small margin is left around the head and somites. This margin will be resected as the central area is seamed onto the extraembryonic area.

The recipient chick blastodisc may be made more discernible by depositing a few particles of neutral red on the vitelline membrane. As neutral red diffuses, it stains the blastodisc evenly. The trimmed donor embryo is transplanted by means of a wide-mouthed pipette onto the recipient blastoderm and is positioned correctly, with respect to the germ layers as well as with respect to the cephalocaudal axis, side by side with the original embryo. Only then is the vitelline membrane of the host blastoderm torn apart and the embryo excised. The transplanted embryo is moved above the cavity, and the edges of the two partner blastodiscs are seamed together by resecting their margins simultaneously with Pascheff scissors. The success of the operation depends on the localization of the blastodisc which, ideally, should be at the center of the egg opening. If the blastodisc is in an oblique position, the suture, submitted to shear stress, may crack open. After the operation, the egg is sealed with tape and reincubated. New blood vessels grow across the seam and the chimeras develop according to a pattern very similar to that of normal quail embryos. The weight of the grafted quail embryo is statistically increased at all ages of incubation, and the retraction of the yolk sac, which is under thyroid control, proceeds more rapidly than in a control chick embryo. Around 10% of the operated embryos continue development and reach day 13 or 14 of incubation. In these chimeras, definitive hemopoietic organs are exclusively colonized by hemopoietic stem cells from the embryo proper, not from the yolk sac (Dieterlen-Lièvre, 1975; Martin *et al.*, 1978), while circulating red blood cells are from the chick species until E6 and become progressively intermixed with erythrocytes from quail thereafter (Beaupain *et al.*, 1979).

This type of chimera has also been made between two chick partners from inbred lines differing by their genetic sex (Lassila *et al.*, 1978), by their presumptive immunoglobin allotypes (Martin *et al.*, 1979), or by their major histocompatability antigens (Lassila *et al.*, 1982). Such chick–chick chimeras were able to hatch and grow to adulthood.

Finally, chick embryos have also been grafted on quail extraembryonic areas, i.e., according to the reverse combination (Cuadros *et al.*, 1992). The principle of the operation is basically the same. It should be pointed out, however, that suturing the transplanted embryonic area onto the recipient blastodisc is very difficult in this configuration because of the small size and the more pronounced curvature of the quail vitelline globe. These chimeras have been raised only until day 5 of incubation.

A variant of the yolk sac chimera consists of replacing part of the embryonic body of one species with the homologous part of the other species. These so-called "complementary chimeras," built either *in vitro* (Didier and Fargeix, 1976) or *in vivo* (Martin *et al.*, 1980; Hajji *et al.*, 1988), have proven useful in studying the development of the kidney and the gonad.

VIII. Results, Discussion, and Perspectives

The quail–chick transplantation technique has been used in many applications. In our own laboratory it has been used to follow the migrations of cells of the neural, hemopoietic, and angiogenic lineages. For the first time, the wide dispersion of cells emerging from the neural crest could be visualized in the embryo itself from the moment they depart from the neural primordium up to when they have homed to their definitive location and have reached a fully differentiated state.

The possibility of labeling selectively small populations of neural crest cells, such as those arising from the vagal region of the embryo which invade the whole gut, gives a striking view of the remarkably invasive capabilities of these cells (see Le Douarin, 1982). The analysis of the fate of the cephalic neural fold performed in the early neurula (Couly *et al.*, 1993) and at later stages of development (see Le Douarin, 1982, and references therein) disclosed the paramount role of this structure in the morphogenesis of the vertebrate head.

The plasticity of the neural crest cell populations arising from each level of the neural axis was revealed by heterotopic transplantations of fragments of the quail neural primordium into chick embryos (Le Douarin and Teillet, 1974). The demonstration followed that the environment in which the neural crest cells migrate is critical in determining their fate.

The experiments which involve the construction of brain chimeras are particularly well suited in detecting the migrations of cells moving within the plane of the neuroepithelium (Le Douarin, 1993). The fact that the ependymal layer of epithelial cells does not mix makes the initial limits of the quail and chick territories permanently visible. Thus, the cells generated by either of them that cross these limits can be recognized even if they have migrated far from their point of origin. Such migrations, tangential in relationship to the surface of the neuroepithelium, cannot be perceived by the conventional radioisotopic method based on pulses of tritiated thymidine, which in contrast reveals radial cell migrations very efficiently.

The quail–chick method has thus clearly revealed the tangential migrations of cells of the rhombic lip in the myelencephalon (Tan and Le Douarin, 1991) and is now being used to study the origin of oligodendrocytes in the spinal cord (Cameron-Curry and Le Douarin, 1996).

Morphogenetic movements affecting large areas of the brain vesicles during neurogenesis can be demonstrated in quail–chick chimeras. This was illustrated for the cerebellum (Hallonet *et al.*, 1990) and was finely analyzed later by transplantation restricted to defined strips of neuroepithelium more or less distant from the sagittal plan (Hallonet and Le Douarin, 1993). The demonstration that mesencephalic areas could induce diencephalic neuroepithelial territories to express the engrailed gene (En2) and to acquire the tectal structure and properties was brought about convincingly by this technique (Itasaki and Nakamura, 1992; Itasaki *et al.*, 1991; Martinez *et al.*, 1991).

Those are only some examples of the results obtained by means of the quail–chick neural chimeras. Clearly this simple method, which can be combined with immunological reagents and molecular probes, still has a large array of future uses for deciphering the complexity of neurogenesis.

Another domain where the quail–chick system has brought important and undisputable data concerns the development of the primary lymphoid organs. Before research began on this subject, the long controversy concerning the embryonic origin of the lymphocytes in the thymus and, in birds, in the bursa of Fabricius was not settled. The hematogenic hypothesis put forward by Moore and Owen (1965, 1967) and the demonstration that all of the lymphocytes and blood cells which develop in the hemopoietic organs have an extrinsic origin have been confirmed. It was also shown that, at least in birds, the hemopoietic precursors that function during adult life originate from the embryo itself and not from the yolk sac as proposed by Moore and Owen (see Metcalf and Moore, 1971). More and more evidence has accumulated indicating that, in mammals as in birds, the intraembryonic mesoderm and not the yolk sac provides the adult with its hemopoietic stem cells (Dieteren-Lièvre, 1975; Dieterlen-Lièvre and Le Douarin, 1993). The origin of intraembryonic hemopoietic stem cells could be located to the mesoderm in the neighborhood of the aorta (Fig. 18) (Dieterlen-Lièvre and Martin, 1981; Dieterlen-Lièvre, 1994).

The quail–chick marker system has shown that the avian embryonic thymus is seeded by successive waves of incoming hemopoietic cells. Figure 18 summarizes the major events in the development of the hemopoietic system, all of which were disclosed by means of interspecific transplantations. The use of species-specific markers of T-cell subpopulations made it possible to precisely determine the type of receptor these T cells produce at different developmental times (Coltey *et al.*, 1989). Moreover, the knowledge thus acquired on thymus ontogeny led to the demonstration that the thymic epithelium plays a major role in tolerance to self (Ohki *et al.*, 1987, 1988). Angiogenesis, the ontogeny of blood vessels, and the differentiation of their constitutive endothelial cells represent a crucial domain of developmental biology that is necessary for understanding several important biological processes such as morphogenesis and growth, as well as for tumor biology (review in Folkman and Shing, 1992). The avian embryo, in which blood vessel development can be easily visualized and followed, has been the elected experimental system for a number of pioneering studies in this field (Péault *et al.*, 1983; Pardanaud *et al.*, 1987, 1989; Pardanaud and Dieterlen-Lièvre, 1993; Noden, 1989; Poole and Coffin, 1989). In particular, it has been

SITES OF ERYTHROPOIESIS AND HEMOPOIETIC CELL PRODUCTION

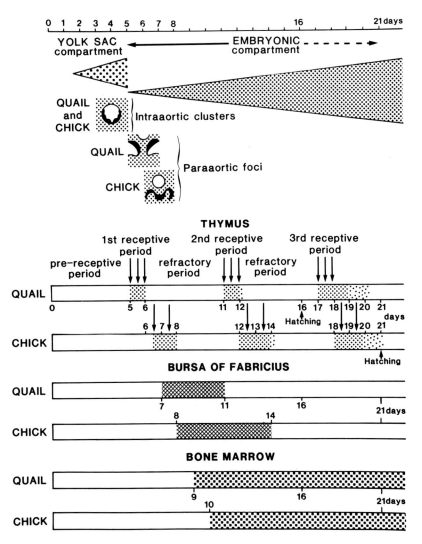

Fig. 18 Timetable of the major events in the ontogeny of the hemopoietic system in quail and chick embryos. During the first phase (symbolized with thick dots) the yolk sac functions with its own stem cells. During the second phase (finer dots) it receives additional stem cells from the embryo, as demonstrated in the chick yolk sac/quail embryo chimeras (Beaupain *et al.*, 1979). The intraaortic and paraaortic hemopoietic processes and the colonization periods of organ rudiments are schematized. This dynamic view of the ontogeny of the hemopoietic system was acquired by means of different quail/chick transplantation schemes; the quail nucleolar marker and the MB1/QH1 monoclonal antibodies were used to identify the species of origin of the component cells.

shown that two different mechanisms are responsible for the emergence of the endothelial tree in the embryo: the body wall is colonized by extrinsic precursors, while the mesenchyme of internal organs gives rise to endothelial cells *in situ* (Pardanaud and Dieterlen-Lièvre, 1993).

To conclude the quail/chick transplantation system has yielded views about the development of the neural and blood-forming systems that are applicable to amniotes. The avian model has also been used to analyze the development of limbs, kidney, and gonads. Further applications still need to be devised, either to follow up initiated investigations or to explore new issues. It is foreseeable that new tools will reinforce already available methods, e.g., probes that will recognize messenger RNAs, or retroviral vectors that will integrate in the genome, in one only of the two species.

Acknowledgments

We thank Marie-Françoise Meunier for expert preparation of the manuscript and reference filing, Yann Rantier and Françoise Viala for photographic work, and Sophie Gournet for line drawings.

References

Alvarado-Mallart, R. M., and Sotelo, C. (1984). Homotopic and heterotopic transplantations of quail tectal primordia in chick embryos: Organization of the retinotectal projections in the chimeric embryos. *Dev. Biol.* **103,** 378–398.

Balaban, E., Teillet, M.-A., and Le Douarin, N. M. (1988). Application of the quail-chick chimera system to the study of brain development and behavior. *Science* **241,** 1339–1342.

Bally-Cuif, L., and Wassef, M. (1994). Ectopic induction and reorganization of Wnt-1 expression in quail-chick chimeras. *Development (Cambridge, UK)* **120,** 3379–3394.

Beaupain, D., Martin, C., and Dieterlen-Lièvre, F. (1979). Are developmental hemoglobin changes related to the origin of stem cells and site of erythropoiesis? *Blood* **53,** 212–225.

Belo, M., Martin, C., Corbel, C., and Le Douarin, N. M. (1985). A novel method to bursectomize avian embryos and obtain quail-chick bursal chimeras. I. Immunocytochemical analysis of such chimeras by using species-specific monoclonal antibodies. *J. Immunol.* **135,** 3785–3794.

Belo, M., Martin, C., Corbel, C., and Le Douarin, N. M. (1989). Thymic epithelium tolerizes chickens to embryonic graft of quail bursa of Fabricius. *Int. Immunol.* **1,** 105–112.

Bucy, R. P., Coltey, M., Chen, C. I., Char, D., Le Douarin, N. M., and Cooper, M. D. (1989). Cytoplasmic CD3+ surface CD8+ lymphocytes develop as a thymus-independent lineage in chick-quail chimeras. *Eur. J. Immunol.* **19,** 1449–1455.

Cameron-Curry, P., and Le Douarin, N. M. (1996). Oligodendrocyte precursors originate from both the dorsal and the ventral parts of the spinal cord. *Neuron,* in press.

Catala, M., Teillet, M.-A., and Le Douarin, N. M. (1995). Organization and development of the tail bud analyzed with the quail-chick chimaera system. *Mech. Dev.* **51,** 51–65.

Catala, M. *et al.* (1996). In preparation.

Chan, M., Chen, C. L., Ager, L., and Cooper, M. (1988). Identification of the avian homologues of mammalian CD4 and CD8 antigens. *J. Immunol.* **140,** 21–33.

Chen, C. H., Ager, L. L., Gartland, G. L., and Cooper, M. D. (1986). Identification of a T3/T cell receptor complex in the chicken. *J. Exp. Med.* **164,** 375–380.

Chen, C. L., Cihak, J., Lösch, U., and Cooper, M. D. (1988). Differential expression of two T cell receptors, TcR1 and TcR2 on chicken lymphocytes. *Eur. J. Immunol.* **18,** 539–543.

Cihak, J., Hoffmann-Fezer, G., Ziegler-Heitbrock, H. W. L., Trainer, H., Schranner, I., Merkenschlager, M., and Lösch, U. (1988). Characterization and functional properties of a novel monoclonal antibody which identifies a T cell receptor in chicken. *Eur. J. Immunol.* **18**, 533–538.

Coltey, M., Bucy, R. P., Chen, C. H., Cihak, J., Lösh, U., Char, D., Le Douarin, N. M., and Cooper, M. D. (1989). Analysis of the first two waves of thymus homing stem cells and their T cell progeny in chick-quail chimeras. *J. Exp. Med.* **170**, 543–557.

Conrad, G. W., Bee, J. A., Roche, S. M., and Teillet, M.-A. (1993). Fabrication of microscalpels by electrolysis of tungsten wire in a meniscus. *J. Neurosci. Methods* **50**, 123–127.

Corbel, C., Belo, M., Martin, C., and Le Douarin, N. M. (1987). A novel method to bursectomize avian embryos and obtain quail/chick bursal chimeras. II. Immune response of bursectomized chicks and chimeras and postnatal rejection of the grafted quail bursas. *J. Immunol.* **138**, 2813–2821.

Couly, G. F., and Le Douarin, N. M. (1985). Mapping of the early neural primordium in quail-chick chimeras. I. Developmental relationships between placodes, facial ectoderm, and prosencephalon. *Dev. Biol.* **110**, 422–439.

Couly, G. F., and Le Douarin N. M. (1987). Mapping of the early neural primordium in quail-chick chimeras. II. The prosencephalic neural plate and neural folds: implications for the genesis of cephalic human congenital abnormalities. *Dev. Biol.* **120**, 198–214.

Couly, G. F., and Le Douarin, N. M. (1988). The fate map of the cephalic neural primordium at the presomitic to the 3-somite stage in the avian embryo. *Development (Cambridge, UK)* **103**, Suppl., 101–113.

Couly, G. F., Coltey, P. M., and Le Douarin, N. M. (1993). The triple origin of skull in higher vertebrates—A study in quail-chick chimeras. *Development (Cambridge, UK)* **117**, 409–429.

Cuadros, M. A., Coltey, P., Nieto, C. M., and Martin, C. (1992). Demonstration of a phagocytic cell system belonging to the hemopoietic lineage and originating from the yolk sac in the early avian embryo. *Development (Cambridge, UK)* **115**, 157–168.

Didier, E., and Fargeix, N. (1976). La population germinale des gonades chez des embryons chimères obtenus par l'association de fragments de blastomères de caille japonaise et de poulet domestique. *Experientia* **32**, 1333–1334.

Dieterlen-Lièvre, F. (1975). On the origin of haemopoietic stem cells in the avian embryo: An experimental approach. *J. Embryol. Exp. Morphol.* **33**, 607–619.

Dieterlen-Lièvre, F. (1984). Emergence of intraembryonic blood stem cells in avian chimeras by means of monoclonal antibodies. *Dev. Comp. Immunol.* **3**, 75–80.

Dieterlen-Lièvre, F. (1994). Hemopoiesis during avian ontogeny. *Poult. Sci. Rev.* **5**, 273–305.

Dieterlen-Lièvre, F., and Le Douarin, N. M. (1993). Developmental rules in the hematopoietic and immune systems of birds: How general are they? *Semin. Dev. Biol.* **4**, 6325–6332.

Dieterlen-Lièvre, F., and Martin, C. (1981). Diffuse intraembryonic hemopoiesis in normal and chimeric avian development. *Dev. Biol.* **88**, 180–191.

Dulac, C., Tropak, M. B., Cameron-Curry, P., Rossier, J., Marshak, D. R., Roder, J., and Le Douarin, N. M. (1992). Structural similarities within the immunoglobulin superfamily. *Neuron* **8**, 323–334.

Eyal-Giladi, H., and Kochav, S. (1976). From cleavage to primitive streak formation: A complementary normal table and a new look at the first stages of the development of the chick. I. General morphology. *Dev. Biol.* **49**, 321–337.

Fadlallah, N., Guy, N., Teillet, M.-A., Schuler, B., Le Douarin, N. M., Naquet, R., and Batini, C. (1995). Brain chimeras for the study of an avian model of genetic epilepsy: Structures involved in sound- and light-induced seizures. *Brain Res.* **675**, 55–66.

Fedecka-Bruner, B., Vaigot, P., Dèsveaux-Chabrol, J., Gendreau, M., Kroemer, G., and Dieterlen-Lièvre, F. (1991). T lymphocyte subsets in the embryonic spleen undergoing a graft-versus-host reaction. *Dev. Immunol.* **1**, 163–168.

Feulgen, R., and Rossenbeck, H. (1924). Mikroskopisch-chemischer Nachweiss einer Nucleinsaüre von Typus der Thymonucleinsaüre und die darauf beruhende elektive Farbung von Zellkernen in microskopischen Präparaten. *Hoppe-Seyler's Z. Physiol. Chem.* **135**, 203–252.

Fitzsimmons, R. C., Garrod, E. M. F., and Garnett, I. (1973). Immunological response following early embryonic surgical bursectomy. *Cell. Immunol.* **9**, 377–383.

Folkman, J., and Shing, Y. (1992). Angiogenesis. *J. Biol. Chem.* **267**, 10931–10934.

Fontaine, J., and Le Douarin, N. M. (1977). Analysis of endoderm formation in the avian blastoderm by the use of quail-chick chimeras. The problem of the neurectodermal origin of the cells of the APUD series. *J. Embryol. Exp. Morphol.* **41**, 209–222.

Fontaine-Perus, J., Chanconie, M., and Le Douarin, N. M. (1985). Embryonic origin of substance P containing neurons in cranial and spinal sensory ganglia of the avian embryo. *Dev. Biol.* **107**, 227–238.

Gabe, M. (1968). "Techniques histologiques." Masson, Paris.

Grapin-Botton, A., Bonnin, M.-A., McNaughton, L., Krumlauf, R., and Le Douarin, N. M. (1995). Plasticity of transposed rhombomeres: Hox gene induction is correlated with phenotypic modifications. *Development (Cambridge, UK)* **121**, 2707–2721.

Guy, N. T. M., Teillet, M.-A., Schuler, B., Le Gal La Salle, G., Le Douarin, N., Naquet, R., and Batini, C. (1992). Pattern of electroencephalographic activity during light induced seizures in genetic epileptic chicken and brain chimeras. *Neurosci. Lett.* **145**, 55–58.

Guy, N. T. M., Batini, C., Naquet, R., and Teillet, M.-A. (1993). Avian photogenic epilepsy and embryonic brain chimeras: Neuronal activity of the adult prosencephalon and mesencephalon. *Exp. Brain Res.* **93**, 196–204.

Hajji, K., Martin, C., Perramon, A., and Dieterlen-Lièvre, F. (1988). Sexual phenotype of avian chimeric gonads with germinal and stromal cells of opposite genetic sexes. *Biol. Struct. Morphol.* **1**, 107–116.

Hallonet, M. E. R., and Le Douarin, N. M. (1993). Tracing neuroepithelial cells of the mesencephalic and metencephalic alar plates during cerebellar ontogeny in quail-chick chimaeras. *Eur. J. Neurosci.* **5**, 1145–1155.

Hallonet, M. E. R., Teillet, M-A., and Le Douarin, N. M (1990). A new approach to the development of the cerebellum provided by the quail-chick marker system. *Development (Cambridge, UK)* **108**, 19–31.

Hamburger, V., and Hamilton, H. L. (1951). A series of normal stages in the development of chick embryo. *J. Morphol.* **88**, 49–92.

Itasaki, N., and Nakamura, H. (1992). Rostrocaudal polarity of the tectum in birds: Correlation of *en* gradient and topographic order in retinotectal projection. *Neuron* **8**, 787–798.

Itasaki, N., Ichijo, H., Hama, C., Matsuno, T., and Nakamura, H. (1991). Establishment of rostrocaudal polarity in tectal primordium: Engrailed expression and subsequent tectal polarity. *Development (Cambridge, UK)* **113**, 1133–1144.

Izpisùa-Belmonte, J. C., De Robertis, E. M., Storey, K. G., and Stern, C. D. (1993). The homeobox gene *goosecoid* and the origin of organizer cells in the early chick blastoderm. *Cell (Cambridge, Mass.)* **74**, 645–659.

Kinutani, M. C., Coltey, M., and Le Douarin, N. M. (1986). Postnatal development of a demyelinating disease in avian spinal cord chimaeras. *Cell (Cambridge, Mass.)* **45**, 307–314.

Lance-Jones, C., and Lagenaur, C. F. (1987). A new marker for identifying quail cells in embryonic avian chimeras: A quail specific antiserum. *J. Histochem. Cytochem.* **35**, 771–780.

Lassila, O., Eskola, J., Toivanen, P., Martin, C., and Dieterlen-Lièvre, F. (1978). The origin of lymphoid stem cells studied in chick yolk sac-embryo chimaeras. *Nature (London)* **272**, 353–354.

Lassila, O., Martin, C., Toivanen, P., and Dieterlen-Lièvre, F. (1982). Erythropoiesis and lymphopoiesis in the chick yolk-sac embryo chimeras: Contribution of yolk sac and intraembryonic stem cells. *Blood* **59**, 377–381.

Le Douarin, N. M. (1969). Particularités du noyau interphasique chez la caille japonaise (*Coturnix coturnix japonica*). Utilisation de ces particularités comme "marquage biologique" dans les recherches sur les interactions tissulaires et les migrations cellulaires au cours de l'ontogenèse. *Bull. Biol. Fr. Belg.* **103**, 435–452.

Le Douarin, N. M. (1971). La structure du noyau interphasique chez différentes espèces d'oiseaux. *C. R. Hebd. Séances Acad. Sci.* **272**, 1402–1404.

Le Douarin, N. M. (1973a). A biological cell labelling technique and its use in experimental embryology. *Dev. Biol.* **30,** 217–222.

Le Douarin, N. M. (1973b). A Feulgen-positive nucleolus. *Exp. Cell Res.* **77,** 459–468.

Le Douarin, N. M. (1982). "The Neural Crest." Cambridge Univ. Press, Cambridge, UK.

Le Douarin, N. M. (1993). Embryonic neural chimaeras in the study of brain development. *Trends Neurosci.* **16,** 64–72.

Le Douarin, N. M., and Jotereau, F. (1975). Tracing of the avian thymus through embryonic life in interspecific chimeras. *J. Exp. Med.* **142,** 17–40.

Le Douarin, N. M., and Teillet, M.-A. (1973). The migration of neural crest cells to the wall of the digestive tract in avian embryo. *J. Embryol. Exp. Morphol.* **30,** 31–48.

Le Douarin, N. M., and Teillet, M.-A. (1974). Experimental analysis of the migration and differentiation of neuroblasts of the autonomic nervous system and of neurectodermal mesenchyme derivatives, using a biological cell marking technique. *Dev. Biol.* **41,** 162–184.

Le Douarin, N. M., Houssaint, E., Jotereau, F., and Belo, M. (1975). Origin of haematopoietic stem cells in the bursa of Fabricius and bone-marrow studied through interspecific chimeras. *Proc. Natl. Acad. Sci. U.S.A.* **72,** 2701–2705.

Le Douarin, N. M., Guillemot, F. P., Oliver, P., and Péault, B. (1983). Distribution and origin of Ia-positive cells in the avian thymus analyzed by means of monoclonal antibodies in heterospecific chimeras. *In* "Progress in Immunology" (Y. Yamamura and T. Tada, eds.), pp. 613–631. Academic Press, New York.

Le Douarin, N. M., Dieterlen-Lièvre, F., and Oliver, P. (1984). Ontogeny of primary lymphoid organs and lymphoid stem cells. *Am. J. Anat.* **170,** 261–299.

Le Lièvre, C., and Le Douarin, N. M. (1975). Mesenchymal derivatives of the neural crest: analysis of chimaeric quail and chick embryos. *J. Embryol. Exp. Morphol.* **34,** 125–154.

Martin, C. (1972). Technique d'explantation *in ovo* de blastodermes d'embryons d'oiseaux. *C. R. Séances Soc. Biol. Ses Fil.* **116,** 283–285.

Martin, C. (1983). Total thymectomy in the early chick embryo. *Arch. Anat. Microsc. Morphol. Exp.* **72,** 107–115.

Martin, C. (1990). Quail-chick chimeras, a tool for developmental immunology. *In* "The Avian Model in Developmental Biology: From Organism to Genes" (N. Le Douarin, F. Dieterlen-Lièvre, and J. Smith, eds.), pp. 207–217. Editions du CNRS, Paris.

Martin, C., Beaupain, D., and Dieterlen-Lièvre, F. (1978). Developmental relationships between vitelline and intra-embryonic haemopoiesis studied in avian "yolk sac chimaeras." *Cell Differ.* **7,** 115–130.

Martin, C., Lassila, O., Nurmi, T., Eskola, J., Dieterlen-Lièvre, F., and Toivanen, P. (1979). Intraembryonic origin of lymphoid stem cells in the chicken. *Scand. J. Immunol.* **10,** 333–338.

Martin, C., Beaupain, D., and Dieterlen-Lièvre, F. (1980). A study of the development of the hemopoietic system using quail-chick chimeras obtained by blastoderm recombination. *Dev. Biol.* **75,** 303–314.

Martinez, S., and Alvarado-Mallart, R.-M. (1989). Rostral cerebellum originates from the caudal portion of the so-called "mesencephalic" vesicle: A study using chick/quail chimeras. *Eur. J. Neurosci.* **1,** 549–560.

Martinez, S., and Alvarado-Mallart, R.-M. (1990). Expression of the homeobox *chick-en* gene in chick/quail chimeras with inverted mes-metencephalic grafts. *Dev. Biol.* **139,** 432–436.

Martinez, S., Wassef, M., and Alvarado-Mallart, R.-M. (1991). Induction of a mesencephalic phenotype in the two-day-old chick prosencephalon is preceded by the early expression of the homeobox gene *en. Neuron* **6,** 971–981.

Metcalf, D., and Moore, M. A. S. (1971). "Haemopoietic Cells." North-Holland Publ., Amsterdam.

Moore, M. A. S., and Owen, J. J. T. (1965). Chromosome marker studies on the development of the haemopoietic system in the chick embryo. *Nature (London)* **208,** 958–989.

Moore, M. A. S., and Owen, J. J. T. (1967). Experimental studies on the development of the thymus. *J. Exp. Med.* **126,** 715–725.

Nakamura, H. (1990). Do CNS anlagen have plasticity in differentiation? Analysis in quail-chick chimera. *Brain Res.* **511,** 122–128.

Nataf, V., Mercier, P., Ziller, C., and Le Douarin, N. M. (1993). Novel markers of melanocyte differentiation in the avian embryo. *Exp. Cell Res.* **207,** 171–182.

New, D. A. T. (1955). A new technique for the cultivation of the chick embryo in vitro. *J. Embryol. Exp. Morphol.* **23,** 79–108.

Noden, D. M. (1989). Embryonic origins and assembly of blood vessels. *Am. Rev. Respir. Dis.* **140,** 1097–1103.

Ohki, H., Martin, C., Corbel, C., Coltey, M., and Le Douarin, N. M. (1987). Tolerance induced by thymic epithelial grafts in birds. *Science* **237,** 1032–1035.

Ohki, H., Martin, C., Coltey, M., and Le Douarin, N. M. (1988). Implants of quail thymic epithelium generate permanent tolerance in embryonically constructed quail/chick chimeras. *Development (Cambridge, UK)* **104,** 619–630.

Pardanaud, L., and Dieterlen-Lièvre, F. (1993). Emergence of endothelial and hemopoietic cells in the avian embryo. *Anat. Embryol.* **187,** 107–114.

Pardanaud, L., and Dieterlen-Lièvre, F. (1995). Does the paraxial mesoderm of the avian embryo have hemangioblastic capacities? *Anat. Embryol.* **192,** 301–308.

Pardanaud, L., Altmann, C., Kitos, P., Dieterlen-Lièvre, F., and Buck, C. (1987). Vasculogenesis in the early quail blastodisc as studied with a monoclonal antibody recognizing endothelial cells. *Development (Cambridge, UK)* **100,** 339–349.

Pardanaud, L., Yassine, F., and Dieterlen-Lièvre, F. (1989). Relationship between vasculogenesis, angiogenesis, and haemopoiesis during avian ontogeny. *Development (Cambridge, UK)* **105,** 473–485.

Péault, B., and Labastie, M.-C. (1990). Surface markers of the hemangioblastic cell lineage: A review of the specificities of MB1 and QH1. *In* "The Avian Model in Developmental Biology: From Organism to Genes" (N. Le Douarin, F. Dieterlen-Lièvre, and J. Smith, eds.), pp. 165–179. Editions du CNRS, Paris.

Péault, B., Thiery, J.-P., and Le Douarin, N. M. (1983). A surface marker for the hemopoietic and endothelial cell lineages in the quail species defined by a monoclonal antibody. *Proc. Natl. Acad. Sci. U.S.A.* **80,** 2976–2980.

Petitte, J. N., Clark, M. E., Liu, G., Verrinder Gibbins, A. M., and Etches, R. J. (1990). Production of somatic and germline chimeras in the chicken by transfer of early blastodermal cells. *Development (Cambridge, UK)* **108,** 185–189.

Poole, T. J., and Coffin, J. D. (1989). Vasculogenesis and angiogenesis: Two distinct morphogenetic mechanisms establish embryonic vascular pattern. *J. Exp. Zool.* **251,** 224.

Rong, P.-M., Ziller, C., Pena-Melian, A., and Le Douarin, N. M. (1987). A monoclonal antibody specific for avian early myogenic cells and differentiated muscle. *Dev. Biol.* **122,** 338–353.

Schoenwolf, G. C., Bortier, H., and Vakaet, L. (1989). Fate mapping the avian neural plate with quail/chick chimeras: Origin of prospective median wedge cells. *J. Exp. Zool.* **249,** 271–278.

Schoenwolf, G. C., Garcia-Martinez, V., and Dias, M. S. (1992). Mesoderm movement and fate during avian gastrulation and neurulation. *Dev. Dyn.* **193,** 235–248.

Simonsen, M. (1985). Graft-versus-host-reactions: The history that never was, and the way things happened to happen. *Immunol. Rev.* **88,** 5–23.

Takagi, S., Toshiaki, T., Kinutani, M., and Fujisawa, H. (1989). Monoclonal antibodies against specific antigens in the chick central nervous system: Putative application as a transplantation marker in the quail-chick chimaera. *J. Histochem. Cytochem.* **37,** 177–184.

Tan, K., and Le Douarin, N. M. (1991). Development of the nuclei and cell migration in the medulla oblongata. Application of the quail-chick chimera system. *Anat. Embryol.* **183,** 321–343.

Tanaka, H., Kinutani, M., Agata, A., Takashima, Y., and Obata, K. (1990). Pathfinding during spinal tract formation in quail-chick chimaera analysed by species specific monoclonal antibodies. *Development (Cambridge, UK)* **110,** 565–571.

Teillet, M.-A., Naquet, R., Le Gal La Salle, G., Merat, P., Schuler, B., and Le Douarin, N. M. (1991). Transfer of genetic epilepsy by embryonic brain grafts in the chicken. *Proc. Natl. Acad. Sci. U.S.A.* **88,** 6966–6970.

Vakaet, L. (1974). Nouvelles possibilités techniques pour l'étude de la gastrulation des oiseaux. *Ann. Biol. Anim. Biochim. Biophys.* **13,** 35–41.

Vasse, J., and Beaupain, D. (1981). Erythropoiesis and hemoglobin in the turtle *Emys orbicularis* L. *J. Embryol. Exp. Morphol.* **62,** 129–138.

Watanabe, M., Kinutani, M., Naito, M., Ochi, O., and Takashima, Y. (1992). Distribution analysis of transferred donor cells in avian blastodermal chimeras. *Development (Cambridge, UK)* **114,** 331–338.

Zacchei, A. M. (1961). Lo sviluppo embrionale della quaglia giaponese. *Archivi Anatomica* **66,** 36–62.

CHAPTER 3

Manipulations of Neural Crest Cells or Their Migratory Pathways

Marianne Bronner-Fraser

Developmental Biology Center
University of California
Irvine, California 92717

I. Introduction
II. Preparation of Avian Neural Crest Cultures
    A. Preparation of Medium
    B. Preparation of Two-Dimensional Substrates
    C. Preparation of Three-Dimensional Substrates
    D. Primary Neural Crest Cultures from the Trunk Region
    E. Primary Neural Crest Cultures from the Cranial Region
    F. Secondary or Clonal Cultures
    G. Whole Trunk Explants
III. Microinjection of Cells and Antibodies into Embryos
    A. Labeling Cells Prior to Microinjection
    B. Microinjection of Cells or Antibodies into Embryos
IV. Labeling of Neural Crest Cells *in Vivo* with Vital Dyes
    A. Whole Neural Tube DiI Injections
    B. Focal Injections of DiI into Neural Folds
V. Grafting techniques
    A. Neural Tube Rotations
    B. Neural Fold Ablations
    C. Notochord Implants
    D. Notochord Ablations
VI. Conclusions
    References

I. Introduction

The formation of the embryo involves intricate cell movements, cell proliferation, and differentiation. The neural crest has long served as a model for the

Copyright © 1996 by Academic Press, Inc. All rights of reproduction in any form reserved.

study of these processes because neural crest cells undergo extensive migrations and give rise to many diverse derivatives. Neural crest cells arise from the dorsal portion of the neural tube. Several unique properties of these cells make the neural crest an ideal system for studying cell migration and differentiation. First, these cells migrate extensively along characteristic pathways. Second, they give rise to diverse and numerous derivatives, ranging from pigment cells and cranial cartilage to adrenal chromaffin cells and the ganglia of the peripheral nervous system. Third, their characteristic position of premigratory neural crest cells within the dorsal portion of the neural tube makes them accessible to surgical and molecular manipulations during initial stages in their development.

This chapter summarizes techniques for the isolation of neural crest cells in tissue culture as well as various manipulations of neural crest cells and some of the tissues with which they interact in the embryo.

II. Preparation of Avian Neural Crest Cultures

Because neural crest cells migrate away from the neural tube, it is possible to isolate them from surrounding tissues by explanting the neural tube or neural folds into culture. The remaining neural tube tissue can then be scraped away, leaving a relatively pure population of neural crest cells. When grown in a rich medium containing embryo extract, these cells differentiate into a number of normal neural crest derivatives, including pigment cells, adrenergic cells, and cholinergic cells. During the first day in culture, this technique makes it possible to examine the migration of neural crest cells on two-dimensional substrates. In addition, the effects of different culture conditions and growth factors on the differentiation of neural crest cells in longer term cultures can be monitored.

A. Preparation of Medium

Standard medium for neural crest cultures:

75% Eagle's minimal essential medium (MEM)
10% horse serum
15% embryo extract

The levels of embryo extract can be varied. In addition, some authors have developed more defined culture conditions for growing neural crest cells (Sieber-Blum, 1991). Although it is possible to purchase powdered embryo extract, it is best to prepare embryo extracts from 10- to 11-day-old chick embryos for optimal neural crest cell differentiation.

The following protocol, adapted from Cohen and Konigsberg (1975), works well as a complete medium for neural crest cells. It is best to collect all of the materials the day before embarking on this procedure as it takes the better part of a day. Note that this procedure is done as cleanly as possible, but that the glassware need not be sterilized since the embryo extract is filtered through a 0.22-μm filter prior to addition to the medium.

Materials

1–2 liters of MEM

100 ml of horse serum

Sterile Millipore filters (0.22, 0.45, 0.8, and 1.2 μm)

Sterile bottles

2 × 250-ml beakers

One large beaker with gauze over the top

Two to three graduated cylinders

Scissors/forceps

Large tubes for ultracentrifugation

Embryo Extract

1. Have ready 10 dozen chicken eggs that have been incubated for 10–11 days. "Candle" eggs by holding them up to a light source so that only viable eggs are visualized and opened. Wipe the eggs with 70% ethanol.

2. With curved sterile scissors, cut a circular opening in the blunt end of the egg. Remove the embryo by sliding one arm of the forceps under the neck of the embryo. The membranes, for the most part, will be left behind. Place the embryos in a large petri dish filled with cold MEM.

3. Using the scissors, remove the eyes and beaks from the embryos and make a few slits in the belly. Then place the embryos into another dish containing cold MEM.

4. To drain excess fluid, place the embryos onto a beaker covered with a double layer of gauze. Rinse with cold MEM to remove excess blood.

5. After draining the embryos, transfer them to a sterile beaker and mince with large scissors.

6. Transfer the minced embryos to a 50-ml plastic syringe and expel into a 500-ml sterile preweighed bottle containing a sterilized stir bar.

7. Weigh the minced embryos and add an equal amount of MEM (1 g = 1 ml). Stir for 1 hr at 4°C.

8. Add hyaluronidase (Worthington Biochemical) for the last 15 min of step 7. The grams of hyaluronidase added equals the number of milliliters of embryo extract times 4×10^{-5}. Chill and filter sterilize the hyaluronidase prior to use.

9. Ultracentrifuge for 30 min at 20,000 rpm at 4°C.

10. Separate supernatant from pellet and ultracentrifuge supernatant at 35,000 rpm at 4°C for 60 min.
11. Collect the supernatant and filter through progressively smaller pore size filters (1.2 μm followed by 0.8 μm followed by 0.45 μm followed by 0.22 μm). After filtration, the embryo extract should have an orange-reddish color and appear slightly cloudy.
12. Combine horse serum (10%), embryo extract (15%), and MEM (75%) to make complete medium and stir for 10 min.
13. Filter the complete medium through sterile 0.22-μm filters into 30-ml sterilized bottles. A bottle holds approximately 20 ml of complete medium and can be kept frozen at -80°C for up to 6 months.

B. Preparation of Two-Dimensional Substrates

Typically, cultures are plated onto substrates coated with extracellular matrix molecules. The protocol for coating dishes with most matrix molecules is similar. Therefore, fibronectin will be used as a typical example.

1. Prepare Howard Ringer's solution (or utilize a saline of your choice). Ringer's solution consists of 7.20 g of NaCl, 0.17 g of $CaCl_2$, 0.37 g of KCl, and 1000 ml of H_2O (distilled).
2. Incubate plastic tissue culture dishes (35 mm diameter or a 15-mm four-well multidish; Nunclon) with 25 μg/ml fibronectin (New York City Blood Bank) in Ringer's solution at 38°C for 1 hr.
3. Remove the excess fibronectin solution and incubate the dish with complete culture medium at 38°C for another hour.

Similar protocols can be used for other matrix components including collagen, laminin, or fragments of these molecules. In addition, the coating concentrations and nature of the salts can be varied to provide distinct types of substrates.

C. Preparation of Three-Dimensional Substrates

For some experiments, it is advantageous to grow neural crest cells or embryonic tissues in three-dimensional substrates. The collagen gels described next are typically used.

Materials

Rat tail collagen (Collaborative Research)

Dulbecco's minimum essential media (DMEM) powder high glucose, no bicarbonate (GIBCO-BRL)

7.5% bicarbonate

Horse serum

F12 nutrient medium (GIBCO); N2 supplement (GIBCO)

L-Glutamine

Penicillin/streptomycin

Four-well multidishes (Nunc)

1. Add 90 μl of rat tail collagen (3.13 mg/ml) to 10 μl of a 10× DMEM solution (pH 4). Vortex to mix. Avoid introducing bubbles. Bring to neutral pH with 7.5% sodium bicarbonate; add approximately 2–4 μl to the mixture. The collagen mixture will turn from a bright yellow to a faint orange color.

2. Place a thin layer of collagen (~ 10 μl) onto the bottom of a four-well Nunc multidish. Spread the collagen around with the tip of a pipette to make a mound about one-third the diameter of the well. This procedure must be done quickly before the collagen polymerizes. Allow it to set at room temperature for 15 to 30 min. Avoid letting the collagen dry.

3. Using a pipetteman or other means of transfer, place the explants onto the gelled collagen. Take care to remove the medium in which the explant was transferred to avoid problems with gelation of the collagen. Overlay it with another layer of collagen. The amount of collagen will vary with the size of the tissue. Make sure that the tissue is covered. Because the explant will often float to the top, use a blunt tunsgsten needle to gently poke the tissue into the liquid collagen and to position the explant in the desired orientation.

4. Allow the gel to set for 15–40 min at room temperature followed by 5 min at 37°C.

5. Gently pipette ~300 μl of complete media, F12 plus N2 or media of choice into the culture dish and incubate at 37°C in a CO_2 incubator.

6. Gels can be fixed and processed for immunostaining or *in situ* hybridization. Peel the gel of the tissue culture dish using watchmaker's forceps.

Another three-dimensional substrate that has been used successfully is Matrigel (Maxwell and Forbes, 1990) which can be made according to the manufacturer's directions.

D. Primary Neural Crest Cultures from the Trunk Region

These methods are essentially those described by Cohen and Konigsberg (1975). For most cultures, quail embryos are used because the neural crest cells from this species differentiate well *in vitro*. However, similar procedures can be followed using other avian embryos and have also been adapted for mammalian embryos. Figure 1 illustrates a typical neural crest explant immediately after plating and after 1 day in culture.

Materials

60-mm glass petri dish filled with black dental wax mixed 1 : 1 with paraffin; sterilize by flaming the surface with a Bunsen burner and cover immediately with a sterilized top

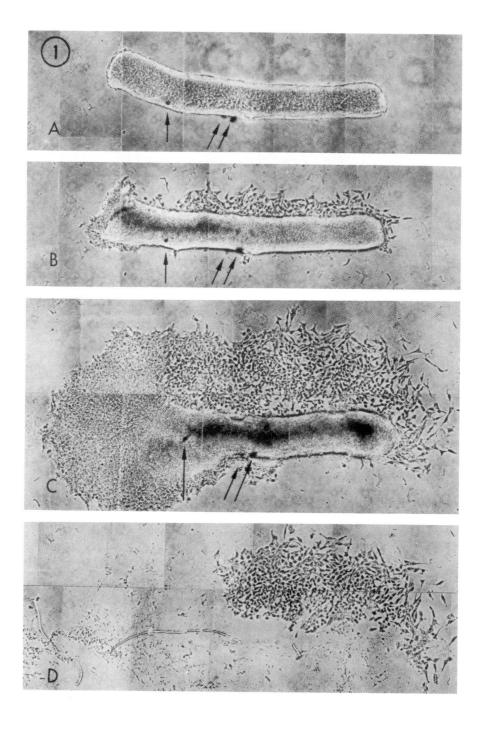

Sterilized fine scissors and forceps

Sterile Pasteur pipettes with a bent end (made by holding over a Bunsen burner until the glass bends); the large end of the pipette should be plugged with cotton

Electrolytically sharpened tungsten needles

Dispase (Worthington, 2 mg/ml in 20 mM HEPES in buffered DMEM)

Sterile three-well dishes

Complete culture medium (as described earlier)

2 × 250-ml sterile beakers

Sterile Ringer's solution

Sterile fibronectin-coated dishes

Quail eggs (*Coturnix coturnix japonica*) incubated at 38°C until they reach stages 13–14 by the criteria of Hamburger and Hamilton (1951); approximately 47 hr of incubation

Procedure

1. In a horizontal laminar flow hood, wash the quail eggs with 70% ethanol. Open the eggs gently with scissors and remove a small piece of the shell, allowing access to the embryo. Grasp the extraembryonic membranes of the embryo, cut it away from the yolk, and place in the black wax dishes filled with Ringer's solution. Embryos can also be put in sterilized dishes without black wax, if desired. Rinse the embryos and replace the Ringer's solution several times until the excess yolk is removed.

2. From each embryo, use sharp tungsten needles to excise the region of the trunk consisting of the six to nine most posterior somites as well as the unsegmented mesenchyme. Dissect by making two longitudinal cuts lateral to the somites and two transverse cuts through the neural tube and adjacent tissue.

3. Remove explants and place them into well dishes containing Ringer's solution for washing. Replace the Ringer's solution with dispase and incubate for 15 min on ice followed by 10 min at 37°C (the exact length of time is empirical and can vary somewhat with age and specific activity of dispase).

Fig. 1 Composite phase-contrast photomicrographs of a single living neural tube after explantation *in vitro*. (A) During the first 2 hr in culture, no neural crest cells emigrate. Arrows indicate carbon particles used to mark the ventral surface of the neural tube. (B) By 8 hr after explantation, some mesenchymal neural crest cells have migrated away from the neural tube. (C) Within 20 hr, hundreds of cells have left the dorsal neural tube. In addition, flattened mesenchymal cells from the neural tube form an epithelial sheet. (D) The nonneural crest cells have been scraped away with a tungsten needle, leaving the neural crest population. From Cohen and Konigsberg (1975).

4. While in dispase, aspirate and expel the explants through a bent sterile Pasteur pipette. This generates shear forces that separate the neural tube from the ectoderm, endoderm, somites, and notochord, although the latter sometimes remains attached.

5. Segregate neural tubes from other tissue and place in a well filled with complete medium, which contains endogenous enzymatic inhibitors that stop the reaction. Rinse with fresh medium.

6. Place isolated neural tubes in a few drops of medium onto prepared tissue culture dishes coated with fibronectin or the substrate of choice (Fig. 1). Incubate for 1 hr at 37°C and fill the culture dish with 1.5 ml of complete medium.

7. After 8 to 24 hr, scrape away the neural tube and any groups of cells with epithelial morphology using the blunt end of a tungsten needle (Fig. 1). Remove the media and debris. Replace with fresh culture medium. Feed the cultures fresh media every other day.

E. Primary Neural Crest Cultures from the Cranial Region

Materials

Same as described earlier

Incubate quail eggs until they reach stage 8 (four to six somites), typically takes about 24 hr

Procedure

1. In a laminar flow hood, wash the eggs with 70% ethanol. Open the eggs as described earlier. Place the embryos in Ringer's solution.

2. Excise midbrain region with sharp tungsten needles. Make two lateral cuts between the neural tube and the ectoderm. Make a longitudinal cut underneath the notochord and two transverse cuts, one between the midbrain and forebrain and a second between the midbrain and hindbrain. Gently tease off the neural folds using a sharp point of the tungsten needle.

3. Wash the neural folds with Ringer's solution and transfer in a few drops of medium onto substrate-coated tissue culture dishes. Incubate at 37°C for 30 to 60 min and then feed with 1.5 ml of complete medium.

F. Secondary or Clonal Cultures

After neural crest cells have migrated away from the explanted neural tube and the neuroepithelial tissue is scraped away, secondary cultures can be prepared by dissociating the neural crest cells and replating them at sparse density. Single cells can be isolated using this procedure, thus making it possible to perform a clonal analysis (Cohen and Konigsberg, 1975; Sieber-Blum and Cohen, 1980; Baroffio *et al.*, 1988, 1991). A simple procedure for preparing secondary cultures is described next. Despite the fact that this procedure is in principle quite straightforward, neural crest cells do not grow well at low density. Therefore, a number of investigators have used more exacting procedures including a more complicated medium (Sieber-Blum, 1991) or have grown clonal neural crest cultures on feeder layers of 3T3 cells (Baroffio *et al.*, 1988).

1. Rinse the primary cultures with Ringer's solution and add a crude preparation of 0.25% collagenase (Worthington CLS) for ~20 min at 37°C. Other enzymes such as dispase or trypsin can be substituted, although the length of treatment must be altered. In addition, cells can be isolated from the substrate by prolonged exposure to calcium-free buffers. Pipette the solution intermittently to dislodge the cells.

2. When the cells are loosened from the substrate, add an equal volume of cold complete medium. Endogenous enzyme inhibitors in the serum will stop the enzyme reaction.

3. Centrifuge the cell suspension at 800 rpm for 5 min. Remove the supernatant by aspiration and resuspend the pellet in ~0.4 ml of complete medium.

4. A Petroff–Heuser bacterial cell counter is used to count the number of cells in the suspension, although other types of hemocytometers can be used. Secondary cultures are typically inoculated with 200 cells per 60-mm Falcon petri dish coated. Various substrates can be used, including fibronectin, polylysine, or a feeder layer of 3T3 cells.

5. For clonal cultures, it is important to verify that single cells have been obtained. This can be accomplished by plating the resuspended cells into multiwell plates and verifying the presence of a single cell per well using an inverted phase-contrast microscope.

6. Cells are fed fresh complete medium every 2–3 days.

G. Whole Trunk Explants

An alternative approach for studying neural crest migration is an explant preparation that allows direct visualization of migrating cells in normal living tissue (Krull *et al.*, 1995). The whole trunk region of the chicken embryo, excised and placed in explant culture, appears to continue normal development for up to 2 days. Neural crest cells migrate in their typical segmental fashion, and the morphological and molecular properties of the somites are comparable to those in intact embryos.

Materials

Similar to those used earlier
Millicell inserts

Six-well Falcon culture plates
Chicken eggs incubated to stage 11

Procedures

1. Cut embryos from egg as described previously and place in Ringer's solution. Using tungsten needles, carefully dissect a region of the trunk, stretching from the fifth to the eleventh most recently formed somites (somites V to XI; Ordahl, 1993). For the dissection, transverse incisions are made just caudal to somite V and just rostral to somite XI. To free the tissue, incisions are made perpendicular to the first, extending longitudinally and lateral to somites V to XI. The resulting explant contains the neural tube, including presumptive neural crest cells, multiple pairs of discrete somites, and other associated structures including the ectoderm and endoderm.

2. Place the ventral surface of the explant onto the Millicell polycarbonate membrane, leaving the dorsal surface of each explant exposed to the atmosphere. Then, underlie the Millicell insert with medium. A defined culture medium composed of Neurobasal medium (GIBCO), supplemented with B27 (GIBCO) and 0.5 mM L-glutamine (Sigma), is used.

These cultures have the advantage of maintaining relatively normal *in vivo* development for 2 days while being readily accessible to both visualization and addition of perturbing reagents.

III. Microinjection of Cells and Antibodies into Embryos

By microinjecting function-blocking antibodies that recognize cell surface, extracellular matrix, or cell adhesion molecules, it is possible to perform *in vivo* perturbation experiments. This approach makes it possible to characterize the nature of cell–cell or cell–matrix interactions required for normal cell migration in living embryos. Antibody perturbation can be done by injecting purified antibodies at selected concentrations or by introducing hybridoma cells that secrete antibody. If introducing hybridoma cells, it is useful to label the cells with a vital dye to allow visualization of the source of antibody.

An additional advantage of this microinjection approach is that any cell type can be injected into selected regions of the embryo. This approach makes it possible to use the embryo as an *in vivo* culture system to examine the differentiation of the microinjected cells. Alternatively, the migratory patterns of these cells can be examined within the embryo.

Similar approaches are used for cell labeling and microinjecting cells/antibodies into chick embryos.

A. Labeling Cells Prior to Microinjection

Cells for microinjection into embryos can be labeled with a variety of vital dyes. Two labeling procedures are described next.

1. *Labeling cells with DiI:* A stock solution of 0.5% 1,1-dioctadecyl-3,3,3',3'-tetramethlindocarbocyanine perchlorate (DiI; Molecular Probes, Junction City, OR) in 100% ethanol (weight/volume) is prepared and can be stored for up to 2 weeks. For cell labeling, the stock is diluted 1:100 in 0.3 *M* sucrose and is centrifuged to remove any crystals that might have precipitated.

Labeling cells with CFSE: An alternative method whereby cells remain labeled for a short time (~24 hr) is the vital dye, 6-carboxyfluorescein diacetate succinimyl ester (CFSE). A stock solution of 10 m*M* CFSE is prepared in dimethyl sulfoxide which is stored at 4°C. For labeling cells, the stock solution is diluted 1:300 in phosphate-buffered saline, pH 7.4.

2. Cells can either be labeled in suspension or on the culture dish. Rinse the cells with Ringer's solution. For cell suspensions, centrifuge the cell suspension at low speed and add 1.5 ml of the DiI or CFSE solution. For cultures, add the vital dye directly to the culture dish. Incubate for 60–90 min at 37°C. Rinse again with Ringer's solution. For cell cultures, remove the cells from the dish by incubating with 0.25% trypsin (GIBCO) for approximately 10 min. The enzyme activity is stopped with the addition of fresh culture medium.

3. Place cells into siliconized centrifuge tubes using siliconized pipettes. Wash and centrifuge three times in Ringer's solution, with the final wash being performed in a microfuge tube to reduce the volume of liquid containing the labeled cells.

B. Microinjection of Cells or Antibodies into Embryos

Essentially identical procedures are used for injecting cells or antibodies into embryos. Only the size of the injection pipette varies since cells need a larger opening than antibody solutions.

Procedures

1. Eggs are windowed as described in Chapter 1. Chicken embryos are incubated at 38°C until they reach the desired stage of development (typically 36 hr for injection onto cranial neural crest migratory pathways and 60 hr for injections onto trunk pathways). A window is cut in the shell over the embryo. India ink (Pelikan Fount) diluted 1:10 in a saline solution is injected under the blastoderm to aid in visualization of the embryo. The vitelline membrane is removed using an electrolytically sharpened tungsten needle.

2. Approximately 5 μl of antibodies and/or labeled cells is backfilled into a pulled micropipette. The micropipette is held in an adapter that is connected to a micromanipulator. The pipette tip is broken off to have an opening of 10–30 μm and the tip is then lowered into the desired region of the embryo (Fig. 2). For cranial injections, the antibodies/cells are typically expelled into the mesenchyme adjacent to the neural tube, whereas for trunk injections they are inserted into one or more somites at the wing level.

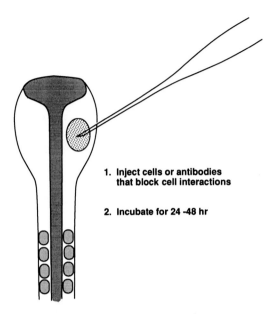

1. **Inject cells or antibodies that block cell interactions**

2. **Incubate for 24 -48 hr**

Fig. 2 The technique used for microinjecting cells or antibodies into the cranial mesenchyme of a 1.5-day-old chick embryo. Cells are labeled prior to injection. Cells and/or antibodies are backfilled into a micropipette having an opening of ~20 μm. The embryo is incubated for an additional 1–2 days and is then fixed and stained.

3. The antibodies/labeled cells are expelled with a pulse of pressure. This is accomplished by connecting the pipette to a pressure source such as a picospritzer or a house air line.

4. Following the injections, the eggs are sealed with cellophane tape (Scotch Magic 3M) and returned to the incubator until the time of fixation. Embryos injected with DiI-labeled cells are fixed in 4% paraformaldehyde or 4% paraformaldehyde/0.25% glutaraldehyde and prepared for cryostat sectioning. Embryos with CFSE-labeled cells are fixed in 4% paraformaldehyde, embedded in paraffin, and sectioned.

IV. Labeling of Neural Crest Cells *in Vivo* with Vital Dyes

A number of useful cell marking techniques are used to examine the pathways of neural crest migration. Classically, neural tube transplantations have provided a wealth of information about migratory pathways and, in particular, neural crest derivatives in avian embryos (see Chapter 2). Neural tubes or neural folds from quail embryos have been transplanted to the same or different axial levels of chick hosts (Le Douarin, 1982). An alternative approach is to label neural crest cells in fixed embryos with antibodies that recognize neural crest cells (HNK-1 and NC-1; Tucker *et al.*, 1984). Although this provides a nonsurgical alternative to grafting paradigms, most antibodies are not entirely specific. They recognize numerous cell adhesion molecules associated with many nonneural crest cells (Kruse *et al.*, 1984) and do not recognize all neural crest populations.

Another cell marking technique for labeling the neural crest is to inject the lipophilic dye DiI (Serbedzija *et al.*, 1989; Sechrist *et al.*, 1993) into the lumen of the neural tube (denoted as whole neural tube injections) or directly into the neural folds (denoted as focal neural fold injections). Because the dye is hydrophobic and lipophilic, it intercalates into all cell membranes that it contacts. Injection into the neural tube marks all neural tube cells including presumptive neural crest cells within its dorsal aspect. Because the time and location of injection can be controlled, this technology provides a direct approach for following migratory pathways. In addition, the dye can be used to follow neural crest pathways in a number of species, including chick, mouse, and frog. Despite the differences in the nature of the techniques involved, DiI labeling, quail/chick chimeras, and antibody staining provide similar pictures of neural crest migratory pathways.

Two techniques for DiI injections to label neural crest cells are provided. For a more detailed discussion of vital dye labeling of other populations of cells in avian embryos, including methods for labeling individual precursor cells, see Chapter 8.

A. Whole Neural Tube DiI Injections

By injecting the DiI into the lumen of the neural tube, the dye intercalates into all neural tube cells, including premigratory neural crest cells. Because DiI is lipophilic and hydrophobic, it is necessary to make up a stock solution of DiI in a nonaqueous solvent. Ethanol (100%) is typically used, although DMSO and other solvents can be substituted. Because ethanol is toxic to cells, the dye must be diluted prior to putting large amounts of ethanol into the embryo. By diluting the stock solution in isotonic sucrose, the dye remains in solution and damage to the embryo is minimal or nonexistent.

1. A 0.05% solution (weight/volume) of DiI (Molecular Probes) is made by diluting the stock solution (0.5% in 100% ethanol) 1:10 in 0.3 M sucrose.

2. The injection micropipette is backfilled with the DiI solution which is then attached to a forced air pressure source (either a picospritzer or a house air line). The tip of the pipette is broken with fine forceps to have an opening of about 10–20 μm. The micropipette is inserted into the lumen of the neural tube using a micromanipulator (Fig. 3, see color insert). Enough dye is expelled to fill most of the neural tube.

3. After injection, the eggs are sealed with cellophane tape and returned to the incubator until the indicated times of fixation. DiI-labeled embryos are

fixed in 4% paraformaldehyde or 4% paraformaldehyde/0.25% glutaraldehyde and prepared for cryostat sectioning (see Chapter 17).

B. Focal Injections of DiI into Neural Folds

Premigratory neural crest cells arise from the dorsal neural folds shortly after
tube closure in the chick embryo. By placing small, focal injections of DiI directly
into the neural folds, one can label a subpopulation of neural crest cells and
examine their subsequent migration over time (Fig. 3). For this method, it is
necessary to use undiluted DiI to produce intense and localized labeling. Because
only a small amount of DiI in ethanol is expelled, ethanol damage to the embryo
is minimal.

1. An undiluted stock solution of DiI (0.5% in 100% ethanol) is backfilled
   into the micropipette as described previously.
2. A small amount of DiI is expelled into the regions of the neural fold. At
   the time of the injection, the injection site is visible as a small red spot
   of dye in the tissue through the epifluorescence microscope (Sechrist *et
   al.,* 1993).
3. DiI can be visualized in living embryos by epifluorescence or after fixation
   in 4% paraformaldehyde. Embryos are prepared for cryostat sectioning as
   described in Chapter 17.

V. Grafting Techniques

A number of embryonic manipulations can be used to alter the rostrocaudal
or dorsoventral position of neural crest cells. In addition, the prospective neural
crest can be removed or the position of the tissue encountered by the neural
crest can be altered, such as the notochord. A few representative manipulations
are described next. For an extensive discussion of other types of embryonic
manipulations, see Chapter 2.

A. Neural Tube Rotations

1. Prepare glass knives by pulling thin glass rods to a sharp tip using an
   electrode puller. Any electrode puller can be used for the preparation of
   glass needles. A needle with a long, slow taper is preferred.
2. Operations can be performed on embryos between 1.5 and 2 days of development. For neural tube rotations, a lateral cut is made between the neural
   tube and the adjacent mesenchyme as well as under the notochord. After
   separating the neural tube/notochord from the adjacent tissue, two transverse cuts are made rostrally and caudally. The whole neural tube, which
   is now loose in the embryo, can be rotated rostrocaudally, dorsoventrally,

or both. An example of dorsoventral neural tube rotation is illustrated in Fig. 4.

3. Eggs are resealed with cellophane tape and returned to the incubator until the time of fixation.

B. Neural Fold Ablations

1. Segments comprising about one-third to one-half of the dorsal neural tube are removed bilaterally with glass needles. Incisions are made perpendicular to the long axis of the neural tube at the rostral and caudal edges of the site to be ablated. Longitudinal cuts are then made at both the boundary between the epidermis and the neural folds and the desired level within the neural tube (Fig. 5).

2. To avoid any possible contribution from the ablated tissue, it is removed from the egg by capillary action through a micropipette.

3. Eggs are resealed with cellophane tape and returned to the incubator until the time of fixation.

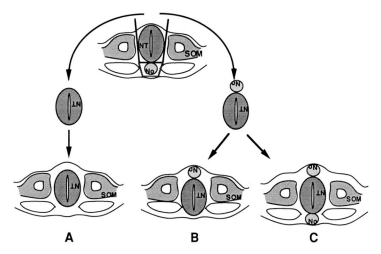

Fig. 4 The neural tube can be rotated in place either rostrocaudally or dorsoventrally. This schematic diagram illustrates dorsoventral rotation either with or without the notochord attached. With a fine glass needle, slits are made between the neural tube (NT) and somites (SOM) and either between the neural tube and notochord (No) or underneath the notochord. The polarity of the tissue is then inverted and it is replaced into the same embryo or into another host prepared in the same way. This makes it possible to produce an embryo in which (A) the neural tube is inverted dorsoventrally in the absence of a notochord, (B) the neural tube is inverted dorsoventrally in the presence of a notochord dorsally, or (C) the neural tube is inverted dorsoventrally in the presence of notochord dorsally and ventrally. For experimental results, see Stern *et al.* (1991).

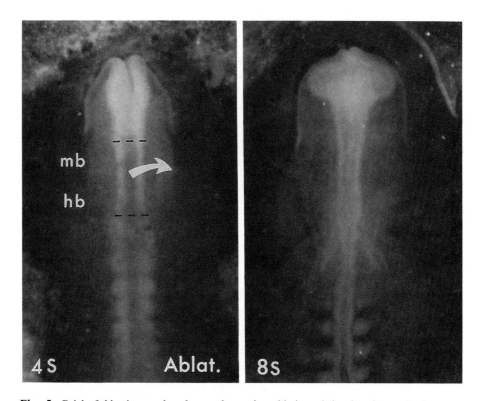

Fig. 5 Bright-field micrographs of an embryo after ablation of the dorsal neural folds in the midbrain and hindbrain region of an embryo operated at the 4 somite stage (left). Using a glass knife, slits are made lateral to the neural tube and the top half to third of the dorsal neural tube is removed. The same embryo several hours later (right) at the 8 somite stage. The neural tube has closed and the embryo appears relatively normal morphologically.

C. Notochord Implants

1. Notochords are isolated using the procedure for isolating neural tubes as described earlier for trunk neural crest cultures. Briefly, a rectangular block of tissue, including the notochord, is dissected out of the embryo at the desired axial level using an electrolytically sharpened tungsten needle. The notochords are isolated from surrounding tissues with dispase treatment. The notochords then are allowed to recover in complete medium for 1 hr prior to implantation.

2. A pulled glass knife is used to make an incision between the neural tube and the adjacent somite.

3. A donor notochord is transferred to the embryo in 2 μl of medium. The notochord is oriented parallel to the incision and is inserted laterally to the neural tube by pushing in with a glass needle.

4. Eggs are resealed with cellophane tape and returned to the incubator until the time of fixation.

D. Notochord Ablations

1. Using a pulled glass needle, an incision is made along both sides of the neural tube of stage 9–10 embryos. A third incision is made perpendicular and posterior to the first incisions, and the neural plate is carefully lifted and folded back (Fig. 6A).

2. The notochord is scraped off the underside of the neural plate, which then is returned to its original position (Fig. 6B). Trypsin (0.15%) (GIBCO) can be added to help separate the notochord from the underlying endoderm. A few drops of complete medium are added to dilute the enzyme and to

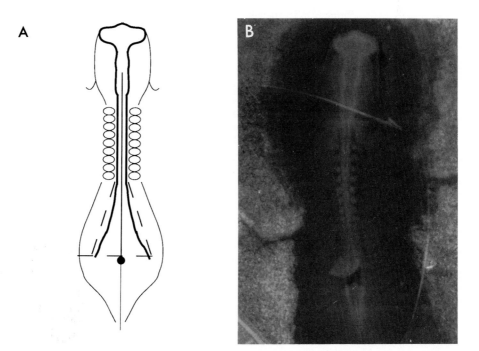

Fig. 6 (A) The microsurgical operation used to ablate the notochord. Incisions were made along the dotted lines as indicated in stage 9 to 10 chick embryos (7–10 somite stage). The neural plate was deflected and the notochord was subsequently removed. The neural plate was then returned to its original position and the embryo was allowed to develop for 1–4 days. (B) Photomicrograph of a stage 9 embryo in which the neural plate has been deflected and the notochord removed. Data from Artinger and Bronner-Fraser (1993).

stop the reaction when the operation is complete. Approximately 100–700 μm of notochord tissue is removed at the time of surgery.

VI. Conclusions

The methods described in this chapter provide a number of techniques that can be applied to the study of neural crest migration and differentiation. Simple adaptations of these techniques make them applicable to other regions of the embryo as well. Because neural crest cells interact with neighboring tissues, it is often useful to combine studies of neural crest development with the development of adjacent structures, including the neural tube, somites, and notochord, as described in other chapters of this volume.

Acknowledgments

The author thanks Drs. Mary Dickinson, Scott Fraser, and Catherine Krull for helpful comments on the manuscript. Development of some of the methods described in this chapter comes from support by NIH Grants HD-25138, HD-15527, and DE-10066.

References

Artinger, K. and Bronner-Fraser, M. (1993). Delayed formation of the floor plate after ablation of the avian notochord. *Neuron* **11**, 1147–1161.

Baroffio, A., Dupin, E., and Le Douarin, N. M. (1988). Clone-forming ability and differentiation potential of migratory neural crest cells. *Proc. Natl. Acad. Sci. U.S.A.* **85**, 5325–5329.

Baroffio, A., Dupin, E., and Le Douarin, N. M. (1991). Common precursors for neural and mesectodermal derivatives in the cephalic neural crest. *Development (Cambridge, UK)* **112**, 301–305.

Birgbauer, E., Sechrist, J., Bronner-Fraser, M., and Fraser, S. (1995). Rhombomeric origin and rostrocaudal reassortment of neural crest cells revealed by intravital microscopy. *Development (Cambridge, UK)* **121**, 935–945.

Cohen, A. M., and Konigsberg, I. R. (1975). A clonal approach to the problem of neural crest determination. *Dev. Biol.* **46**, 262–280.

Hamburger, V., and Hamilton, H. L. (1951). A series of normal stages in the development of the chick embryo. *J. Morphol.* **88**, 49–92.

Krull, C. E., Collazo, A., Fraser, S. E., and Bronner-Fraser, M. (1995). Dynamic analysis of trunk neural crest migration. *Development (Cambridge, UK)* **121**, 3733–3743.

Kruse, J., Mailhammer, R., Wenecke, H., Faissner, A., Sommer, I., Goridis, C., and Schachner, M. (1984). Neural cell adhesion molecules and myelin-associated glycoprotein share a common carbohydrate moiety recognized by monoclonal antibodies L2 and HNK-1. *Nature (London)* **311**, 153–155.

Le Douarin, N. M. (1982). "The Neural Crest." Cambridge Univ. Press, Cambridge, UK.

Maxwell, G. D., and Forbes, M. E. (1990). Exogenous basement membrane-like matrix stimulates adrenergic development in avian neural crest cultures. *Development (Cambridge, UK)* **101**, 767–776.

Ordahl, C. (1993). "Myogenic lineages within the developing somite." Wiley-Liss, New York.

Sechrist, J., Serbedzija, G. N., Fraser, S. E., Scherson, T., and Bronner-Fraser, M. (1993). Segmental migration of the hindbrain neural crest does not arise from segmental generation. *Development (Cambridge, UK)* **118**, 691–703.

Serbedzija, G., Bronner-Fraser, M., and Fraser, S. E. (1989). Vital dye analysis of the timing and pathways of avian trunk neural crest cell migration. *Development (Cambridge, UK)* **106,** 806–816.

Sieber-Blum, M., and Cohen, A. (1980). Clonal analysis of quail neural crest cells: They are pluripotent and differentiate in vitro in the absence of non-neural crest cells. *Dev. Biol.* **80,** 96–106.

Sieber-Blum, M. (1991). Role of the neurotrophic factors BDNF and NGF in the commitment of pluripotent neural crest cells. *Neuron* **6**(6), 949–955.

Stern, C. D., Artinger, K. B., and Bronner-Fraser, M. (1991). Tissue interactions affecting the migration and differentiation of neural crest cells in the chick embryo. *Development (Cambridge, UK)* **113,** 207–216.

Tucker, G. C., Aoyama, H., Lipinski, M., Tursz, T., and Thiery, J. P. (1984). Identical reactivity of monoclonal antibodies HNK-1 and NC-1: Conservation in vertebrates on cells derived from the neural primordium and on some leukocytes. *Cell Differ.* **14,** 223–230.

CHAPTER 4

Manipulation of the Avian Segmental Plate *in Vivo*

Brian A. Williams and Charles P. Ordahl

Department of Anatomy and
Cardiovascular Research Institute
University of California, San Francisco
San Francisco, California 94143

I. Introduction
II. Materials
    A. Host and Donor Embryos
    B. Solutions
    C. Pipettes and Pipette Tips
    D. Microscalpels
    E. Microdissection Dishes
    F. Sealing Tape
    G. Antibodies
III. Methods
    A. Preparation of Donor Embryo
    B. Removal of Donor Segmental Plate
    C. Preparation of Host Embryo
    D. Removal of Host Segmental Plate
    E. Implantation of Donor Segmental Plate
    F. Harvesting Experimental Embryos
IV. Critical Aspects of the Procedure
V. Results and Discussion
VI. Conclusions and Perspectives
    References

I. Introduction

The avian embryo provides a useful experimental system for the investigation of vertebrate development (Le Douarin and McLaren, 1984). Early events in avian development, such as axis specification, mesoderm induction, and gastrulation, are usually studied in culture systems outside of the egg (Eyal-Giladi *et al.,* 1992; New, 1955; Spratt, 1946; Vakaet, 1984). However, once gastrulation is complete and the cells have begun to organize themselves into a recognizable, bilaterally symmetric vertebrate embryo, *in ovo* surgical experimentation can be carried out. In order to track the fate of experimentally manipulated cells in the embryo, cell-labeling techniques are required. When combined with the tools of molecular biology, lineage tracing is a powerful tool for analyzing the mechanisms of cell specification and morphogenesis.

The quail–chick grafting method developed by Le Douarin (1973) has been successfully used as a cell-labeling technique in the avian embryo. Organ anlagen in the chick embryo are marked by surgical replacement with the corresponding anlage from a quail embryo. The cells generated by the grafted quail anlage can be identified in Feulgen-stained tissue sections by the presence of bright crimson nucleoli, which are absent from the pale-staining nuclei of host chick cells. This method allows long-term analysis of the contribution of the graft since the marker is transmitted faithfully to all descendant cells. An improvement in the resolution of the method has been introduced by the production of a monoclonal antibody (J. A. Carlson and B. M. Carlson, personal communication) which allows the identification of individual graft-derived cells that are located in areas populated primarily by chick host cells.

The method presented in this chapter describes the transplantation of fragments of the segmental plate (Ordahl and Le Douarin, 1992), the precursor to the somites, which are the embryonic anlagen of skeletal muscle and the axial skeleton. Replacement of the chick segmental plate with that of quail allows one to trace the development of skeletal muscle and the axial skeleton and to design experiments to analyze the specification of the cell types giving rise to these organs. Several different methods are presented, involving whole segmental plate replacement and extirpation as well as transplantation of selected fragments of the segmental plate.

II. Materials

A. Host and Donor Embryos

Quail eggs can be obtained in the United States from Strickland Quail Farm (Pooler, GA). Chick eggs can be obtained from local producers. Eggs are stored at 4°C for up to 1 week and are then incubated at 37–39°C in a humidified (60–80%) incubator.

B. Solutions

Tyrode's solution is available from Sigma Chemical Co. (Catalog No. T-2145) in powdered form, which should be stored at 4°C until reconstituted for use.

Pancreatin is a crude enzyme preparation (Sigma Cat. No. P-3292) used to digest extracellular matrix in donor and host embryos. It is usually supplied at 4× concentration and should be stored in single-use aliquots at −20°C as a 1× stock after dilution with Tyrode's solution. A 2% solution of fetal bovine serum (any supplier) diluted in Tyrode's solution is used to hold donor tissue fragments prior to implantation in hosts. Fetal bovine serum is stored in single-use aliquots at −20°C until dilution with Tyrode's solution. Collagenase is stored in single-use aliquots at a 1% concentration in Tyrode's solution at −20°C and is available from Sigma in powdered form (Catalog No. C-0130).

C. Pipettes and Pipette Tips

Mouth-operated micropipettes are prepared by pulling borosilicate (not flint) glass microcapillary tubes (100 μl size; Fisher No. 21-164-28) over a small Bunsen burner flame. The tips of pulled pipettes are broken off to achieve the desired diameter, typically about 50–100 μm or occasionally larger. Micropipettes are connected to a mouthpiece using rubber or plastic hosing. For transporting donor tissue fragments, a P-20 pipetteman or a comparable tool is fitted with a narrow pipette tip (Phenix Research Products, Cat. No. T-010BR).

D. Microscalpels

A method for creating tungsten microscalpels by electrolysis has been published by Conrad et al. (1993). Tungsten wire can be ordered from Goodfellow (Cat. No. 005155; 0.38 mm diameter, 99.95% purity). During surgery, if the tip of the microscalpel becomes coated with cellular debris from the incisions, it can be cleaned off by brief immersion in a small sonication bath. This method preserves the shape of the blade while removing the adherent debris that dulls the microscalpel. Other microtools useful for embryo surgery, such as forceps, microscissors, insect pins, and perforated spoons, can be obtained from Fine Science Tools (Foster City, CA).

E. Microdissection Dishes

Small glass concave embryological culture dishes (Cat. No. 910B; Variety Glass) are filled halfway with black Dow Corning Sylgard (KR Anderson Co., Cat. No. 170, black). The black Sylgard provides contrast for visualizing the white/translucent tissues of the embryo.

F. Sealing Tape

Windows and other holes in egg shells can be sealed with Scotch book mending tape available from Kielty and Dayton (Cat. No. R8-191-CR).

G. Antibodies

The antibodies developed by D. Bader (MF20) and J. and B. Carlson (QCPN) were obtained from the Developmental Studies Hybridoma Bank maintained by the Department of Biological Sciences, University of Iowa, Iowa City, Iowa.

III. Methods

A. Preparation of Donor Embryo

Quail eggs are incubated, round end facing up, in a forced draft incubator at 37°C until stage 11–12 HH (approximately 48 hr). The egg is removed from the incubator and is gently swabbed with 70% ethanol. Albumen is decanted through a small circular hole cut in the pointed end of the egg using a pair of curved scissors. After albumen decantation has lowered the embryo, the opening may be enlarged to facilitate further albumen decantation. The white stringy chalazae can also be cut with the scissors to facilitate decantation. The yolk, with the embryo on its surface, is then floated in Tyrode's solution contained in a small bowl (Fig. 1A). The blastodisc is cut away from the yolk using a serrated forceps and iridectomy scissors. The embryo is removed to a small dissection dish with a perforated spoon, rinsed free of yolk platelets, and pinned to the Sylgard with 0.15-mm insect pins, ventral side up. The first pin is inserted through the area opaca and then the opposite corner of the area opaca is pinned, after lightly stretching the embryo. Additional pins are then similarly inserted until the embryo is pinned in at least four corners (Fig. 1B).

B. Removal of Donor Segmental Plate

Figures 1C and 1D illustrate the sequence of steps used to prepare the donor segmental plate. The notochord and underside of the early somites and segmental plate should be visible. A midline incision is made in the endoderm (Fig. 1C) parallel to the notochord using a short snipping stroke, where the scalpel tip is inserted into the endoderm and sharply lifted upwards (Ordahl and Christ, 1995). A small amount (<5 μl) of 1× pancreatin is pipetted onto the incision using a micropipette. Only a minimal amount of enzyme should be used to prevent overdigestion of the donor tissue (see Section IV). The digestive action of the pancreatin allows the endoderm, and any other tissues such as the aorta, to be teased away from the underlying segmental plate mesoderm. Once fully exposed, an orientation mark should be placed on the segmental plate using fine animal carbon or a vital dye or other method (Ordahl and Christ, 1995).

The first incision in the mesoderm is begun at the rostral tip of the segmental plate between its lateral margin and the medial margin of the Wolffian duct (Fig. 1D, step 1). The incision is extended caudally for a length equivalent to approximately 5 somites, using a slashing motion with either a microneedle or

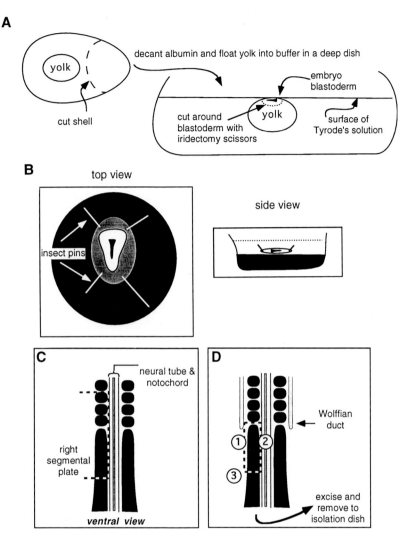

Fig. 1 Preparation of donor (quail) embryo. (A) Removal of the donor embryo from the egg. (B) Donor embryo staked out in Sylgard dish. (C) Ventral view of the paraxial mesoderm of the donor embryo pinned in a Sylgard dish. An incision is made in the endoderm along the midline (pictured as a dotted line), and the endoderm is reflected away from the paraxial mesoderm after the application of pancreatin. (D) Ventral view diagramming the cuts in the donor mesoderm (pictured as dotted lines). The first cut (1) is made between the segmental plate and the intermediate mesoderm, for a length of about 5 somites. The second cut (2) is made between the segmental plate and the neural tube, and mainly involves teasing the segmental plate away from the neural tube. The third cut (3) is made transversely, approximately 5 somites distance caudal to the anterior tip of the segmental plate.

a broad, flat-bladed microscalpel (Ordahl and Christ, 1995). This incision separates the segmental plate from the intermediate and lateral plate mesoderm, and gives a smooth lateral edge to the donor tissue. Next, the segmental plate is separated from the neural tube, first by scoring between the medial margin of the segmental plate and the neural tube, and then by teasing the segmental plate laterally away from the neural tube (Fig. 1D, step 2). Finally, a caudal transverse incision is made in the segmental plate at a point approximately 5 somites distance caudal to the rostral tip of the segmental plate (Fig. 1D, step 3). The segmental plate donor fragment can then be lifted away from the underlying ectoderm with the flat edge of the scalpel blade. If necessary, additional pancreatin can be introduced to speed release of the segmental plate from the ectoderm.

The donor segmental plate is transferred to a holding dish using a P-20 pipetteman. The pipetteman allows the tissue fragment to be contained in a small, manageable volume of transfer solution. The pipette tip is first fully charged with 2% fetal calf serum to prevent tissue fragments from sticking to the internal surface of the tip. The tissue should not be drawn deeply into the pipette tip so that it can be easily moved in and out of the pipette by action of the plunger. The tissue fragment is then ejected into a droplet of 2% fetal calf serum in a small plastic culture dish, covered, and stored at room temperature until transplantation into the host embryo (Fig. 2E).

If the medial and lateral halves of the segmental plate are to be transplanted separately, the first incision should be made directly through the longitudinal midline of the segmental plate (Figs. 3A and 3B), using the same slashing stroke described earlier, thereby dividing the medial and lateral halves of the segmental plate. After orientation marking, the lateral and medial halves are excised, respectively, using the scalpel strokes described in Figs. 3A and 3B. The donor half-segmental plate fragments are then separated from the ectoderm and placed in holding dishes as described earlier.

C. Preparation of Host Embryo

Chick host eggs are incubated on their sides for 42–54 hr to stage 11–12 HH (Hamburger and Hamilton, 1951) and are carefully maintained in this orientation thereafter. The top of the egg shell is marked to indicate the location of the embryo. The egg is removed from the incubator, swabbed with 70% ethanol, and a small puncture is made in the pointed end by tapping with blunt forceps. An 18-gauge needle fitted to a 10-ml syringe is used to withdraw 0.5–2 ml of albumen through this hole, taking care not to puncture the yolk (Fig. 2A). The removal of albumen lowers the embryo away from the egg shell, allowing a window to be cut in the shell over the embryo with curved scissors. At this stage of development, the embryonic blood cells have begun to form and should be barely visible as a small red crescent at the posterior margin of the embryo. Ideally, the embryo will be centrally located on the surface of the yolk; if it is located grossly eccentrically, it is not a good candidate for surgery, it should be discarded, and another host prepared. These steps are summarized in Fig. 2A.

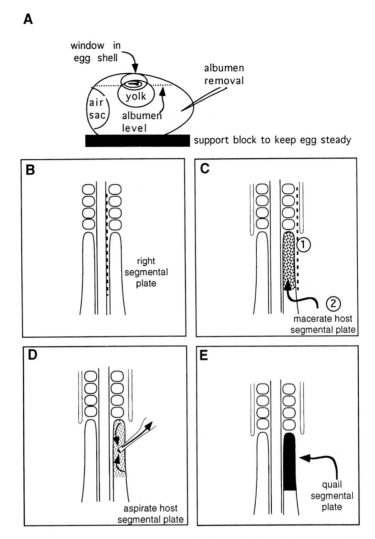

Fig. 2 Preparation of host (chick) embryo. (A) Scheme for lowering the host embryo from the shell. (B) The first incision in the host ectoderm is made between the neural tube and the segmental plate, as indicated by the dotted line. (C) Incisions in the host mesoderm. A longitudinal incision (1) is made lateral to the segmental plate; the tissue is then macerated (2) using a microscalpel. (D) The macerated fragments are aspirated with a small mouth pipette. (E) The donor tissue is moved into place with a microscalpel.

Under the dissecting microscope, the translucent embryo is almost invisible against the yellow background of yolk. A contrast medium prepared by mixing Pelikan No. 17 black ink 1 : 1 with Tyrode's solution is therefore injected between the embryo and the underlying yolk using a fine-tipped mouth pipette. The pipette, preloaded with contrast medium, is inserted through the vitelline membrane and the area opaca. After positioning the pipette tip under the embryo, a minimal amount of ink is expressed by mouth pressure. Once visible, the embryo can be staged precisely by counting the number of somites (Ordahl and Christ, 1995).

A small incision or puncture is made in the vitelline membrane near the head region of the embryo. It is then moistened with a few drops of Tyrode's solution applied with a Pasteur pipette. As the Tyrode's solution flows down through the incision, the vitelline membrane will float away from the embryo proper and can be removed with forceps or a few strokes of the broad microscalpel, without damaging the embryo below.

D. Removal of Host Segmental Plate

The sequence of incisions made in the host embryo is outlined in Figs. 2B through 2E. The first incision is made by snipping the ectoderm between the segmental plate and the neural tube. This incision should extend farther cranially and caudally than the intended target site in the mesoderm (Fig. 2B). A small amount of pancreatin is pipetted onto the longitudinal incision, and the flap of ectoderm is teased away from the underlying mesoderm.

Incisions in the mesoderm are then made to circumscribe the portion of the segmental plate to be removed (Fig. 2C, step 1). The region to be excised is then macerated using a microscalpel, taking care not to puncture the endoderm and blood vessels residing immediately below (Fig. 2C, step 2). A minimal amount of pancreatin (<5 μl) can be introduced to loosen the fragments. The macerated tissue fragments of the segmental plate are removed by aspiration (Fig. 2D), and the area is quenched with about 20 μl 10% fetal calf serum and rinsed three times with 20 μl of Tyrode's solution. When removal of the host segmental plate fragment is complete, the smooth surface of the endoderm should be visible at the bottom of the excavated area. If any bits of host segmental plate adhere to the surface of the endoderm, they should be removed by aspiration.

If only medial or lateral halves of the segmental plate are to be replaced with quail donor fragments, the sequence of incisions is copied from Figs. 3A and 3B. The figures show the approach from the ventral side of the donor, whereas the removal of host tissue is performed from a dorsal approach. The temporal sequence of incisions is the same.

E. Implantation of Donor Segmental Plate

The quail donor segmental plate fragment is transferred from the holding dish onto the surface of the host embryo blastodisc using a P-20 pipetteman. The pipetteman tip should be precharged with Tyrode's solution to avoid the cotransfer of excess serum which can cause tissue fragments to "float" in the host environment.

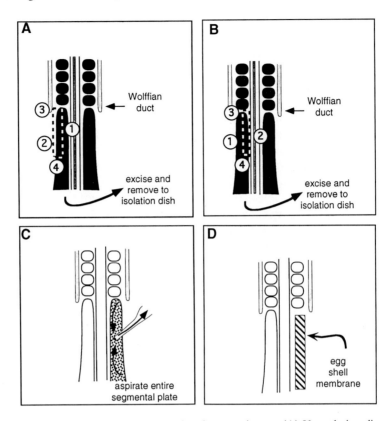

Fig. 3 Half-segmental plate grafts and extirpation experiments. (A) Ventral view diagramming cuts in the donor mesoderm for a lateral half graft. After reflection of the endoderm as in Fig. 1C, a longitudinal incision is made in the center of the segmental plate for 5 somites distance. Next, a longitudinal incision is made between the intermediate mesoderm and the segmental plate (2), followed by transverse (3 and 4) incisions which define the cranial and caudal extent of the graft. (B) To prepare a medial half graft, the first incision (1) is again made in the middle of the segmental plate, followed by (2) an incision between the plate and neural tube, and finally transverse (3 and 4) incisions. (C) Dorsal view diagramming preparation of the host for segmental plate extirpation. After incision of the ectoderm as in Fig. 2B and maceration of the segmental plate as in Fig. 2C, the entire segmental plate is aspirated with a mouth pipette. (D) A stuffer fragment prepared from either the host egg shell membrane or lateral plate tissue from a quail donor is used to replace the extirpated segmental plate.

As necessary, the donor tissue fragment can be sized and trimmed to fit the excavated area of the host using a thin microscalpel. Taking care to preserve the orientation of the tissue as marked previously, the donor graft is then gently tucked into position using the flat edge of a microscalpel (Fig. 2E). The ectoderm is replaced, and the egg is sealed with a pliable brand of tape (see Section II). Taping the window closed on the spherical surface of the egg shell will cause pleats to form in the tape that should be sealed together tightly and pressed tightly to the egg shell to prevent loss of moisture from the embryo in the incubator. After a tight seal has been produced, the egg is returned to the incubator.

If ablation of the segmental plate is to be performed (summarized in Figs. 3C and 3D), a "stuffer fragment" should be inserted into its place to prevent the remaining posterior portions of the segmental plate from expanding into, and compensating for, the extirpated region. Stuffer fragments derived from both the lateral plate mesoderm and the acellular egg shell membrane have been used. These provide a partial block to the invasion of cells from other regions of the mosoderm. Lateral plate mesoderm is the more difficult of the two to prepare for grafting because it has an "elastic" quality that makes it difficult to slice with a microscalpel. It is most easily cut by slashing with a microneedle or a broad, flat microscalpel. The lateral plate fragment is then bathed in a few microliters of 0.5% collagenase to separate the ectoderm from the mesoderm. Once the ectoderm has been removed, the enzyme action is quenched with fetal calf serum, as described earlier, and the mesoderm is trimmed to fit.

The egg shell membrane can be prepared from the shards around the window in the host embryo shell. This tissue is impossible to cut with a scalpel and should be trimmed using iridectomy scissors. It should be kept soaked in Tyrode's solution at all times to aid in positioning it into the excavated host site. After implantation of either type of stuffer fragment, the ectoderm is replaced over the operated site, and the egg is sealed as described earlier and returned to the incubator.

F. Harvesting Experimental Embryos

The reincubation period (a few hours to several days) for chimeric embryos depends on the research objective. The embryo is harvested by first carefully opening the window and irrigating the embryo with fresh Tyrode's solution. The embryo can then be cut away from the underlying yolk using a pair of serrated forceps and iridectomy scissors. It is then lifted out of the egg shell with a perforated spoon, removed to Tyrode's solution in a dissection dish, and rinsed free of yolk platelets. The Tyrode's solution is then withdrawn and replaced with fixative. The embryo is then processed for histological examination using standard procedures.

IV. Critical Aspects of the Procedure

Host selection is an important factor for the survival of segmental plate grafts for long incubation periods. Embryos that are centered on the yolk, have evidence of blood island development at the posterior margin of the blastodisc, and a vigorously beating heart are the best candidates. The host should be out of the incubator for a minimum amount of time during surgery, ideally no longer than 20 min.

A thorough rinsing of the areas treated with enzymes is esssential for good survival. Such areas are first quenched with 20 μl of fetal calf serum and then rinsed at least three times with 20 μl Tyrode's solution. Rinsing is performed by flooding the surgery area with Tyrode's solution, followed by immediate removal by aspiration. If large holes inexplicably appear in the endoderm or if the host has the appearance of being split apart in the region of the incision and excavation, it is possible that too much (or too long a duration of) enzyme has been used.

Finally, it is crucial that the window in the egg shell be resealed tightly with tape prior to reincubation. Dehydration in the forced draft incubator is the major cause of death in postoperative embryos; this usually results from the tape not being adequately secured to the egg shell. If necessary, a second layer of tape can be placed over regions that are poorly sealed.

V. Results and Discussion

Figure 4 (see color insert) shows the distribution of quail cells in a chimeric embryo 3 days after the thoracic segmental plate of a chick host was replaced by that of quail. The contralateral side was unoperated and served as a control. Fig. 4A shows a section with dark blue quail nuclei stained with the anti-quail antibody, QCPN (J. A. Carlson and B. M. Carlson, personal communication). Since the section is viewed from its cranial aspect, the quail cells appear on the left side of Fig. 4A. The entire paraxial mesoderm compartment is populated with quail nuclei on the operated side but none appear on the unoperated side, indicating that cells do not cross the midline of the embryo (Fig. 4A, arrowheads).

Figure 4B shows an adjacent section stained with the antimuscle myosin antibody MF20 to show developing muscles. The myosin positive cells (Fig. 4B, arrow) on the operated side of the section contain quail nuclei as shown in Fig. 4A. This type of analysis allows for the evaluation of the fate of cells derived from the grafted segmental plate.

VI. Conclusions and Perspectives

The paraxial mesoderm of the avian embryo undergoes several morphological transitions during development, each of which has significance for the production of specified cell types and for the organization of the body plan. A method for manipulation of the paraxial mesoderm after it has been divided into somites has been published by Ordahl and Christ (1995). The methods described in this chapter allow analysis of the paraxial mesoderm prior to segmentation and invasion by neural crest cells from the neural tube and prior to events thought to be involved in the specification of cell lineages, as determined both by previous experimentation (Aoyama and Asamoto, 1988; Christ et al., 1992; Ordahl and

Le Douarin, 1992) and by *in situ* hybridization studies (Pownall and Emerson, 1992; Williams and Ordahl, 1994). The paraxial mesoderm imposes a pattern on the central nervous system and therefore contains significant information for producing the segmented nature of the vertebrate body plan. In addition, the elements of the axial skeleton, as well as the entire musculature of the body, are produced from this tissue. Cell marking experiments allow the researcher to assess the contribution of marked cells to the future organs formed from the segmental plate, whereas the extirpation technique allows an evaluation of the effect of the segmental plate on surrounding tissues.

Acknowledgments

The authors acknowledge the training and support received from Drs. Nicole Le Douarin and Marie-Aimée Teillet of the Institut d'Embryologie in Paris in whose laboratories these procedures were first developed. This work was supported by grants to C.P.O. from the Muscular Dystrophy Association of America and the National Institutes of Health (HL 43821).

Dedication

C.P.O. dedicates this paper to the memory of his mother, Grace Swanson Ordahl, August 7, 1908–April 5, 1995.

References

Aoyama, H., and Asamoto, K. (1988). Determination of somite cells: Independence of cell differentiation and morphogenesis. *Development (Cambridge, UK)* **104,** 15–28.

Christ, B., Brand-Saberi, B., Grim, M., and Wilting, J. (1992). Local signalling in dermomyotomal cell type specification. *Anat. Embryol.* **186,** 505–510.

Conrad, G., Bee, J., Roche, S. M., and Teillet, M.-A. (1993). Fabrication of microscalpels by electrolysis of tungsten wire in a meniscus. *J. Neurosc. Methods* **50,** 123–127.

Eyal-Giladi, H., Debby, A., and Harel, N. (1992). The posterior section of the chick's area pellucida and its involvement in hypoblast and primitive streak formation. *Development (Cambridge, UK)* **116,** 819–830.

Hamburger, V., and Hamilton, H. (1951). A series of normal stages in the development of the chick embryo. *J. Morphol.* **88,** 49–92.

Le Douarin, N. (1973). A Feulgen-positive nucleolus. *Exp. Cell Res.* **77,** 459–468.

Le Douarin, N., and McLaren, A., eds. (1984). "Chimeras in Developmental Biology." Academic Press, Orlando, FL.

New, D. A. T. (1955). A new technique for the cultivation of the chick embryo *in vitro. J. Embryol. Exp. Morphol.* **3,** 326–331.

Ordahl, C. P., and Christ, B. (1995). Avian somite transplantation: A review of basic methods. *Methods Cell Biol.* (in press).

Ordahl, C. P., and Le Douarin, N. (1992). Two myogenic lineages within the developing somite. *Development (Cambridge, UK)* **114,** 339–353.

Pownall, M. E., and Emerson, C. P. (1992). Sequential activation of three myogenic regulatory genes during somite morphogenesis in quail embryos. *Dev. Biol.* **151,** 67–79.

Spratt, N. T. J. (1946). Formation of the primitive streak in the explanted chick blastoderm marked with carbon particles. *J. Exp. Zool.* **103,** 259–304.

Vakaet, L. (1984). The initiation of gastrula ingression in the chick blastoderm. *Am. Zool.* **24,** 555–562.

Williams, B. A., and Ordahl, C. P. (1994). Pax-3 expression in segmental mesoderm marks early stages in myogenic cell specification. *Development (Cambridge, UK)* **120,** 785–796.

CHAPTER 5

Somite Strips: An Embryo Fillet Preparation

Kathryn W. Tosney, Robert A. Oakley, Mia Champion, Lisa Bodley, Rebecca Sexton, and Kevin B. Hotary★

Department of Biology
The University of Michigan
Ann Arbor, Michigan 48109

★ Department of Internal Medicine and Comprehensive Cancer Center
The University of Michigan Medical School
Ann Arbor, Michigan 48109

I. Introduction
II. Fillet Preparation
    A. Overview
    B. Substrata
    C. Dissection
    D. Culture
    E. Neurons
    F. Fixing and Labeling
III. Critical Aspects
    A. Tissue Architecture
    B. Temporal–Spatial Concerns
    C. Contaminating Populations
    D. Borders
    E. Neurons
IV. Analyzing Neurites to Assess Guidance Interactions
    A. Neurite Lengths
    B. Neurite Trajectories
V. Conclusions and Perspectives
    A. Assessing Additional Populations
    B. Assessing Molecular Cues
    C. Utility and Limitations
References

I. Introduction

In the past decade, somites have (deservedly) received intense experimental interest. They are a focus for analyzing such diverse developmental processes as segmentation, determination, differentiation, and axonal guidance (e.g., Bellairs *et al.,* 1986; French *et al.,* 1988). The heightened scrutiny reaps the harvest of information gleaned from previous *in vivo* studies that establish somites as model systems for studying processes such as axonal guidance, which is the focus of this chapter. Anatomical studies have shown that differences between anterior and posterior somite guide axons and neural crest cells, both of which traverse anterior but not posterior somite to form segmental arrays corresponding to the segmentally repeated somites (e.g., Keynes and Stern, 1984; Bronner-Fraser and Stern, 1991). The somitic tissue responsible for the permissive and inhibitory subdivisions is the sclerotome; the dermatome and the myotome are not essential for segmental outgrowth patterns (Tosney, 1987). However, though it is known which tissues carry the guidance cues, the molecules or the cellular interactions that mediate the responses to these tissues have yet to be identified.

This chapter describes an assay, the somite strip, that can be used to study somitic guidance cues at cellular and molecular levels. This assay confers the benefits of studying a semi-intact system in a culture setting. It is a hybrid *in vivo–in vitro* assay that exposes anterior and posterior sclerotomes to view and yet retains in culture both the segmental architecture and typical molecular characteristics such as differential binding to peanut agglutinin lectin (PNA; see Oakley and Tosney, 1991). Dissociated, labeled neurons sprinkled onto the strip have direct access to sclerotomal guidance cues and extend neurites accordingly. The neurites are visible and provide the diagnostic tools which are neurite length, trajectory, and orientation relative to somitic populations and borders. The neurite lengths provide a quantitative measure of relative permissiveness that can be used to monitor the effects of treatments designed to block the activity of guidance molecules. The orientations and trajectories distinguish positive from inhibitory interactions and also discriminate between long-distance and contact-mediated interactions. The assay supports a variety of investigations into the inhibitory and permissive properties of anterior and posterior sclerotome.

II. Fillet Preparation

A. Overview

The embryo is filleted by removing the viscera, notochord, neural tube, and limbs, leaving only the somites and covering ectoderm. This strip of tissue is placed ectoderm side down on a laminin substratum. The ectoderm spreads on the laminin, but the somite does not spread on the ectodermal undersurface and therefore retains its integrity. The neurons to be assessed are labeled with a nontoxic fluorescent dye, dissociated, sprinkled over the somite strip, and allowed to extend neurites overnight. Guidance mechanisms are deduced from the relative lengths and the trajectories of neurites. Each section below first gives an orienting overview and then describes the procedure in detail.

B. Substrata

Prepare coverslips the night before and incubate them overnight. The next morning, wash, dry, and place the coverslips in four-well plates. Since only one side of the coverslip is coated with laminin, keep the orientation of the coverslip in mind as it is washed and dried.

1. Set Up

Use acid-washed 12-mm-round coverslips (Clay Adams, Gold Seal). With forceps, dip each coverslip in 95% ethanol, dab off excess fluid against the lip of the beaker, and ignite the ethanol in a flame. Do not hold the coverslip in the flame longer than it takes to ignite it. If the coverslip has excess ethanol or is held in the flame, it will crack. Briefly pause to allow the coverslip to cool and place it in a sterile 35-mm petri dish. Add 25 μl of laminin (100 μg/ml in 50 mM carbonate buffer, pH 9.6) to each coverslip. Place a second flamed coverslip on each drop of laminin to make a laminin–coverslip sandwich. Cover the dish and place it in a CO_2 incubator at 37°C overnight.

2. Wash

Wash coverslips the next day, at least 30 min before placing the somite strips in culture, to allow them adequate time to dry. First, place sterile filter paper in a fresh 35-mm petri dish. With sterile forceps, pick up and discard the top coverslip from the sandwich. Dip the bottom coverslip several times in a small beaker of sterile distilled water. Change forceps and dip again. The forceps must be changed because the first forceps will take up some solution by capillary action and then, when opened, deposit it on the coverslip again. Place the coverslip laminin-side up in the petri dish containing sterile filter paper and allow to dry. Do not expose the laminin to UV light which would render the laminin inadhesive.

C. Dissection

Embryos are removed from the egg, washed extensively to limit contamination, and eviscerated. The notochord, spinal cord, and mesonephros are then removed to expose the somites, and the strips are cleaned and trimmed to size. Do all manipulations in a laminar flow hood or other aseptic environment. Have an

open flame (Bunsen burner or alcohol lamp) and a beaker of 95% ethanol at
hand to flame (sterilize) instruments between steps.

1. Select the Correct Stages

Strips are best prepared from lower thoracic and upper lumbar levels of stage
17–18 (3-day-old) embryos. Somites at these levels/stages have developed enough
to have distinct boundaries between sclerotome populations. In more mature
somites, contaminating populations such as the mesonephros are less readily
removed and portions of the anterior sclerotome will have begun to develop
inhibitory properties (see Tosney, 1991, and below).

2. Prepare Dishes

Fill three 35-mm petri dishes and one 60-mm Sylgard-bottomed dish with
Hanks balanced saline (GIBCO). Sylgard (Dow Corning; available from Brown-
ELL-Electro, Wood Dale, IL) is an optically clear, autoclavable polymer. A
layer 1 cm deep is polymerized in the bottom of a glass dish according to
manufacturer directions; pins can be stuck in it. Add 750 units pen-strep (GIBCO)
to each of the three 35-mm dishes and 2500 units of pen-strep to the Sylgard dish.

3. Remove Embryos from Eggs

Candle the eggs: hold an egg adjacent to a light source to determine where
the embryo lies. Trace a circle around the embryo. Swab the eggs thoroughly
with 70% ethanol. Use an 18-gauge needle attached to a 10-ml syringe to remove
5–10 ml of albumin from the egg: insert the needle through the shell at the fat
end of the egg, angling the needle down and toward the side to avoid piercing
the yolk. With the albumin removed, the embryo will fall away from the shell
and can be removed with less chance of damage or contamination. Using curved
forceps like scissors, cut out the penciled circle of egg shell. Using dissecting
scissors, cut a circle around the embryo through the blastodisc and yolk sac. Lift
the embryo out by scooping it up with curved forceps; do not try to grasp the
embryo or it will be crushed. Transfer the embryo to a prepared 35-mm dish
and gently swirl to wash away as much yolk as possible.

4. Remove Embryonic Membranes

Place the petri dish on a dissecting scope stage and observe at low magnification
for all further steps. Grasp membranes on either side of the midline at the leg
bud level using two sterile forceps. Gently pull laterally to open a hole, and then
continue opening the membranes toward the head. Pull the membranes from
both sides to the ventral midline, where they attach to the body wall. Sever the

attachment. Decapitate the embryo using Vannas scissors (Fine Science Tools, Foster City, CA) and discard the head. Cut off and discard the heart.

5. Wash Embryos

Using curved forceps, transfer the embryos to the second and then the third prepared petri dishes. Each time, gently swirl the dish for a minute to wash the embryos. After the final wash, transfer the embryos to the Sylgard-coated dish.

6. Pin Embryos

Gently hold an embryo on its back using sterile forceps. Insert a minutien pin (2 mm Fine Science Tools, Foster City, CA) through the notochord in the neck and push it securely into the Sylgard. Now push a pin through the tail and gently *stretch* the embryo in the anterior–posterior direction as you secure the tail pin into the Sylgard. If the embryo is not stretched, it will flop around while the ventral tissues are removed, making the task difficult. Use four pins to pin back the body wall and expose the ventral tissues. Because the body wall is thin, pin it through the limb buds on each side, applying gentle tension to stretch the body cavity. If more than one embryo is being dissected, pin them down like spokes in a wheel, with their necks toward the hub.

7. Remove the Gut

The midgut may be attached by a thin, membrane-like extension to the ventral body wall. Free the midgut from the body wall using forceps. Remove the entire gut by grasping the tubular foregut in the neck region with the forceps and peeling it posteriorly. Exert force only along the anterior–posterior axis; pulling laterally will often tear the embryo in two.

8. Remove the Notochord

Use forceps to sever the notochord at the upper forelimb level. Grasp the notochord just posterior to the break and carefully peel it toward the tail. If the notochord is difficult to remove, use two forceps: work the tips of one pair of forceps between the notochord and neural tube and use the second pair to pull toward the posterior. Pull the notochord free just past the leg buds and then cut it off. Trying to pull it away from the tail usually results in pulling off the entire tail, and sometimes the limbs as well.

9. Remove the Spinal Cord

Using forceps, pick up a minutien pin. Use the sharp end of the pin to split the neural tube at the midline. As the neural tube is opened, each half will fold laterally to cover the medial aspect of the somites. Now remove one-half of the spinal cord by grasping it at the forelimb level with forceps and peeling it posteriorly. Repeat for the other side. Be gentle: remember that the neural tube contacts sclerotome and that somites can be easily damaged with this manipulation. Also, carefully leave intact the ectoderm overlying the neural tube to hold the bilateral strip together.

10. Remove the Mesonephros

The mesonephros lies at the ventral–lateral edge of the somites and has vascular connections with the centrally lying aorta; the aorta itself generally comes out when the notochord is removed. Use forceps to slightly elevate the mesonephros while working a minutien pin between it and the sclerotome. Start at the forelimb region and work posteriorly. At most posterior, least mature somite levels, it will be harder to separate the mesonephros without damaging somites and more care will be needed. Now go back and carefully clean off any remaining tissue that obscures the surface of the sclerotome or that is attached to the sides of the somite strips. Once the dissection is complete, the prominent borders between somites as well as the less prominent division between anterior and posterior sclerotomes should be easily visible.

11. Place Orienting Marks

Unless the strip is going to be labeled after fixation with a marker for posterior (e.g., peanut agglutinin lectin, below; see Oakley and Tosney, 1991), a marker should be applied now to distinguish the anterior from the posterior after incubation. Carbon particles can be used or 1,1′-dioctadecyl-3,3,3′,3′-tetramethylindocarbocyanine perchlorate (DiI; Molecular Probes, Eugene, OR) can be injected into a posterior segment at one end of the strip. To prepare DiI stock, dissolve 2.5 mg DiI in 1 ml 100% ethyl alcohol. Stock solution may be kept refrigerated for up to 2 weeks. Just before use, dilute 200 μl of stock in 800 μl of 10% sucrose in distilled water and filter with a 0.5-μm syringe-type filter. Pull micropipettes from electrode glass to give a long tapered end. Break off the tip at a diameter of about one-tenth the diameter of a somite, as determined by eye. For injection, use an assembly with a 1-cc syringe inserted into a 0.22-μm filter with an 18.5-gauge needle at its tip. Attach polypropylene tubing between the needle and the micropipette. Suck DiI into the pipette and inject a very small amount into an anterior or posterior sclerotome.

12. Trim Strip

Remove all pins except for those securing the neck and tail. Use Vannas scissors to remove limb buds and to trim the strip into a clean rectangle. Do not separate the bilateral pairs of somites; single rows of somites may curl up laterally, preventing the ectoderm from contacting and spreading on the substratum.

D. Culture

The strips are placed ectoderm-side down on the laminin-coated coverslips and are held in place with sterile tungsten wire. A variety of simple culture media are appropriate, but F12 culture medium supplemented as in Chapter 6 of this volume is commonly used. Avoid serum which promotes overgrowth by contaminating cells and which may block growth cones' access to some surface molecules.

1. Transfer Strips to Culture Plates

Add 0.9 ml of culture medium to each 15-mm-diameter well of a four-well plate (Nunc). Culture each strip in a separate well. Place one laminin-coated coverslip in each well, laminin side up, making sure it settles to the bottom without trapping bubbles. If bubbles are trapped, gently push the coverslip down with sterile forceps until the bubbles pop out. Prewet a sterile Pasteur pipette with medium to prevent the tissue from sticking to the glass. Carefully suck up a somite strip by placing the pipette tip at one end of the strip and slightly releasing the bulb. When done correctly, the strip will enter the pipette readily (it tends to fold along its midline) and will lie close to the tip of the pipette. Now transfer the strip to one of the wells with a minimum of fluid transfer. Transfer additional strips in the same manner.

2. Secure Strips

Use a dissecting scope to examine the strips in the wells. If necessary, use forceps to flip the somite strip over to get the ectodermal side facing the laminin. Use forceps to dip small pieces (0.5 cm) of tungsten wire (0.005 in. diameter; R. D. Mathis, Long Beach, CA) in 95% ethanol and flame. Hold the wire out of the flame for a minute to cool. Place a wire across a strip at the posterior end, along the border between the anterior and posterior halves of the last somite pair. Once the wire is positioned correctly, push it down into the tissue to secure the posterior end. Be gentle to avoid severing the tissue. Repeat for the anterior end, stretching the strip as flat as possible.

3. Incubate

Carefully move the plate into a 5% CO_2 incubator at 37°C. Incubate for 2–4 hr before adding neurons. This period allows the ectoderm to attach and begin to spread on the laminin.

E. Neurons

Neurons are labeled with DiI, dissociated, sprinkled on the adherent strips, and cultured overnight. Any neural population that can be labeled with DiI and dissociated can be assessed in this assay. This section describes preparing sensory neurons (DRG) and labeling them after dissociation. A method for labeling cell bodies by injecting nerves in intact preparations is described in the original publication on DiI by Honig and Hume (1986).

1. Dissect

Remove a 5- to 6-day (stages 24–26) embryo from its egg, rinse, decapitate, and remove membranes as described earlier. At these stages, thoracic and lumbar sensory neurites have yet to reach their targets. Transfer embryo to a Sylgard-bottomed glass dish with 10 ml of Hanks' saline and 750 units of pen-strep. Pin the embryo on its back, cut a slit along the body wall along the anterior to posterior axis, spread the flaps of tissue, and pin them down. Eviscerate and clean the body cavity of loose tissue. Near the embryo's neck, use iridectomy scissors to cut transversely through the ventral vertebrae. Then place the scissors parallel with the bottom of the dish and cut the vertebral processes to each side. Pick up the flap of vertebral tissue and pull it toward the posterior. If the tissue stops separating easily, snip the lateral vertebral processes as it is pulled. When the tail is reached, cut off the vertebral strip. Remove the neural tube to expose the DRG. Pluck out 20–30 DRG using forceps and clean off any debris. Collect the ganglia in one area of the dish. Prewet the tip of a pipette with Hanks' (to prevent tissue from sticking) and use it to transfer the DRG into a 35-mm petri dish containing 5 ml of Hanks'.

2. Dissociation Label

Mince each DRG and transfer the pieces into a 10-ml plastic tube containing 4.5 ml modified Puck's glucose and 0.5 ml of 10× trypsin (GIBCO). Incubate for 20 min in a water bath at 37° C. Add 5 ml of medium containing 5% horse serum to quench the trypsin reaction, mix, and then centrifuge to pellet the cells. Use medium with 5% serum for all the following steps except the last resuspension. Triturate the pellet in 1 ml of medium. Resuspend in 9 ml of medium and centrifuge. Decant fluid. Resuspend pellet in 1900 μl of medium and 100 μl of DiI stock solution (2.5 mg DiI in 100 μl dimethyl sulfoxide and 900 μl 100% ethyl alcohol, sonicated, and filtered). Triturate and incubate for 40 min at 37°C in a 5% CO_2 tissue culture incubator. Add 9 ml of medium and centrifuge. Repeat trituration and rinsing step two more times and then resuspend in 1 ml of medium without serum. Add 150–200 μl to each culture well, adjusting the cell density so that only a few neurons adhere to each strip.

F. Fixing and Labeling

Strips are fixed and then labeled with PNA, a marker for inhibitory tissues.

Wash cultures with a room temperature wash solution (5.0 ml 4× Kreb's buffer, 5.0 ml 1.6 M sucrose in distilled water, 10 ml distilled water) to remove floating cells that could otherwise be deposited on the strip. For each wash, gently remove medium until the somites are just covered with fluid. Gently rinse the wash solution over the somites until the wells are almost full. Let sit 10 min. Repeat three times. Fix overnight in 4% paraformaldehyde (5 ml of 8% paraformaldehyde, 2.5 ml 4× Kreb's buffer, 2.5 ml 1.6 M sucrose in distilled water). For 10–15 min each, rinse three to five times in phosphate-buffered saline (PBS), twice in PBS containing 0.2 M glycine, and twice in HEPES-buffered saline containing 1% bovine serum albumin (BSA) and 0.1 mM calcium. Label for 1 hr with PNA–FITC (Vector, Burlingame, CA; 10 μl/ml in HEPES-buffered saline with 1% BSA). Wash three times in PBS. Place a small (ca. 12 mm) circle of silicon grease on a microscope slide. Remove a coverslip from its well, place it on the circle with the strip side up, add PBS, and cover with a larger coverslip.

III. Critical Aspects

The virtue of this assay is that it exposes sclerotomes in a repeated spatial array and yet retains both the physical relations among somitic populations and the molecular characteristics such as differential PNA-binding activity. Moreover, the borders between permissive (anterior) and inhibitory (posterior) populations are easily seen (Fig. 1). Attention must therefore be paid to elements that can disrupt relevant tissue relationships, obscure borders, or prevent neurons from interacting with the sclerotome.

A. Tissue Architecture

To maintain tissue relations, the strips must appear somewhat flattened on the spread ectodermal sheet. If the ectoderm is torn and allows the somite to touch the substratum, the somitic cells will spread onto the substratum as a monolayer and there will no longer be an obvious border between populations. If the edge of the ectodermal sheet fails to contact the substratum, the somites will ball up, making it difficult to see borders or deposited neurons. Such slices assume an hourglass-like shape, being curled away from the substratum between the flat areas held down by the pins. They are suboptimal for analysis. If the strips curl in this fashion, incubate them longer before adding neurons to allow the ectoderm greater time to adhere and handle them more gently to prevent dislodgment. Since the ectodermal sheet appears to adhere only at its cut edges, it is easily dislodged. Strips of six to eight somite pairs tend to curl less than longer strips.

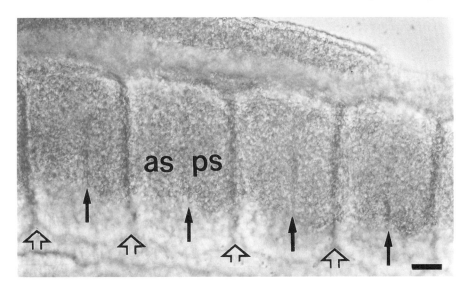

Fig. 1 Half of a bilateral somite strip after 18 hr of culture. Open arrows mark the borders between somites whereas dark arrows mark the border between sclerotome halves. The ectodermal edge is visible at top right. as, anterior sclerotome; ps, posterior sclerotome. Bar: 50 μm.

In our hands, tissue architecture in strips has not been compromised by necrosis. Cell death within the somite has been restricted to its normal site, within dorsal–anterior sclerotome. Nevertheless the health of cultures should be periodically monitored using indicators such as acridine orange or typan blue exclusion.

B. Temporal–Spatial Concerns

The stage and axial level of somites are crucial. Somites change in two ways during development that complicate the simple dichotomy between anterior and posterior functional domains. Unless you are alert to these development features, you could be confounded by apparently inhibitory qualities within anterior sclerotome. These complexities are circumvented using thoracic and lumbar somites from stage 17–18 embryos; they are monitored by looking for PNA-binding activity within the anterior sclerotome. First, anterior sclerotome normally becomes less permissive as somites mature. Second, the ventral portion of the sclerotome assumes an inhibitory character upon interacting with the notochord; removing the notochord early prevents this interaction and allows the ventral–anterior sclerotome to retain its permissive qualities (see Tosney and Oakley, 1990). If strips are prepared from more mature somites (e.g., from stage 19 or older embryos), the notochord will be removed only after the interaction has commenced. In culture, the ventral sclerotomes display inhibitory qualities to varying degrees. These resulting inhibitory qualities can be studied in the assay.

However, note that the PNA label must be used to distinguish between dorsal permissive and ventral inhibitory populations within anterior sclerotome since no independently visible border like that between anterior and posterior marks these domains.

C. Contaminating Populations

The most pernicious source of contamination is vascular endothelial cells. These cells can be detected with Nomarski or phase optics by their large size, spread morphology, and tendency to form strands or sheets on the surface of the somite. They can be eradicated only by honing the dissection technique. Avoiding serum reduces the magnitude of such contamination.

Neural crest cells can be considered as a second "contaminant" or as a natural component of the somitic environment. Strips can be constructed with minimal crest cells by focusing on the last six somites to form. In these most posterior somites, crest cells may lie between the somite and neural tube but have yet to penetrate sclerotome (Bronner-Fraser and Stern, 1991; Tosney *et al.*, 1994). Cleaning this surface before explanting the strip usually eridicates these cells. Invasion of crest cells can be monitored using HNK-1 antibody after fixation.

Cells accompanying the neural populations of interest should be considered contaminants. There are two solutions for this problem: visualizing the contamination and minimizing its effect. If, as with DRG, the population is dissociation labeled with DiI, then the contaminating cells (Schwann cells) will be also be labeled and will be visible. Central nervous system (CNS) neurons require additional steps. For instance, motoneurons can be labeled by injecting spinal nerves with DiI and allowing time for DiI to diffuse to the cell bodies (see Honig and Hume, 1986). The ventrolateral spinal cord is then dissected and labeled with DiO after dissociation. With this protocol, motoneurons are double-labeled while contaminating cells are labeled with DiO alone. An additional precaution is vital for reducing the possibility of analyzing interactions with introduced cells or with other neurons rather than with sclerotome cells. Seed all cultures at a density (empirically determined for your conditions) in which only a few labeled neurons adhere per strip.

D. Borders

In well-spread strips, borders between sclerotome populations are remarkably visible with either phase or Nomarski optics (Fig. 1). Borders can be obscured by contaminating endothelial cells or by curling of the strip (see earlier discussion). The fluorescent PNA label is less useful for precisely delineating borders: since it labels deep layers as well as superficial layers, the glow from out of focus areas can obscure the exact boundary. PNA is useful for identifying putative inhibitory domains rather than borders (Fig.4A).

E. Neurons

In this assay, neurites extend predominantly on the surface of the strip; they seldom penetrate to any depth and they are easily visualized with epifluorescence using an upright microscope. Note that fewer neurons will adhere to the strip than to the substratum, perhaps because the somites are like a small mountain range in the dish—many deposited neurons simply roll down its slope. The sprouting efficiency and lengths can be compared to the neurons on laminin in the same dish. The sprouting efficiency for sensory and motor neurons is similar on the dish and on both scerotome populations, whereas neurite length varies dramatically. This observation is expected if the assay displays differences relevant to guidance rather than to neurite initiation.

IV. Analyzing Neurites to Assess Guidance Interactions

A. Neurite Lengths

Neurite lengths can be used to deduce relative "permissiveness" but do not, by themselves, distinguish among possible guidance interactions (below). For instance, sensory and motor neurites are shorter on posterior than on anterior sclerotome, in accord with the demonstrated differential permissiveness of these tissues in the embryo. Neurites do extend even on posterior sclerotome, showing that this tissue is neither totally unpermissive nor toxic. However, even on anterior sclerotome the neurites are much shorter than on laminin, suggesting that even anterior sclerotome is a suboptimal environment for advance.

B. Neurite Trajectories

The direction and orientation of neurites are diagnostic for different guidance mechanisms, as diagrammed in Fig. 2. In contact-mediated mechanisms, trajectories are expected to alter only on contact. In long-distance (putative chemotactic) mechanisms, trajectories are expected to alter before direct contact. For instance, examine the trajectories of neurites from neurons on anterior sclerotome in Figs. 2A and 2B. If posterior sclerotome repulsed growth cones from a distance, neurites should consistently turn away from posterior sclerotome before contacting it (Fig. 2A). If posterior sclerotome inhibited only on contact, neurites should turn to avoid posterior sclerotome only after contact with a posterior border (Fig. 2B). To assure that such a contact-mediated mechanism was valid, it would have to be shown that the border itself did not physically impede crossing, i.e., that growth cones cross freely from posterior to anterior. To distinguish long-distance mechanisms, measure the orientation of neurites relative to borders (Fig. 2C). Our results with motor and sensory neurons implicate two mechanisms of guidance. Both populations avoid posterior sclerotome on contact and both orient toward anterior sclerotome from a distance (Figs. 3 and 4B).

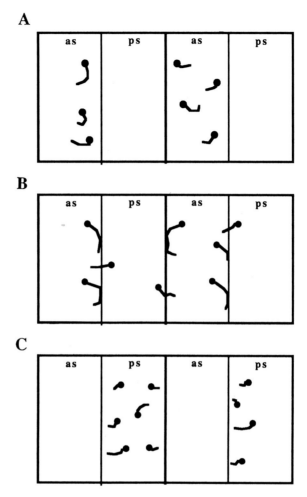

Fig. 2 Neurite trajectories predicted by three different interactions. (A) Repulsion at a distance: neurites on anterior sclerotome (as) turn away from posterior (ps) sclerotome before contacting it; neurites are oriented away from the closest posterior half. (B) Contact-mediated avoidance: Growth cones turn only upon contact with a posterior border but cross freely from posterior to anterior sclerotome. (C) Long-distance attraction: neurites on posterior sclerotome are oriented toward the closest anterior sclerotome; neurites turn toward anterior sclerotome before contacting it.

V. Conclusions and Perspectives

A. Assessing Additional Populations

As described earlier, any neuronal populations that can be selectively labeled and dissociated can be assessed in this assay. Testing a variety of CNS neurons could show, for instance, whether select CNS populations are able to detect and

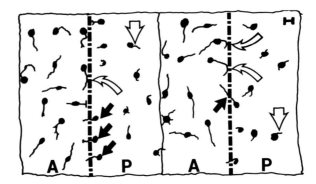

Fig. 3 Typical results. Schematic from combined camera lucida tracings of sensory neurons deposited on somite strips. Hollow curved arrows indicate examples of avoidance on contact with the posterior (P) border. Dark arrows indicate examples of crossing from posterior (P) to anterior (A) sclerotome. Hollow straight arrows indicate examples of orientation toward the nearest anterior sclerotome. Bar: 10 μm.

respond to either the inhibitory or the permissive guidance cues present in somites. Such studies would reveal the extent to which the navigational cues resident in somites might be relevant to other populations. Assessing neural crest interactions would be more complicated since these cells leave no trail showing where they have been in culture, unlike neurons, in which the trajectory is inferred by the position of the neurite. Given time, neural crest cells might differentially accumulate on anterior sclerotome. However, distinguishing their behavior at borders is impossible without directly visualizing them as they move. Live interactions could be videotaped in this assay if the assay were appropriately modified (see below). Alternatively, embryos could be sliced horizontally and videotaped as in Chapter 6 (this volume).

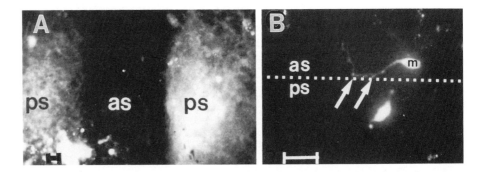

Fig. 4 Typical results (A) PNA binds to posterior sclerotome (ps) but not to anterior sclerotome (as) in somite strips after 18 hr in culture. (B) Motor neuron (m) labeled with DiI extends a neurite on anterior sclerotome that turns on contact with posterior sclerotome (arrows). The dotted line indicates the border between anterior and posterior sclerotome halves. Bars: 10 μm.

B. Assessing Molecular Cues

With some modifications, this assay is suitable for investigating the molecular nature of both the attractive chemotactic and the contact-mediated inhibitory cue by adding blocking antibodies, enzymes, or metabolic inhibitors to the culture medium. For instance, in preliminary studies it has been demonstrated that neurites no longer respect an anterior–posterior boundary when PNA is added to the medium. For some treatments, it may be necessary to prefix and wash strips to avoid directly damaging the somitic cells. If so, the outgrowth on prefixed strips as a control must be analyzed; it is not yet known if both contact-mediated and chemotactic mechanisms are retained in fixed preparations. To assess how treatments affect guidance mechanisms, the same measures that implicate mechanism, e.g., turning at borders for contact-mediated avoidance, must be used. The neurite lengths provide an easily quantifiable measure of effects on relative permissiveness.

C. Utility and Limitations

This assay uses neurite responses to detect guidance cues, as in a similar slice assay (Chapter 6, this volume). Unlike the slice assay, which allows access to all guidance cues from the spinal cord to the limb, the somite strip focuses on a representative subset of permissive and inhibitory cues that are repetitively arrayed in a single preparation. The analysis is simplified since it is based on rectangular sets of tissues rather than on the often irregular shape of tissues in slices. It is simpler to measure neurite orientation relative to borders that are arrayed as rectangles. The borders can also be visualized independently in strips without using the PNA label that is required to detect putatively inhibitory domains in slices. Strips are thus more suitable for many molecular analyses than are slices. Neurites deposited on the surface of either preparation can also be filmed. However, the surface of the slice is relatively flat whereas the somites in strips slope down toward the coverslip on both sides. This difference matters to an investigator who would have to refocus more often to follow a growth cone or cell on somite strips. The slice preparation is obviously better adapted to a time-lapse analysis of neuronal populations that are labeled *in situ* and extend within the slice rather than on its surface. Each assay thus has somewhat different applications but one significant similarity. In both assays, portions of embryos that are big enough to simulate the real internal environment of the embryo are used, but they are placed in a culture setting that is much more accessible than the embryo to intervention, to exogenous chemicals, to visualization, and to analysis.

References

Bellairs, R., Ede, D. A., and Lash, J. W., eds. (1986). "Somites in Developing Embryos." Plenum, New York.

Bronner-Fraser, M., and Stern, C. (1991). Effects of mesodermal tissues on avian neural crest cell migration. *Dev. Biol.* **143,** 213–217.

French, V., Ingham, P., Cooke, J., and Smith, J., eds. (1988). "Mechanisms of Segmentation," Development, Vol. 104 Supplement. Company of Biologists Limited, Cambridge, UK.

Honig, M. G., and Hume, R. I. (1986). Flourescent carbocyanine dyes allow living neurons of identified origin to be studied in long term cultures *J. Cell Biol.* **103,** 171–187.

Keynes, R. J., and Stern, C. (1984). Segmentation in the vertebrate nervous system. *Nature (London)* **310,** 786–789.

Oakley, R. A., and Tosney, K. W. (1991). Peanut agglutinin and chondroitin-6-sulfate are molecular markers for tissues that act as barriers to axon advance in the avian embryo. *Dev. Biol.* **147,** 187–206.

Tosney, K. W. (1987). Proximal tissues and patterned neurite outgrowth at the lumbosacral level of the chick embryo: Deletion of the dermamyotome. *Dev. Biol.* **122,** 540–588.

Tosney, K. W. (1991). Cells and cell interactions that guide motor axons in the developing chick embryo. *BioEssays* **13,** 1–7.

Tosney, K. W., and Oakley, R. A. (1990). The perinotochordal mesenchyme acts as a barrier to axon advance in the chick embryo: Implications for a general mechanism of axonal guidance. *Exp. Neurol.* **109,** 75–89.

Tosney, K. W., Dehnbostel, D. B., and Erickson, C. A. (1994). Neural crest cells prefer the myotome's basal lamina over the sclerotome as a substratum. *Dev. Biol.* **163,** 389–406.

CHAPTER 6

Embryo Slices

**Kevin B. Hotary, Lynn T. Landmesser,★
and Kathryn W. Tosney†**

Department of Internal Medicine and Comprehensive Cancer Center
The University of Michigan Medical School
Ann Arbor, Michigan 48109

★ Department of Neuroscience
Case Western Reserve University School of Medicine
Cleveland, Ohio 44106

† Department of Biology
The University of Michigan
Ann Arbor, Michigan 48109

I. Introduction
II. Cutting and Culturing Embryo Slices
    A. Embryo Preparation
    B. Cutting Slices
    C. Culturing Slices
    D. Fixing and Mounting Slices
    E. Peanut Agglutinin Lectin Labeling
    F. Media and Solutions
III. Embryo Slice Characteristics
IV. Experimental Results Using Embryo Slices
    A. The Slice as an Assay for Neurite Guidance Mechanisms
    B. *In Situ* Studies with Embryo Slices
V. Conclusions and Perspectives
    References

I. Introduction

Two approaches have generally been taken in attempting to answer the question of how motile cells and neuronal processes navigate in the embryo. Surgical

Copyright © 1996 by Academic Press, Inc. All rights of reproduction in any form reserved.

manipulations, such as tissue grafts or deletions, have long been used and provide much of the framework upon which modern developmental biology is built. Surgical approaches are particularly common with avian embryos because they are easily accessed and manipulated, and because reliable cell markers are available (Le Douarin, 1973; Tucker *et al.,* 1984). Cell culture techniques provide insights into the interactions, molecules, and intracellular mechanisms behind directed cell movements in a greatly simplified environment (reviewed by Levi *et al.,* 1990; Kapfhammer and Schwab, 1992).

While both surgical and culture approaches have provided a wealth of important information, each also has limitations. For example, while embryonic surgeries have shown which tissues are necessary for motor axon outgrowth (reviewed by Tosney, 1992), such manipulations cannot conclusively identify the mechanisms by which these tissues provide directional cues. In addition, it is difficult or impossible to deduce accurately the temporal sequence and mode (i.e., continuous or saltatory) of cell movements from static sections. Cell cultures have the advantage of being simple and so are relatively easy to manipulate and analyze. But cell cultures also have the disadvantage of being simple and so cannot replicate the complexity of the embryonic milieu and the numerous factors that affect guidance.

An important tool in studying central nervous system (CNS) development and function is the tissue slice (reviewed by Gahwiler, 1988). CNS slices maintain many physical and molecular characteristics of the tissues from which they were cut and allow developmental and physiological events to be directly observed and manipulated in a more normal environment. Up until now, there was no comparable system for studying biological processes in peripheral tissues.

This chapter describes a chick embryo slice preparation that was originally developed by Landmesser (1988) to study motor axon guidance through peripheral tissues. Like CNS slices, chick embryo slices maintain many characteristics of the intact embryo and allow a detailed study of neurite outgrowth in an environment neurites normally encounter *in vivo.* Embryo slices also provide the ability to study other developmental processes that are not easily examined in intact embryos. In addition, embryo slices can be manipulated relatively easily both physically and chemically. Thus, this preparation provides many of the advantages of both whole embryo manipulations and cell cultures while also overcoming many of the limitations of these approaches.

II. Cutting and Culturing Embryo Slices

The following protocols describe how to prepare transverse slices of the caudal half of chick embryos. Slices can be made in any orientation from any region of the embryo, but slight modifications of the procedures will be necessary depending on the age of the embryo and the specific hardware used to cut slices. These modifications are usually trivial.

Slices are used to study how dissociated cells sprinkled on the slice surface interact with different tissues and how cells endogenous to the slice progress. For either preparation, embryos should first be rinsed free of loose yolk granules, eviscerated, and cleaned of loose bits of tissue and skin. The region to be sliced is then isolated and embedded in agarose, which provides the necessary stiffness for sectioning on a vibratome. Slices are cultured either adhered to a substratum or free floating, depending on the experiment.

A. Embryo Preparation

1. Candle eggs and mark the position of the embryo. Lower the level of the embryo by withdrawing 5–10 ml of albumin through an 18-gauge needle attached to a 10-ml syringe. The lower level of the embryo minimizes the risk of damage when removing the overlying shell. Remove the shell over the embryo using blunt forceps.

2. Cut through the yolk sac around the outside of the embryo with Vanna's scissors (Fine Science Tools, Foster City, CA) or with fine dissecting scissors and lift the embryo out of the shell using curved, blunt forceps as a ladle. Place the embryo in a petri dish filled with a sterile physiological saline (e.g., Hanks' balanced salts or Tyrode's solution) containing penicillin–streptomycin (50–100 U/ml; GIBCO).

3. Rinse the embryo in the sterile saline to remove adherent yolk granules by gently rocking the petri dish. Remove extraembryonic membranes using jeweler's forceps and Vanna's scissors.

4. Transfer the embryo through three successive washes in sterile saline containing penicillin–streptomycin (50–100 U/ml). After the last wash, transfer the embryo to a glass petri dish coated with a 5- to 7-mm layer of silicone elastomer (Sylgard; Dow Corning, Midland, MI: available from Brown-ELL-Electro, Wood Dale, IL) and filled with sterile saline/penicillin–streptomycin (50–100 U/ml).

5. Decapitate the embryo by firmly grasping the neck just rostral to the heart with a pair of jeweler's forceps and squeezing.

6. Pin the embryo ventral side up using insect pins cut to a length of 5–10 mm. Insert one pin through the neck and another through the tail, pulling the embryo taut, but not so taut as to tear it.

7. Remove the heart and make a slit in the ventral body wall from the neck to the tail using Vanna's scissors.

8. Pin the loose flaps of skin laterally to expose the body cavity and internal organs. Again, pull the embryo tightly, but not so tightly as to tear it. The tension produced will ease evisceration of the embryo in the succeeding step. The most secure attachment is usually achieved by placing pins through the lose ectoderm and the limb buds; however, if the limb buds are to be included in the culture, pin only through the loose ectoderm.

9. Eviscerate the embryo. With jeweler's forceps, grasp the foregut rostrally and pull toward the tail (the pinning through the neck is usually sturdier than that at the tail, so pulling the viscera caudally minimizes the risk of tearing the embryo in the process). In older embryos (stage 20+) it is usually possible to remove the gut and most other organs in one piece. The mesonephros can then be removed in one strip from each side of the embryo. In younger embryos the gut and mesonephros usually must be removed in several small pieces (for more detail on eviscerating younger embryos, see Chapter 5).

10. Remove the dorsal aorta with jeweler's forceps and clean off any remaining bits of loose tissue. Also, trim off loose ectoderm, as fragments will later stick in the embedding agarose, making removal of the slices difficult.

B. Cutting Slices

1. Embed the embryo in 2% low melting-point agarose (GIBCO ultrapure LMP agarose) made up in sterile physiological saline in a plastic boat of the type commonly used for paraffin embedding (available from VWR Scientific). Place the embryo in the boat once the agarose has sufficiently cooled but has not yet started to set. Use forceps to move the embryo into the desired slicing orientation.

2. Once set, cut out a block of agarose containing the embryo and mount on the vibratome specimen platform with cyanoacrylate adhesive (Krazy Glue, Borden Inc., Columbus, OH).

3. Mount the platform on the vibratome and cut slices. Clean and semisterilize the chamber in which slices are cut by washing in 70% ethanol followed by several rinses with sterile distilled water and then several rinses in sterile saline. To keep the agarose stiff throughout slicing, keep the bath solution on ice until use and keep the slicing chamber cold. We cut slices 150–250 μm thick on an EMCorp (Chestnut Hill, MA) Model H1200 vibratome.

4. Remove slices to a petri dish containing ice-cold sterile saline and remove any adhering bits of agarose or remaining loose pieces of tissue.

5. Transfer cleaned slices to a petri dish containing culture medium (see later). Slices can be easily transferred with minimal damage using a wide-bore plastic pipette that has been prewetted with culture medium (to prevent the slices from sticking to the pipette walls). Slices can be kept in these dishes for several hours at 37°C in 5% CO_2 until transferred to their final culture dishes.

C. Culturing Slices

Slices may be cultured either adhered to a substratum or free floating, depending on the experiment. For experiments in which fixed and stained slices are analyzed (e.g., when cells are seeded on slices), it is often advantageous to have the slices adhere to a substrate, as this makes observations and processing significantly easier. The length of the culture period is also a factor, as limb buds that are not attached to a substrate tend to curl upon themselves. Occasionally, this curling will be so severe that the limb covers most or all of the slice surface. Cultures in which slices are grown attached to a substrate will be referred to as "adherent" cultures. "Floating" cultures are often used when it is beneficial to be able to move or reorient the slices, e.g., when making time-lapse recordings of endogenous cell movements.

1. Adherent Cultures

Acid-washed coverslips (Clay Adams Gold Seal) coated with type IV collagen (200 μg/ml in carbonate buffer; Sigma) provide good slice adhesion without promoting excessive spread onto the coverslip. Other substrates tested (laminin, polylysine, and several commercially prepared substrata) were either not adhesive enough, resulting in poorly attached or free-floating slices, or promoted migration of cells out of the slice, resulting in a loss of structure. We use 12-mm-diameter coverslips placed in 15-mm- diameter four-well dishes (Nunc). Transfer slices from the holding dish (step 5 above) to the culture wells using a prewetted wide-bore pipette and manipulate them into the desired position with forceps. Culture slices in medium (see later) without serum. When slices are cultured with serum, the ectoderm tends to overgrow the slice surface rapidly, covering the internal tissues and dislodging or covering any cells sprinkled on the slice.

The number of slices the coverslips can accommodate will vary with the size of the region cut. A maximum of six stage 17–26 hindlimb slices are cultured per coverslip. The slices, if undisturbed, will adhere lightly to the coverslip within an hour and firmly within a few hours. The slices will remain stuck down throughout most fixation and labeling procedures if handled carefully.

2. Floating Cultures

For the experiments described later, floating cultures were prepared in specially constructed chambers. These chambers are made by first drilling a 12-mm-diameter hole in the bottom of a 35-mm plastic petri dish. This hole is then covered from the outside with a glass coverslip attached with silicone cement. This chamber allows the viewer to clearly visualize and record labeled cells and cell processes in the living slices when the slices are held firmly in place on the coverslip. Slices are held still using a small piece of coverslip that has been stuck to the coverslip on the dish bottom with a small bead of silicone grease. The grease acts as a hinge, allowing the coverslip segment to be gently lowered onto the slice. The slice is thus held firmly against the dish bottom and is easily accessible for observation with an inverted microscope. Slices can be easily moved or reoriented at any time by lifting the coverslip segment.

A variety of other chambers can be used for floating cultures as long as the slices are not allowed to settle in one place for long periods, as they will eventually adhere to nearly any substrate, including the plastic surface of a petri dish. Long-term floating cultures may require gentle rocking. Floating cultures are prepared in the same medium as that used for adherent cultures with some possible modifications (see below) depending on the experiment.

D. Fixing and Mounting Slices

The following protocol is written specifically for fixing adherent cultures in their culture wells and for mounting them on slides for observation on an upright microscope. The same solutions and procedures are used for floating cultures, except the slices are usually transferred in a wide-bore pipette from one solution to the next.

1. Rinse slices three times for 10 min each in Kreb's buffer/sucrose (see below). At each rinse, withdraw one-half of the volume of fluid in the well and replace with fresh buffer. Avoid draining the wells completely in this and all subsequent steps, as air–water interfaces tend to dislodge the slices.
2. After the final rinse, replace one-half of the fluid in the well with 4% paraformaldehyde (in Kreb's/sucrose) and let stand for 10 min.
3. Replace one-half of the fluid with fresh 4% paraformaldehyde and fix the cultures for 30 min to overnight.
4. Rinse the fixed slices three to five times (10 min each) in phosphate-buffered saline (PBS). The slices are now ready for further specific processing, such as antibody or lectin labeling or mounting. A protocol for peanut agglutinin lectin (PNA) labeling is given in Section II,E.
5. To mount adherent slices for observations on an upright microscope, make a ring of silicone grease of about 20 mm diameter on a microscope slide. This grease ring should be higher than the thickness of the slices on the coverslip. With jeweler's forceps, gently lift the coverslip containing the slices out of the culture well (at this point the slices should remain attached) and place them slice-side up in the middle of the grease ring. Flood this well with PBS or some other mounting solution and cover with a clean coverslip. Push the second coverslip down until it is just above the surface of the slice, but avoid squashing the slice. Mount floating slices and the inevitable occasional detached adherent slice on 24 × 60-mm or 25 × 75-mm coverslips. Ring the periphery of the coverslip with silicone grease and transfer the loose slices to the ringed well with a wide-bore pipette. Cover the coverslip with a second like-sized coverslip and press together to hold the slices stationary. The slices can then be viewed from either side on an upright microscope.

E. Peanut Agglutinin Lectin Labeling

Chick embryo tissues that inhibit peripheral neurite outgrowth preferentially bind PNA (Oakley and Tosney, 1991). This binding activity can be used to identify tissues in a slice. The following protocol describes how to label fixed slices with fluorescein-conjugated PNA.

1. Rinse slices (that have been fixed as described earlier and are presently in PBS) twice for 15 min each in PBS containing 20 mM glycine.
2. Rinse slices twice (15 min each) in HEPES-buffered saline (HBS: 150 mM NaCl, 10 mM HEPES) containing 1% bovine serum albumin (BSA) and 0.1 mM CaCl$_2$.
3. Replace HBS with HBS (as just described with BSA and CaCl$_2$) containing FITC-PNA (Vector Research, Burlingame, CA) at 5–10 μl/ml. Incubate for 1 hr at room temperature.
4. Rinse three times in PBS (10 min each) and mount as described previously.

F. Media and Solutions

1. Culture Medium

The basic medium used for both adherent and floating cultures consists of F-12 supplemented with:

33 mM glucose
22 mM glutamine
5 μg/ml insulin
6 ng/ml progesterone
1.6 μg/ml putrescine
8 ng/ml sodium selenite
5 μg/ml transferrin
100 U/ml penicillin–streptomycin

All of these ingredients are available from Sigma or GIBCO. When sensory neurons are added to the slices, the culture medium is further supplemented with 100 ng/ml 7S nerve growth factor. F-12 medium is formulated to equilibrate in an atmosphere containing 5% CO_2. In cases when slices will be out of a CO_2 atmosphere for prolonged periods (e.g., when sitting on a microscope stage during time-lapse recording), 10–20 mM HEPES can be added to the medium to buffer pH changes. Alternatively, Leibovitz's L-15 medium, which buffers pH in an ambient atmosphere (Banker and Goslin, 1991), can be used in place of F-12.

2. Kreb's Buffer/Sucrose

The following final concentrations of Kreb's buffer/sucrose are used during slice fixation. In practice, separate 4× solutions of both buffer and sucrose are made up and then the two are mixed with distilled H$_2$O in a 1:1:2 (Kreb's: sucrose:water) ratio for use in the initial rinses. The fix solution (4% paraformaldehyde) is made up in the same ratio, replacing the water with 8% paraformaldehyde.

145 mM NaCl
5 mM KCl
1.2 mM CaCl$_2$
1.3 mM MgCl$_2$
1.2 mM NaH$_2$PO$_4$
10 mM glucose
20 mM HEPES
400 mM sucrose

III. Embryo Slice Characteristics

For the embryo slice preparation to be useful in a variety of experimental situations, it must meet several criteria. The slices must remain viable in culture for a period of time ranging from a few hours to days. During the culture period the slices should retain the normal morphology and tissue relationships of the embryo and should support normal developmental processes. Finally, the slices should retain the normal molecular characteristics of the embryo.

We have characterized slices and have found that they meet these criteria. Slices retain the essential embryonic morphology and tissue relationships for up to 2 days in culture. After this period, differential tissue growth disrupts the structure of the slice and the ectoderm begins to overgrow and obscure the surface. An example of typical slice development after 1 day in culture is shown in Fig. 1. The dorsal root ganglia can be seen in their normal position lateral to the neural tube. The apical ectodermal ridge is clearly visible at the tip of the limb, which itself has matured so that the dorsal and ventral muscle masses and the closely packed precartilaginous cells of the developing femur are distinguishable from the surrounding mesenchyme. The skin has not spread to cover the slice surface, leaving the internal tissues exposed, and the slice surface is relatively free of dead cells and cell debris. Slice cells that have migrated onto the coverslip serve to anchor the slice to the coverslip.

One obvious concern with any large tissue explant is necrosis. With embryo slices, the trauma of slicing itself is not overly deleterious since the surface is not covered with dead cells or cell debris (Fig. 1A). Likewise, in order to confirm that slices are not necrotic internally (e.g., due to hypoxia), slices are stained with acridine organe or calcein-AM/ethidium homodimer-1 (live/dead cell assay; Molecular Probes, Eugene, OR). Dead cells are common in slices, but they are generally clustered only in embryonic regions that normally display cell death, such as the anterior and posterior necrotic zones of the limb and the plexus region. Most slice regions show only occasional and widely dispersed dead cells.

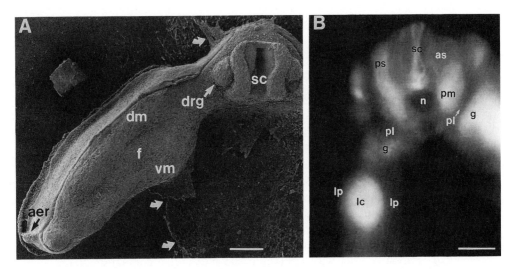

Fig. 1 (A) Scanning electron micrograph of a stage 22 chick embryo slice after 20 hr in culture. The slice surface is free of debris, leaving internal tissues exposed (ventral tissues have been removed in this slice). Embryonic structures and tissue relationships are normal, and the dorsal (dm) and ventral (vm) muscle masses as well as the femur (f) are beginning to form in the limb. Cells that have migrated out of the slice (arrows) anchor the slice to the coverslip. aer, apical ectodermal ridge; drg, dorsal root ganglion; sc, spinal cord. (B) Fluorescence micrograph of the PNA-labeling pattern in a stage 26 slice after 20 hr in culture. The section was made obliquely so both posterior (ps, labeled) and anterior (as, unlabeled) sclerotome are visible. Other tissues inhibitory to axon advance (pm, perintochordal mesenchyme; g, pelvic girdle; lc, limb core) are labeled while other permissive tissues (pl, plexus; lp, limb path) are not. n, notochord. Scale bars: 150 μm.

In addition to cell death, cell differentiation, and tissue morphogenesis, other developmental processes appear to proceed fairly normally in embryo slices. For example, in time-lapse recordings, motor axons within slices (Section IV,B; Fig. 5) progress at a rate comparable to that calculated for *in vivo* outgrowth. At the molecular level, slices show an identical pattern of PNA binding as that seen in normal embryos (Oakley and Tosney, 1991); PNA binds strongly to tissues inhibitory to axon advance and weakly or not at all to permissive tissues (Fig. 1B)

IV. Experimental Results Using Embryo Slices

The easiest way to describe the utility of the embryo slice preparation is through examples of experiments done using slices. This section briefly summarizes some experimental procedures and presents some typical results. The first part of this section describes using adherent slices as an assay for sensory and motor neurite guidance mechanisms. The second part of the section describes using floating slices to analyze endogenous motor axon outgrowth with time-lapse videomicroscopy. An overview of the basic procedures used in these experiments is shown schematically in Fig. 2.

A. The Slice as an Assay for Neurite Guidance Mechanisms

We used embryo slices to start defining the cellular mechanisms of peripheral neurite guidance. Adherent slices are seeded with dissociated, DiI-labeled (see Honig and Hume, 1986) sensory or motor neurons (see Chapter 5 for a protocol on preparing labeled, dissociated neuron populations). On slices, the neurons and their processes have free access to embryonic tissues and to the guidance cues they provide. By analyzing the lengths and trajectories of neurites relative to various slice tissues, the nature of peripheral guidance cues can be determined, as different cues predict distinctly different neurite responses. (1) The absence of neurite extension indicates a nonpermissive substratum. (2) Neurite turning upon contact with another tissue indicates a contact-mediated avoidance cue. (3) A consistent extension or turning toward a tissue indicates the emission of

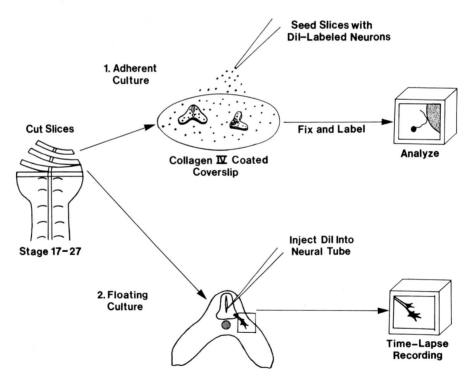

Fig. 2 The basic procedures for experiments using either adherent slices with seeded cells or floating cultures in which motor axons have been labeled for time-lapse videomicroscopy.

a diffusible attractant while (4) a consistent turning away from a tissue outside the range of direct contact indicates a diffusible repellent.

Both sensory and motor neurons will extend neurites on any slice tissue at all developmental stages that we have examined (stages 17–26 using the criteria of Hamburger and Hamilton, 1951); however, different neurite lengths clearly reflect the relative permissiveness of a tissue (Fig. 3A). On permissive tissues through which peripheral neurites normally extend (dorsal anterior sclerotome, pelvic plexus, and limb path), neurites attain much greater lengths than on inhibitory tissues (posterior sclerotome, perinotochordal mesenchyme, pelvic girdle, and limb core). In addition, neurites on permissive tissues turn to avoid inhibitory tissues (Fig. 3B). This avoidance response is not due merely to a physical barrier at the tissue border, since neurites on inhibitory tissue freely cross onto permissive tissue.

The slice assay can detect diffusible cues. Both sensory and motor neurites show directed outgrowth toward dorsal anterior sclerotome when on adjacent tissues. This response is detected outside the range of possible contact mediation and decreases with distance from dorsal anterior sclerotome. This long-distance attraction to dorsal anterior sclerotome is also displayed in a collagen gel assay developed specifically for the detection of diffusible cues [for a description of collagen gel cultures see Lumsden and Davies (1983)] and in "somite-strip" cultures (see Chapter 5).

The embryo slice has allowed us to define some of the cellular mechanisms that guide peripheral neurite extension. A clear demonstration of neurite guidance

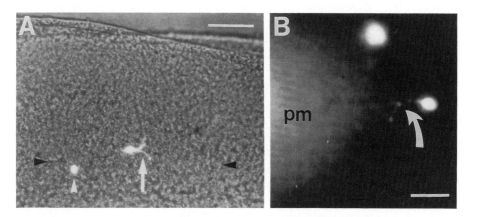

Fig. 3 DiI-labeled motor (A) and sensory (B) neurons deposited on slices and cultured for 18 hr. Two motor neurons deposited on the slice limb are shown in A. One neuron (arrowhead) landed on precartilaginous femur tissue (limb core) and only a very short neurite sprouted. A second neuron (arrow) on the nearby limb path has extended two longer neurites. The black arrowheads indicate the boundary between path and core. In B, a neurite (curved arrow) from a sensory neuron in the plexus contacts the border of the PNA-labeled perinotochordal mesenchyme (pm) and turns. Scale bars: 25 μm.

mechanisms acting within the embryo was previously lacking due to the absence of a suitable assay. Neurites orient toward the first peripheral tissue which they traverse, the dorsal anterior sclerotome, via an attractant emitted by this tissue. Once peripherally directed, neurites are restricted to pathways via contact-mediated cues; nonpathway (inhibitory) tissues repel neurites on contact, while pathway tissues permit advance. Somewhat surprisingly, inhibitory tissues were found not to be absolutely nonpermissive, as both motor and sensory neurons can extend neurites on any tissue at any stage of development. It is only when the neurite is given a choice between tissues at borders that permissive tissues are invariably selected for continued extension and inhibitory tissues are avoided.

B. *In Situ* Studies with Embryo Slices

Most of what is known about development comes from examinations of dead tissue. Observations of developmental processes in living tissue have been difficult because of the physical and optical constraints embryos impose upon such observations. Because embryo slices continue to develop in culture and are easily visualized microscopically, they are amenable to direct observation and manipulations.

We have used slices together with time-lapse videomicroscopy to study motor axon outgrowth. Motor neurons were labeled in slices by pressure injecting a small bolus of DiI into the lumen or ventrolateral wall of the neural tube (Fig. 4). After 2 to 4 hr, the DiI had labeled some motor neurites so that even some growth cone filopodia were clearly visible (Fig. 4, inset). The slices were then mounted as described earlier for floating cultures, and time-lapse recordings were made on an inverted microscope equipped with a computerized imaging system (Image-1, Universal Imaging Corp., Media, PA). Since DiI can be phototoxic, images were collected only every 1 to 5 min with each collection period requiring only about 1 sec of illumination. Illumination was further reduced with neutral density filters and the images were background subtracted and contrast enhanced. Thus far, we have followed axon outgrowth continuously for up to 8 hr.

Our time-lapse recordings have shown that motor growth cones follow their usual trajectory from the neural tube toward the limb, progressing at an average rate of about 10–20 μm/hour. Advance was sometimes, but not always, steady (Fig. 5). Some growth cones remained stationary or even partially regressed over periods ranging from just a few minutes to several hours. These growth cones were clearly alive and active during these periods, as evidenced by their frequent filopodial movements and protrusive activity. These stationary periods were often followed by periods of rapid progress before another stationary period. Prolonged stationary periods were also often seen in regions where the growth cones were required to choose between two or more possible alternative pathways (the "decision regions" of Tosney and Landmesser, 1985) and often preceded growth cone turning.

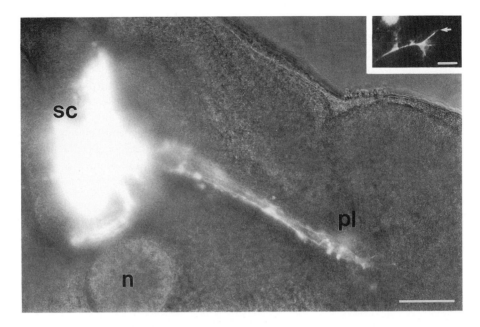

Fig. 4 DiI-labeled motor neurons within slices. A bolus of DiI was pressure injected into the spinal cord (sc) of a stage 22 slice. After about 3 hr, a group of motor axons, some of which extend as far as the plexus (pl), are brightly labeled. n, notochord. Scale bar: 50 μm. The inset shows a higher magnification view of a motor axon growth cone from a different slice labeled in the same way. The DiI label allows clear visualization of individual filopodia (arrow) in growth cones. Scale bar: 20 μm.

We have thus far limited our observation periods to a maximum of about 8 hr. There is no apparent reason why, with the proper precautions to maintain pH and temperature, these observation periods could not be significantly extended. Nonetheless, these relatively short-term recordings of embryo slices have already

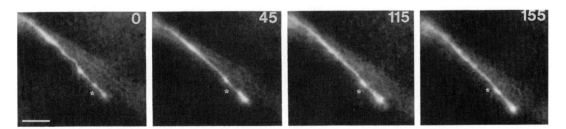

Fig. 5 Time-lapse series of DiI-labeled motor axon advancing within a stage 23 slice. Over a total recording period of 4.5 hr this axon advanced steadily at an average rate of about 12 μm/hr. Numbers indicate elapsed time in minutes. Asterisks mark a fixed reference point in the slice. Scale bar: 25 μm.

provided information that could not have been obtained with other methods. In particular, the saltatory movement of many growth cones as they advance, and the frequent active stationary periods that often precede turns could not be realized in fixed sections. It seems unlikely that these stationary periods were caused by damage to the growth cones (e.g., through DiI phototoxicity) since the growth cones were always active during these periods. In addition, stationary periods often preceded rapid advance or turning, and stationary periods were most often evident in growth cones in decision regions. This suggests that the growth cone during these stationary periods is processing information in preparation for its next movement. Similar saltatory growth cone movement has been described in brain slices (Halloran and Kalil, 1994) and may be a typical mode of axonal advance.

V. Conclusions and Perspectives

This chapter described an embryo slice preparation that can be used to gain insights into development that cannot be obtained using fixed tissue or dissociated cell cultures. These slices are relatively easy to prepare and culture, and require only a minimal investment of time and money. More importantly, these slices remain alive and support normal developmental processes in culture, retaining the normal morphology and tissue relationships of the embryo in addition to those molecular characteristics we have so far assessed. We thus feel confident that results obtained with slices are representative of normal development.

Since we now know many of the cellular mechanisms by which embryonic tissues direct sensory and motor neurites, slices can be used to determine the molecular components of these guidance cues, e.g., by applying function-blocking antibodies or other inhibitors in the same assay. Likewise, the mechanisms by which guidance signals are transduced at the growth cone can be determined using either slices or other culture methods based on the information obtained with slices. Questions about the universality of guidance cues can also be addressed by seeding slices with different cell populations (e.g., central nervous system neurons) or even cells from different species.

Embryo slices are open to the environment, and all of the internal tissues that are normally difficult or impossible to access in the intact embryo are freely accessible in the slice. These tissues can be relatively easily and quite specifically manipulated either physically (Fig. 6) or (less specifically) chemically. For example, one population of motor neurons (the epaxials) send axons dorsolaterally, directly to their target, the myotome. The nature of the cue that specifically guides this motor population is not known. Physical manipulations (e.g., partial or complete deletions) of the myotome will allow this specific guidance cue to be defined and will pave the way to determining its molecular components.

This chapter has concentrated primarily on using embryo slices to study peripheral neurite guidance. Clearly, however, there are many other uses for slices.

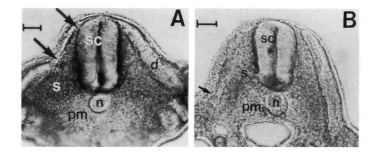

Fig. 6 Slices in which the dermamyotome has been removed (A) The dermamyotome (d) has just been removed from the region between the two arrows. The overlying ectoderm and the sclerotome (s) remain intact. After a few hours in culture, the wound made by removing the dorsal dermamyotome is no longer visible following a similar operation in a different slice (B). The arrow indicates the remaining dermatome and myotome on the operated side. Other labels are the same as Fig. 1. Scale bars: 50 μm.

Central nervous system cells are clearly visible in slices in which DiI has been injected into the neural tube. Preliminary time-lapse recordings show great movement among and within these cells. Axonal migration along different early spinal cord tracts can also be studied and manipulated in slices, particularly in longitudinal slices in which a length of neural tube several segments long is isolated and splayed open to display the inner walls. In addition, we find that neural crest cells migrate normally from DiI-injected slice neural tubes, allowing neural crest formation and cell migration to be studied in an essentially normal environment.

References

Banker, G., and Goslin, K., eds. (1991). "Culturing Nerve Cells," pp. 41–73. MIT Press, Cambridge, MA.

Gahwiler, B. H. (1988). Organotypic cultures of neural tissue. *Trends Neurosci.* **11**, 484–489.

Halloran, M. C., and Kalil, K. (1994). Dynamic behaviors of growth cones extending in the corpus callosum of living cortical brain slices observed with video microscopy. *J. Neurosci.* **14**, 2161–2177.

Hamburger, V., and Hamilton, H. L. (1951). A series of normal stages in the development of the chick embryo. *J. Morphol.* **88**, 49–92.

Honig, M. G., and Hume, R. I. (1986). Fluorescent carbocyanine dyes allow living neurons of identified origin to studied in long term culture. *J. Cell Biol.* **103**, 173–187.

Kapfhammer, J. P., and Schwab, M. E. (1992). Modulators of neuronal migration and neurite growth. *Curr. Opin. Cell Biol.* **4**, 863–868.

Landmesser, L. (1988). Peripheral guidance cues and the formation of specific motor projections in the chick. *In* "From Message to Mind" (S. E. Easter, Jr., K. F. Barald, and B. M. Carlson, eds.), pp. 121–133. Sinauer Assoc., Sunderland, MA.

Le Douarin, N. M. (1973). A biological cell labeling technique and its use in experimental embryology. *Dev. Biol.* **30**, 217–222.

Levi, G., Duband, J.-L., and Thiery, J. P. (1990). Modes of cell migration in the vertebrate embryo. *Int. Rev. Cytol.* **123**, 201–252.

Lumsden, A. G. S., and Davies, A. M. (1983). Earliest sensory nerve fibres are guided to peripheral targets by attractants other than nerve growth factor. *Nature (London)* **306**, 786–788.

Oakley, R. A., and Tosney, K. W. (1991). Peanut agglutinin and chondroitin-6-sulfate are molelcular markers for tissues that act as barriers to axon advance in the avian embryo. *Dev. Biol.* **147,** 187–206.

Tosney, K. W. (1992). Growth cone navigation in the proximal environment of the chick embryo. *In* "The Nerve Growth Cone" (P. C. Letourneau, S. B. Kater, and E. R. Macagno, eds.), pp. 387–403. Raven Press, New York.

Tosney, K. W., and Landmesser, L. T. (1985). Growth cone morphology and trajectory in the lumbosacral region of the chick embryo. *J. Neurosci.* **5,** 2345–2358.

Tucker, G. C., Aoyama, H., Lipinski, M., Tursz, T., and Thiery, J. P. (1984). Identical reactivity of monoclonal antibodies HNK-1 and NC-1: Conservation in vertebrates on cells derived from the neural primordium and on some leukocytes. *Cell Differ.* **14,** 223–230.

CHAPTER 7

Operations on Limb Buds of Avian Embryos

John W. Saunders, Jr.
Department of Biological Sciences
State University of New York
Albany, New York 12222

I. Introduction
II. Preparing to Operate
    A. Incubating the Egg
    B. Tools and Solutions
    C. Making a Window to Expose the Embryo
III. Extraembryonic Membranes
    A. Uncovering the Embryo
IV. Making Various Kinds of Grafts
    A. Chorioallantoic Grafts
    B. Flank Grafts
    C. Intracoelomic Grafts
    D. Grafts to the Somites
    E. Limb-to-Limb Grafts
V. Manipulations Involving the Apical Ectodermal Ridge
    A. Excision of the AER
VI. Grafts to Test Polarizing Activity
    A. Grafting the ZPA
    B. Other Tests of Polarizing Activity
VII. Enzymatic Dissociation and Recombination of Limb Tissues
    A. Ectoderm−Mesoderm Recombinations
References

I. Introduction

Intraembryonic operations involving avian species are used to investigate many problems in the field of vertebrate embryology. The early embryo of the bird

Copyright © 1996 by Academic Press, Inc. All rights of reproduction in any form reserved.

floats on at the upper surface of the yolk, which is held relatively motionless by the albuminous coats that envelop it. This fact enables the investigator to carry out microsurgical procedures on the embryo by operating through a "window" in the shell of the egg. Also, the coelom of the early embryo and its vascular chorioallantoic membrane, which appears later on, are particularly useful as culture sites for analyzing the morphogenetic potentials of putative organ-forming tissues.

There are various methods by which investigators may gain access to an avian embryo in order to carry out experiments on it. The method chosen is determined by the objectives of the experiment. For some studies it is necessary for the embryo to survive to late postoperative stages: to study the control of feather structure, for example, the operated chick is required to hatch and for questions relating to development of the skeletal, muscular, and nervous systems, the embryo must develop for several days after operation. For other kinds of questions, particularly those relating to cellular movements in the early blastoderm, the embryo needs to survive the operator's insults for only a few hours or for only a day or two.

In what follows, the presumption is that the embryo is to be exposed and so handled as to promote its chances of survival to the "fetal" stage, or even to hatch. Accordingly, procedures for exposing the embryo in such a way as to retain as much as possible its normal relationships to its physical environment are outlined first followed by procedures for carrying out various grafting experiments that are extensively used in solving problems relating to the development of the limbs.

II. Preparing to Operate

A. Incubating the Egg

Fertile eggs to be operated on are best incubated in a forced draft incubator at a temperature of 38.5–39.0°C and at about 95% relative humidity. Eggs should be rotated during incubation prior to operation so that the embryo and its membranes will not adhere to the shell membranes. In preparation for operation, eggs should be removed from the incubator and placed on individual "nests." A suitable nest consists of a bit of cotton padding in a Syracuse dish, but a fragment of egg carton or other suitable holding device may be used.

The incubation age of the embryo, and its corresponding stage of development, is customarily designated according to the Hamburger–Hamilton (HH) stage seriation (Hamburger and Hamilton, 1951). For the most part, procedures described in this chapter are carried out on embryos from about 72 to 96 hr of incubation. During this time, embryos normally develop from HH stage 17 to HH stage 24. The HH series is illustrated in a number of publications. (Hamilton, 1952; Schoenwolf, 1995).

B. Tools and Solutions

Simple tools and chemical solutions suffice to carry out the operations described in this chapter. Clean instruments dipped or swabbed in 70% ethanol usually provide adequate protection against bacterial contamination. Glass pipettes used for transferring salt solutions and organ rudiments should be sterilized by autoclaving and be kept sterile prior to use. Glass or plastic containers used for storing tissues to be grafted should also be sterile.

Several kinds of isotonic salt solutions are used for bathing, embryos, organ rudiments, and tissues. Ringer's and Tyrode's solutions are simple, easily prepared, and in common use. These solutions should be prepared in advance, sterilized, and stored in small vessels for dispensing during operations.

Ringer's solution		Tyrode's solution	
NaCl	9.0 g	NaCl	9.0 g
$CaCl_2$	0.25 g	$CaCl_2$	0.24 g
KCl	0.42 g	KCl	0.42 g
H_2O	1000 ml	$NaHCO_3$	0.30 g
		Glucose	1.0 g
		H_2O	1000 ml

Chick embryos are remarkably resistant to bacterial and fungal infection if reasonable precautions are taken to avoid gross contamination. Nevertheless, it is wise to have solutions of antibacterial drugs in appropriate saline solutions available, two or three drops of which may be added to the embryo after operation. A useful solution is a penicillin–streptomycin mixture.

"Pen–strep"	
Penicillin	12 mg
Streptomycin	20 mg
Tyrode's solution	100 ml

C. Making a Window to Expose the Embryo

The embryo is exposed by making an opening in the shell, a procedure called "windowing," "fenestration," or, in laboratory jargon, "opening the egg." Eggs may be opened at the time of operation or some hours or a day earlier, as convenient for the operator. Eggs opened early are returned to the incubator to develop to the desired HH stage or, if embryonic development is to be slowed, they may be left at room temperature for some hours and then reincubated as needed.

1. Locating the Window

The window is preferably opened directly over the embryo, which normally lies uppermost on the yolk, directly under the shell (Fig. 1). Its position is determined by "candling." When white-shelled eggs are transilluminated from below (candled), the heart and blood vessels of the embryo can be seen through the shell and the position of the embryo can then be marked by a penciled rectangular outline. A rectangle 1.5×0.75 cm is usually of sufficient size. When eggs with pigmented shells are used, the position of the embryo must be approximated from knowing that it will occupy the uppermost part of the yolk. Usually it is well to plan for a somewhat larger window when eggs with opaque shells are operated on.

2. "Dropping" the Embryo

The upper surface of the egg in its nest is gently swabbed with cotton soaked in 70% ethanol before opening. Next, measures are taken such that creating the window will not damage the embryo or its vasculature (Fig. 1). Either of the following procedures is appropriate: (1) the air space between the two layers of the shell membrane at the blunt end of the egg is collapsed by penetrating the shell and outer shell membrane by means of any sharpened instrument such as the tip of a pointed scalpel blade, closed tines of a sharpened forceps, or the tip of a syringe needle; or (2) a sterile 18-gauge needle attached to a 5-ml disposable syringe is inserted into the lowermost portion of the egg through the acute end

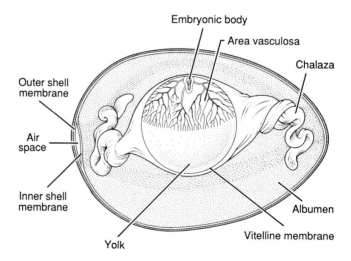

Fig. 1 Fertilized egg of the chick. The embryo lies at the upper part of the yolk. The blastoderm, with area vasculosa, is beginning to spread over the yolk beneath the vitelline membrane.

and 2 or 3 ml of liquid albumen is withdrawn. The second of these procedures is probably the better (a bit of albumen that oozes out the hole soon solidifies and plugs the opening made by the needle). The result of either of these procedures is that once the shell and shell membranes over the embryo are pierced, the embryo will drop away from the overlying shell and the subsequent opening of the window will not damage the embryo or its associated blood vessels.

3. Cutting the Window

The window is cut along the previously marked lines by means of a dental separating saw or by using a piece of hacksaw blade (Fig. 2). The separating saw consists of a diamond-rimmed aluminum disc rotated by means of the hand-piece of a dental machine or a small hand tool, such as the Dremel Moto Tool. A suitable saw blade may be made from half of a hacksaw blade, 24 teeth to the inch, that has been sharpened on a grinding wheel to remove the "set" from the teeth. The saw thus prepared is held in the hand and is used to cut through the shell by means of a gentle back and forth motion. Regardless how the cut

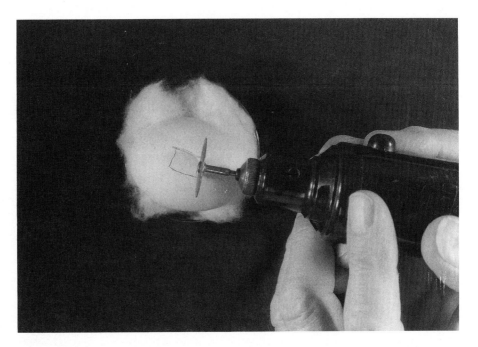

Fig. 2 Preparation for making a window in the hen's egg. The egg was candled, the position of the embryo was marked by means of a penciled rectangle, and the marked egg was placed in a nest of cotton batting. A cut through the shell along one side of the rectangle was made using a dental separating saw, which is shown poised over the egg in preparation for a second cut.

is made, it should pass through the shell without penetrating the double-layered shell membrane overlying the embryo. After the outline of the window is cut, the sawdust is rinsed away by gently squirting a few drops of Ringer's by means of a glass pipette. The shell is then lifted away, and the shell membranes over the embryo are then removed using fine forceps (Fig. 3). As this is being done, or before, the embryo will sink away from the edges of the opening. A drop of sterile Ringer's solution is then gently layered over the embryo. The embryo is then ready for operation or the egg may be sealed and returned to the incubator.

4. Sealing the Egg

The egg may be sealed in any of several ways. The saved piece of shell may be replaced over the hole and the rim sealed with melted paraffin. Many investigators find it most convenient to cover the opening with transparent cellulose tape. Alternatively, a rectangle of Parafilm may be laid over the window and its edges sealed with a wood-burning tool whose temperature is controlled by means of a variable voltage transformer. However done, the covering must be carefully sealed to prevent dehydration of the egg.

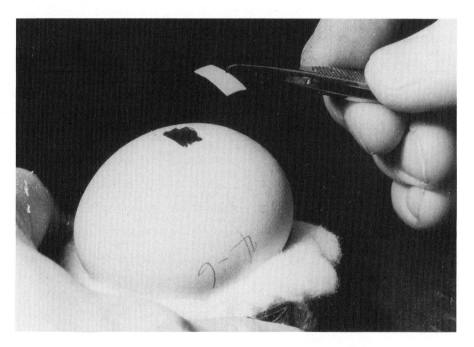

Fig. 3 Windowed egg. The cut-away portion of shell is poised over the open window. Shell membranes have been removed except for small portions near the edges of the window, thus providing a shelf to which the excised shell may be returned and sealed in place.

III. Extraembryonic Membranes

At early stages, the blastoderm (embryo plus vascular extraembryonic tissue) lies beneath and somewhat adherent to the vitelline membrane, which is the membrane that is continuous with the bounding membrane of the yolk (Fig. 1). Beneath the embryo proper is a somewhat fluid yolk, the subgerminal fluid. As development proceeds through the second day of incubation, the embryonic body rotates progressively, beginning at its anterior end, so that it comes to lie on its left side. Nonvascular folds of extraembryonic tissue, the amniotic folds, envelop the embryo, first from the head, then progressively along right and left sides, and from the tail. These folds meet in the midline, forming a recognizable suture, the seroamniotic raphe. Then meeting and fusion of the folds create a dual membranous covering of the embryo: an inner double membrane called the amnion and a double outer layer called the chorion. The space between the amnion and chorion is the extraembryonic coelom, which is continuous with the future body cavity, or coelom, of the embryo. Within the confines of the amnion, the embryo floats with the right side uppermost in a compartment of amniotic fluid.

By the third day of incubation, the amniotic folds have cut beneath the emerging embryonic body, progressing toward the ventral midline at the future umbilicus. Through the umbilicus, blood vessels enter and exit the body of the embryo from the area vasculosa, the portion of the blastoderm from where the first blood supplies of the embryo arise. During the fourth day of development, a vascular outpocketing of the embryonic hindgut emerges through the umbilicus into the space between the amnion and chorion. This outpocketing is the allantois, or allantoic vesicle. The allantois expands greatly, filing the extraembryonic coelom. Fusing with the chorion as it expands, it creates the highly vascular chorioallantoic membrane (CAM), which eventually fills the inner surface of the egg and serves as the respiratory and excretory organ of the embryo (Fig. 4).

A. Uncovering the Embryo

In order to operate on the 3- to 4-day embryo, the membranes that protect it must be removed. The vitelline membrane normally remains intact through the fourth day of operation and must be pierced in order to get at the embryo. The vitelline membrane, chorion, and amnion must then be opened over the embryo at least to the extent of exposing the prospective operative field.

The vitelline membrane is almost invisible as viewed by means of the dissecting microscope, but its presence can be detected by gently probing with a fine needle or forceps. Better still, it can be made visible by staining with a vital dye, such as Nile blue sulfate, applied by means of a ball-tipped glass needle, the end of which has been coated with agar and soaked in a solution of the dye (Fig. 5). The dye-tipped staining needle is moistened in Ringer's solution and is touched to the membrane, which takes up the dye where the needle is applied. The

John W. Saunders, Jr.

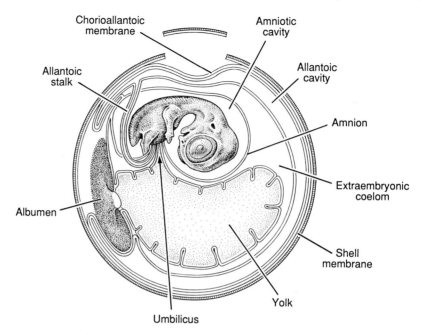

Fig. 4 A fertilized egg at about 9 days of incubation after prior fenestration. Relationships of the chorioallantoic membrane to shell and shell membranes, and to the embryo and extraembryonic membranes are shown. The chorioallantoic membrane is uppermost beneath the open window.

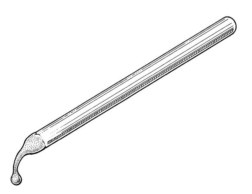

Fig. 5 Staining needle. A soft glass rod or tubing is flamed and drawn to create a handle with a ball-tipped end. The tip is dipped in hot 2% agar, previously solubilized by boiling. It is withdrawn, cooled briefly, and dipped two or three more times with intervals of cooling. The instrument is air dried overnight and then the tip is immersed in sterile 0.5% Nile blue sulfate in the bottom of a stoppered sterile test tube, where it may remain indefinitely. Before use, the staining needle should be air dried, preferably under a quartz UV-sterilizing lamp, for several hours. Alternatively, agar-tipped needles may be stained and stored in 0.5% Nile blue sulfate in 30% ethanol. Air dried and protected from dust, they can then be used without sterilization, usually with success.

vitelline membrane thus made visible can be torn open by means of a fine glass or tungsten needle; or, perhaps better still, it may be grasped and torn by means of finely ground and polished watchmaker's forceps.

In a similar manner the chorion and amnion are removed from over the operative field. In embryos of stages 18 to 24, these membranes can be easily separated at the seroamniotic raphe using a sharp needle for whatever craniocaudal length may be desired. Otherwise, the membranes may be torn away by means of watchmaker's forceps. Regardless how the opening is made, the chorion and amnion heal the opening with 24 hr restoring the appropriate extraembryonic compartments.

IV. Making Various Kinds of Grafts

Avian embryos provide host sites to test the developmental performances of organ rudiments under a variety of experimental conditions. The chick embryo is the host of choice for the most part, but techniques described here can be used for preparing hosts of other avian species such as quail, duck, pheasant, and goose, and for implanting tissues from various amniote species.

The following sections deal with techniques of isolation and grafting that have been used successfully for analyzing morphogenesis of the limb. These techniques involve grafts to the embryonic body, which are carried out at young stages, and to the vascular chorioallantoic membrane at advanced stages.

A. Chorioallantoic Grafts

Hosts to chorioallantoic grafts are typically chick embryos incubated for 9 to 10 days, by which time the chorioallantoic membrane is heavily vascularized, thus providing an excellent blood supply to a graft (Fig. 4). At the 9- to 10-day stage, the chorioallantois is closely applied to the shell membranes and may be damaged severely during opening of the egg. It is best, therefore, to window the egg between 72 and 96 hr of incubation, dropping the embryo so that, at the appropriate stage for receiving a graft, the chorioallantois will not adhere to the shell membranes.

1. Preparing the Site and Placing the Graft

Prior to making chorioallantoic grafts, samples of donor tissue should be collected and held in a covered dish of an appropriate sterile salt solution such as Ringer's. The cover is removed from the window to expose the CAM. A desirable graft site on the membrane is a rich capillary bed near a branch in a major vitelline artery. The tip of a sharpened tungsten or stainless-steel needle is then used to abrade the surface of the CAM over the capillary bed in such a manner as to cause slight bleeding. The tissue to be grafted is then transported in a small amount of Ringer's solution via a glass pipette and is carefully placed over the abraded area of the CAM by means of a fine probe. The window is then resealed and gently shifted to the incubator. After a few hours, or the next day, the window may be uncovered and the graft examined to determine if it has been vascularized.

2. Recovering the Graft

Grafts may be allowed to develop until about the 18th day of incubation. The cover of the window is then removed and the graft site is located. The graft may not be visible immediately, for it may have been encapsulated by the CAM and sunk below the surface. If necessary, the entire content of the egg may be emptied into a large dish of saline and the extraembryonic membranes carefully searched for the graft, which may need to be freed from encapsulating membranes.

The CAM is a very useful site for culturing a variety of avian organ primordia and for propagating mammalian tumors. (cf. Levi-Montalcini and Hamburger, 1953; Rawles, 1936; Saunders, 1948; Willier, 1933). CAM grafts have been employed to analyze potentialities for self-differentiation of limb bud rudiments, as described next.

3. Grafts of the Chick Wing Bud to the CAM

The technique for testing the ability of the tip of the embryonic limb bud to form its terminal parts away from the influence of the embryonic body is described here. Hosts for CAM grafts should be at the desired stage and have been previously windowed. Several donor embryos should be prepared to provide adequate material to assure that there will be successful grafts.

A donor embryo of about 80 hr of incubation is windowed (or the window is opened if an opening has been made earlier) and the membranes are gently torn away to expose the wing bud. This process may be facilitated using the staining needle, as described earlier. The wing bud is then severed at whatever level is desired and transferred by means of a fine glass pipette to a dish of sterile Ringer's solution. Before the operation, the bud may be stained lightly with Nile blue applied by means of a staining needle to enhance visibility. To sever the limb or its tip, a glass (Saunders, 1948) or tungsten (Dossel, 1958) needle with a fine L-shaped tip is used (Fig. 6). The sharp tip of the L is repeatedly hooked into the bud and drawn upward through the tissue in such a way as to disconnect completely the tip from the base of the bud. This procedure preserves the cross-sectional shape of the bud, thus providing a broad mesodermal surface for the entry of blood vessels at the graft site. Scissors (e.g., irididectomy scissors) should not be used, for their shearing action compresses the bud and causes the ectodermal surfaces of the graft to be apposed.

If several buds are to be grafted, they should be stored in Ringer's solution until ready for use (in fact, they may be stored overnight in the refrigerator at

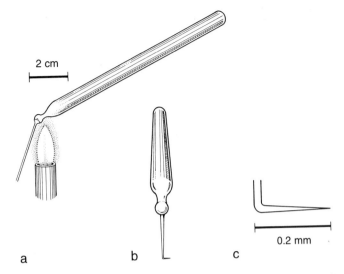

Fig. 6 Glass operating needle. A ball-tipped soft glass rod is heated over a small flame until the tip is cherry red. (a) A fine filament of colored glass is then fused to the ball. The end of the filament (b) is then drawn out and given an L-shaped tip (c) by manipulating it against an electrically heated nichrome wire on the stage of the dissecting microscope. Because glass needles are very fragile, many operators prefer to use needles made from tungsten wire. Wire may be fused to a glass handle or glued to a wooden dowel. The needles can be shaped by means of a flame (Dossel, 1958) or by electrolysis (Hubel, 1957).

4°C and remain perfectly viable). The bud to be grafted is transported from its storage site by means of glass pipette and is gently placed on the graft site. If possible, the bud is oriented so that its cut surface is apposed to the abraded surface of the CAM. Extra salt solution carried over with the graft is gently withdrawn by suction via micropipette. The window is then covered and the egg is placed in the incubator.

B. Flank Grafts

For a variety of reasons, one may wish to make grafts of the limb bud, or a part thereof, to the flank. A classical reason is to determine effects of an extra limb on the differentiation of sensory and motor nerves of the host (Hamburger and Levi-Montalcini, 1949; Lance-Jones and Dias, 1991). For flank grafts, hosts and donors should be prepared in advance by windowing, with incubation continued to the desired stage of development. Donor limb buds or parts thereof are removed as described previously and held in Ringer's solution for subsequent grafting. To make a graft, first prepare the host by removing the membranes over the flank area, and then transfer the donor limb by means of pipette to a position on the chorion next to its torn edge. Next make a longitudinal incision in the flank using a glass or tungsten needle having an L-shaped tip, as described earlier. The incision should be about 1 mm in length and should pass completely through the body wall and into the coelom. Care should be exercised not to penetrate the posterior cardinal vein whose course can be seen dimly through the body wall at the base of the somites. The incision will tend to remain closed, more so in older embryos. The graft is then manipulated toward the slit using a slender but slightly blunted steel or tungsten needle. Inserting the graft into the slit may seem almost impossible at the first attempt. If one is particularly dexterous, the slit may be held open by means of a needle grasped in one hand, while a needle held in the other hand is used to push the graft into the opening. For a one-handed operation, it is best to try to push one end of the cut surface of the graft into the slit, thus forcing it open, and then easing the rest of the graft in, leaving the top of the limb protruding to the exterior. Once the graft is in place, the window is sealed over and the egg is returned to the incubator. The window should be opened an hour or two later to determine if the graft has healed to the host. At this time a drop or two of pen–strep should be added to inhibit infection.

C. Intracoelomic Grafts

Various organ rudiments, including limb buds, have been grafted to the coelom of the chick embryo to test their developmental potentialities in relative isolation or to determine effects on the host embryo of diffusible agents emanating from the graft (Levi-Montalcini and Hamburger, 1953; Saunders, 1948). There are two simple ways to make coelomic grafts. The first of these is initiated according to the procedure outlined for flank grafts. After a slit is made in the flank, the graft of the limb bud, or of whatever tissue is to be tested, is merely pushed through the slit into the body cavity of the embryo.

A second method is equally simple, but is best carried out on embryos of stage 24, when the allantoic vesicle protrudes prominently into the extraembryonic coelom. For this procedure, the chorion is torn away from the region overlying the allantois. This opening provides access to the extraembryonic coelom, which is continuous with the embryonic coelom through the umbilicus. After the graft is transferred to the host, it is simply pushed through the umbilicus into the embryonic coelom (Dossel, 1954).

Following either of these procedures, the host is allowed to develop to a total of ~18 days of incubation and is then removed from the egg. The abdomen is opened by ventral incision and the viscera inspected for the presence of the graft. In the case of limb bud grafts, the tip of the limb often protrudes through the umbilicus of the host and is visible without dissection.

D. Grafts to the Somites

It is often easier to graft a limb bud to the dorsal surface of the host embryo at the flank level than it is to make a flank graft (MacCabe et al., 1973). Host embryos of stages 23–24 are the best for this purpose. The host is exposed at the flank level by removal of membranes, as before. The ectoderm is then removed from the right side over the region of four or five adjacent somites. Then the needle is used to tear away the dorsal surface of the somites, injuring the myotome, and thus creating a wound bed into which there is a small amount of bleeding from ruptured capillaries.

The donor limb bud is then transferred to the host and its mesodermal surface is apposed to the surface of the wound bed. Surface tension of the amniotic fluid usually suffices to hold the graft in place for the 30 min or so required for a degree of healing to occur. Once the operator is relatively certain that the graft is safely in place, the egg may be sealed and returned to the incubator.

Embryos at stages 23 and 24 often show a good deal of spontaneous movement, which might be expected to dislodge the graft. The fact is, however, that the embryo cools during the time of operation and its movements are greatly diminished. Also, the host embryo may be precooled at room temperature prior to operation, but too much cooling causes the embryo to sink deeply into the subgerminal space and to rotate in such a way as to make operation difficult.

E. Limb-to-Limb Grafts

Tissue grafts from one limb bud to another or manipulations involving the deletion or interchange of parts within a limb bud have been made in order to solve a number of problems involving morphogenesis of the skeletal, muscular, nervous, and integumentary systems (Amprino and Camosso, 1963; Saunders *at el.*, 1958; Stirling and Summerbell, 1988). How some of these manipulations are carried out is described next.

1. Reorienting the Apex of a Limb Bud

The apex of the wing or leg bud is severed, rotated about its proximodistal axis, and restored to the stump. This operation is most easily performed on the wing bud of an embryo of stage 22 or 23. The windowed egg is reopened at the desired stage and the membranes overlying the bud are removed. Before severing the limb tip, one or two small glass or tungsten "microtacks" (Fig. 7) previously prepared, sterilized, and held in sterile Ringer's solution are deposited by means of fine forceps on the chorion near its torn edge. The tip of the limb bud is then severed by repeated hooking through the tissue with the L-shaped tip of an operating needle. The loosened tip will then be free in the amniotic fluid and will tend to sink beneath the embryo. It may be rescued by gentle manipulation with a fine needle or, better still, by guiding it with the tip of a microtack held in the tines or fine forceps and pressed gently against the distal part of the isolate. The limb tip is positioned against the bleeding stump of the bud with its anteroposterior axis in the opposite of normal orientation, and the sharp end of the microtack is pushed through the tip and deeply into the base of the bud.

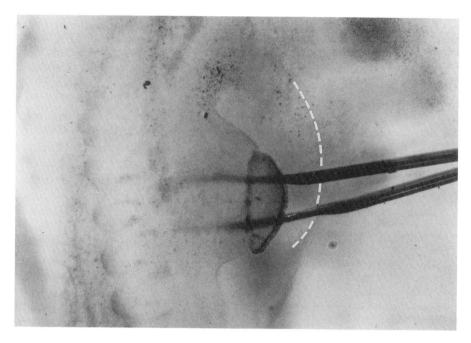

Fig. 7 Chick embryo of stage 22 showing microtacks securing a reoriented wing tip (operation APDV). The anterior is uppermost in the figure. The microtacks are inserted deeply into the stump of the operated bud and their blunt ends rest on the chorion, whose torn outline is indicated by a dashed line. Adapted from Saunders *et al.* (1958).

One or more additional tacks may be added to secure the rotated tip in place. Again, use caution not to push the tip of a tack into the postcardinal vein.

Glass microtacks used for this procedure should be long enough (2.5 to 3 mm) that the blunt end rests atop the chorion at the margin of its tear. After the operation, the window is covered and the egg is gently removed from the operating stage of the microscope and is held without further disturbance for about 30 min before being transported to the incubator. After 2 to 3 hr, the rotated tip will have healed sufficiently that the glass tacks can be removed. Tungsten microtacks are generally made much smaller and are left in place during postoperative development. For determining effects of the operation on the pattern of skeletal, muscular, and cutaneous parts of the limb and their innervation, incubation should be continued to a total of 10 days.

A reorientation operation of this type is classified as APDV, meaning that anterioposterior and dorsoventral axes of the graft and stump are apposed. A left limb tip may be grafted to the stump of a right limb bud either with its anteroposterior axis corresponding to that of the stump (operation AADV) or with its dorsoventral axis corresponding (operation APDV). Such an operation requires, of course, that a donor left limb tip be procured in advance of the operation and be transported by pipette to the host whose own limb tip is to be removed. Because embryos of limb bud stages lie on the left side, the donor embryo must be removed from the egg, washed free of yolk, and, with membranes removed, suffer the removal of the requisite limb tip.

2. Wing–Leg Exchanges

Using essentially the same techniques as just described, one may exchange tips of wing and leg buds between the same or different embryos, using hosts and donors of the same or different ages depending on the particular developmental questions asked.

3. Creating Intercalary Deficiencies or Excesses

One may ask whether the limb bud can regulate after the deletion or addition of intercalary limb parts (Kieny and Pautou, 1976, 1977). To create an intercalary deficiency, an intermediate proximodistal segment of the limb bud is excised using a hooked operating needle. First a distal cut is made behind the apex of the bud, reserving the tip. Second, another cut is made nearer the base of the stump. The isolated tip is then manipulated against the abbreviated stump and is tacked as described earlier for the reorientation operation.

In a somewhat more difficult procedure, an intercalary segment, removed as just described, may be transported to a host embryo and inserted between a freshly severed tip and its stump. Tacks are used to manipulate and fasten the limb parts as before.

V. Manipulations Involving the Apical Ectodermal Ridge

The limb buds first appear as swellings of the somatopleure, whose ectodermal component soon thickens apically forming a ridge called the apical ectodermal ridge (AER). The AER of the wing bud is asymmetrical in the sense that its thickness is greater posteriorly than anteriorly, whereas that of the leg bud tends to be more symmetrical, particularly at early stages. Numerous experiments carried out since 1948 have been undertaken to determine the significance of the AER.

A. Excision of the AER

The AER may be removed by means of a tungsten or glass needle having an L-shaped tip. Before undertaking the operation it is advantageous to stain the AER using an agar-tipped Nile blue staining needle. Staining is most useful for the neophyte and is often used by the experienced operator. The structure of the AER also shows up relatively well if a bit of reflective aluminum foil is placed beneath the bud. A bolus of diluted India ink injected beneath the blastoderm also serves to make the AER more visible, but the ink may compromise long-term development.

India ink for injection
1 ml Pelikan "Fount" India ink 9 ml sterile Ringer's solution

The AER has a nipple-like cross-sectional configuration whose base makes a well-defined border with the dorsal and ventral ectoderm (Fig. 8). To remove

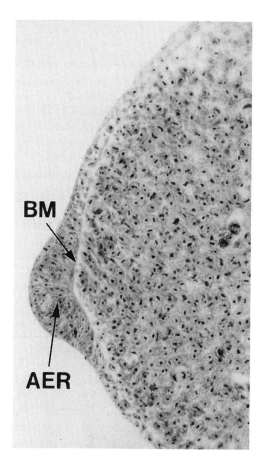

Fig. 8 Cross section through the tip of a chick wing bud of stage 21. The apical ectodermal ridge (AER) consists of a pseudostratified columnar epithelium and a covering layer of flattened periderm cells. A well-defined basement membrane (BM) separates the ectoderm from the mesoderm. Adapted from Saunders (1948).

the ridge, the operator preferably starts at its anterior end, hooking the tip of the operating needle beneath the ridge at its junction with the ventral ectoderm and pulling dorsally and posteriorly. This process is repeated along the perimeter of the bud until the entire ridge is removed piecemeal. The tip of the bud should be inspected carefully to check that all scraps of the ridge have been removed.

Control operations include removing equivalent quantities of ectoderm from the dorsal side of the limb bud and deliberate wounding of the mesoderm subjacent to the intact AER.

Similar experiments may be carried out in which only a part of the AER is removed (Saunders, 1948). After all operations, eggs should be sealed promptly, returned to the incubator, and incubation continued to day 10.

VI. Grafts to Test Polarizing Activity

When the wing bud first appears, a zone in which the coordinated expressions of a number of genes create what has been called the zone of polarizing activity (ZPA) (MacCabe *et al.*, 1973; Saunders and Gasseling, 1968, 1983; Tabin, 1995; Tickle, 1980; Tickle and Eichele, 1994) is present in the mesenchyme at its posterior edge near the body wall (Fig. 9a). When a small block of cells from this zone is placed under the loosened AER of the right wing bud preaxially, tissues adjacent and distal to the implant proliferate and form a supernumerary set of wing parts mirror twinned with respect to the normal limb tip (i.e., parts of left-hand asymmetry). A similar implant placed subjacent to the AER at the

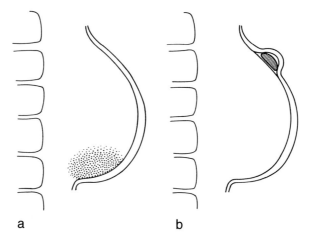

a   b

Fig. 9 Graft to detect polarizing activity. Outlines of the wing bud as seen in dorsal view at stage 21: (a) the stippled area is the approximate location of the ZPA, which is the site of interaction of several gene products that convey the polarizing property; and (b) a graft to be tested for polarizing activity is inserted beneath the loosened AER of the wing bud preaxially.

distal end of the bud causes the formation of a supernumerary right wing tip from preaxial tissue proximal to the graft. Since the discovery of the ZPA, many efforts have been made to elucidate the mechanism of its effects and to identify other sources of similar activity (Yang and Niswander, 1995; Tabin, 1995).

A. Grafting the ZPA

To demonstrate the ZPA, host and donor embryos of stage 20 should be prepared. From the donor, excise a small block of mesoderm (about 0.50 to 0.75 μm on a side), with or without its covering dorsal and/or ventral ectoderm, from the posterior side of the host and transfer it by means of a small-bore glass pipette to the surface of the chorion next to an exposed host wing bud. Using the L-tipped needle, gently loosen the AER along the anterior edge of the host wing bud by severing its connections to dorsal and ventral ectoderm for a distance of about 100 mm, but without breaking its connections to the intact ridge proximally or distally. The donor tissue may then be guided to the operative site using a fine needle, gently inserting it between the loosened ridge and the underlying mesoderm (Fig. 9b). Contraction of the loosened AER usually holds the graft in place in short order. The operated embryo is then sealed and returned to the incubator to be opened again at the ninth or tenth incubation day.

Notably, to test for "polarizing" activity, it is essential that little or no mesoderm intervene between the implant and the AER. Sometimes, however, it is necessary to excavate a bit of mesoderm from beneath the AER to provide a site in which an implant can remain. This method is less desirable, however.

B. Other Tests of Polarizing Activity

Using the just-described method, tests for polarizing activity in the embryonic chick limb bud have been carried out with tissues from other avian species, from mammalian sources, including human material, and from reptilian material. Nonlimb tissues can be tested in a similar manner.

It is also possible to implant ion-exchange beads carrying test chemicals beneath the AER as described here. Notably, it has been shown that such beads, heparin-treated and soaked in all-*trans*-retinoic acid, have the ability to elicit a sequence of events leading to the formation of mirror-twinned wing tips. For such tests, beads 200 to 250 μm in diameter should be chosen for appropriate pretreatment, followed by grafting beneath the loosened AER (Tickle *et al.*, 1982; Eichele *et al.*, 1984).

VII. Enzymatic Dissociation and Recombination of Limb Tissues

One may separate the ectodermal and mesodermal components of the limb and test them in various combinations. For example, one may wish to examine the effects of reversing the axial relationships of ectoderm and mesoderm in the wing or leg bud, or to test the behavior of leg bud ectoderm in combination with wing bud mesoderm. To carry out such programs, one must first separate the components of the limb by means of enzymatic digestion.

A. Ectoderm–Mesoderm Recombination

1. Combining Wing Bud Ectoderm and Leg Bud Mesoderm

For this experiment, wing and leg buds must be harvested from the same or different donors and treated separately. The limb buds may be cut from embryos that have been removed from the egg and dissected in Ringer's solution or they may be removed from embryos *in ovo* in the event that the donors are to be held for further study. After harvesting, both buds are rinsed by flushing via pipette through two or three changes of Ca^{2+}- and Mg^{2+}-free Tyrode's solution (CMF) and are then treated separately, as described in what follows.

After flushing in CMF, ectodermal donor buds are removed to a cold solution of 2% trypsin (Difco 250) in CMF and are held at 4°C in the refrigerator for approximately 3 hr. During this period the basement membrane at the ectodermal–mesodermal interface is broken down and the ectoderm becomes loosened from the mesoderm. [Alternatively, a solution of 2% trypsin plus 1% pancreatin (4 × USP) may be prepared in CMF and incubated at 37°C for approximately 30 min. Enzyme solutions should be sterilized by filtration prior to use and stored refrigerated or frozen in sterile containers.]

Prior to completion of the trypsinization procedure, mesodermal donors are transferred to a sterile solution of 1% EDTA in CMF and incubated at 37°C for 20 to 25 min, by which time the ectoderm can usually be removed without damaging the mesoderm. The ectoderm itself is damaged by this procedure and is discarded. It can sometimes be removed intact, but usually comes off piecemeal. The mesoderm, which remains quite firm during EDTA treatment, is then rinsed briefly in Tyrode's solution and is then transferred to a sterile solution of horse serum–Tyrode's (one part sterile horse serum and one part Tyrode's) and held on a cold stage at 2–4°C (or over ice).

The ectoderm donor is then transferred to the same cold dish and its ectodermal jacket is manipulated free and intact from the mesoderm using fine needles, forceps, or a fine scalpel—whatever works best for the operator. The ectodermal isolate is then slid over the host mesoderm with the aid of steel or tungsten needles.

After the operation the combined specimen should be allowed to warm gradually to room temperature. During warming, the ectodermal covering shrinks tightly about the mesoderm, and the preparation takes on the appearance of a freshly isolated limb bud. The recombinant may now be pipetted into a dish of fresh Tyrode's or Ringer's solution and held at room temperature for 3 to 4 hr as necessary or convenient. It is then grafted to the flank or, preferably, to the somite region of a newly prepared host embryo.

2. Other Possibilities

The fact that ectodermal and mesodermal components of the limb buds can be safely separated and recombined offers many possibilities for other experiments. For example, the ectodermal jacket can be placed on a host mesoderm after being turned inside out (Errick and Saunders, 1974); the ectoderm can be combined with limb bud mesoderm with its axial relationships reversed (MacCabe et al., 1974); ectoderm from nonlimb sources can be interposed between the limb ectoderm and mesoderm (Errick and Saunders, 1976; Murphy et al., 1983); and trypsinized mesodermal limb bud cores can be dissociated into single-cell suspensions, pelleted centrifugally, placed in ectodermal jackets, and grafted (MacCabe et al., 1973).

References

Amprino, R., and Camosso, M. E. (1963). Effects of exchanging the AP-reoriented apex between wing and hind-limb bud. *Acta Embryol. Morphol. Exp.* **6**, 241–259.

Dossel, W. E. (1954). A new method of intracoelomic grafting. *Science* **120**, 262–263.

Dossel, W. E. (1958). Preparation of tungsten micro-needles for use in embryologic research. *Lab. Invest.* **7**, 171–173.

Eichele, G., Tickle, C., and Alberts, B. M. (1984). Microcontrolled release of biologically active compounds in chick embryos: Beads of 200 μm diameter for the local release of retinoids. *Anal. Biochem.* **142**, 542–555.

Errick, J., and Saunders, J. W. (1974). Effects of an "inside-out" limb bud ectoderm of development of the avian limb. *Dev. Biol.* **41**, 338–351.

Errick, J. E., and Saunders, J. W. (1976). Limb outgrowth in the chick embryo induced by dissociated and reaggregated cells of the apical ectodermal ridge. *Dev. Biol.* **50**, 26–34.

Hamburger, V., and Hamilton, H. L. (1951). A series of normal stages in the development of the chick embryo. *J. Morphol.* **88**, 49–92.

Hamburger, V., and Levi-Montalcini, R. (1949). Proliferation differentiation and degeneration in the spinal ganglia of the chick embryo under normal and experimental conditions. *J. Exp. Zool.* **111**, 457–502.

Hamilton, H. H. (1952). "Lillie's Development of the Chick," 1st ed. Henry Holt, New York.

Hubel, D. H. (1957). Tungsten microelectrode for recording from single units. *Science* **125**, 549–550.

Kieny, M., and Pautou, M.-P. (1976). Régulation des excédents dans le développement du bourgeon de membre de l'embryon d'oiseau. Analyse expérimental de combinaisons xénoplastiques caille/poulet. *Wilhelm Roux's Arch Dev. Biol.* **179**, 327–338.

Kieny, M., and Pautou, M.-P. (1977). Proximo-distal pattern regulation in deficient avian limb buds. *Wilhelm Roux's Arch. Dev. Biol.* **183**, 177–191.

Lance-Jones, C., and Dias, M. (1991). The influence of presumptive limb connective tissue on motoneuron axon guidance. *Dev. Biol.* **143**, 93–110.

Levi-Montalcini, R., and Hamburger, V. (1953). A diffusible agent of mouse sarcoma, producing hyperplasia of sympathetic ganglia and hyperneurotization of viscera in the chick embroy. *J. Exp. Zool.* **123**, 233–288.

MacCabe, J. A., Saunders, J. W., and Pickett, M. (1973). The control of the anteroposterior and dorsoventral axes in embryonic chick limbs constructed of dissociated and reaggregated limb-bud mesoderm. *Dev. Biol.* **31**, 323–335.

MacCabe, J. A., Errick, J., and Saunders, J. W. (1974) Ectodermal control of the dorso-ventral axis of the leg bud of the chick embryo. *Dev. Biol.* **39**, 69–82.

Murphy, M. J., Gasseling, M.T., and Saunders, J. W. (1983). Formation of a functional apical ectodermal ridge from nonridge ectoderm in limb buds of chick and quail embryos. *J. Exp. Zool.* **226**, 391–398.

Rawles, M. E. (1936). A study in the localization of organ-forming areas in the chick blastoderm of the head-process stage. *J. Exp. Zool.* **72**, 271–315.

Saunders, J. W. (1948). The proximodistal sequence of origin of the parts of the chick wing and the role of the ectoderm. *J. Exp. Zool.* **108**, 363–403.

Saunders, J. W., and Gasseling, M. T. (1968). Ectodermal-mesodermal interactions in the origin of limb symmetry. *In* "Epithelial-Mesenchymal Interactions" (R. E. Fleischmajer and R. Billingham, eds.). pp. 78–97. Williams & Wilkins, Baltimore.

Saunders, J. W., and Gasseling, M. T. (1983). New insights into the problem of pattern regulation in the limb bud of the chick embryo. *In* "Limb Development and Regeneration: Part A" (J.F. Fallon and A. I. Caplan, eds.), pp. 67–76. Alan R. Liss, New York.

Saunders, J. W., Gasseling, M. T., and Gfeller, M. D., Sr. (1958). Interactions of ectoderm and mesoderm in the origin of axial relationships in the wing of the fowl. *J. Exp. Zool.* **137**, 39–74.

Schoenwolf, G. C. (1995). "Laboratory Studies of Vertebrate and Invertebrate Embryo," 7th ed. Prentice-Hall, Englewood Cliffs, NJ.

Stirling, R. V., and Summerbell, D. (1988). Specific guidance of motor axons to duplicated muscles in the developing amniote limb. *Development (Cambridge, UK)* **103**, 97–110.

Tabin, C. (1995). The initiation of the limb bud: Growth factors, *Hox* genes, and retinoids. *Cell (Cambridge, Mass.)* **80**, 671–674.

Tickle, C. (1980). The polarizing region and limb development. *In* "Development in Mammals" (M. H. Johnson, ed.), pp. 101–137. North-Holland Publ., Amsterdam.

Tickle, C., and Eichele, G. (1994). Vertebrate limb development. *Annu. Rev. Cell. Biol.* **10**, 121–152.

Tickle, C., Alperts, B. M., Wolpert, L., and Lee, J. (1982). Local application of retinoic acid to the limb bond *(sic)* mimics the action of the polarizing region. *Nature (London)* **296**, 564–565.

Willier, B. H. (1933). Potencies of the gonad-forming area in the chick as tested in chorio-allantoic grafts. *Wilhelm Roux' Arch. Entwicklungsmech. Org.* **130**, 616–649.

Yang, Y., and Niswander, L. (1995). Interaction between the signaling molecules WNT7a and SHH during vertebrate limb development: Dorsal signals regulate anteroposterior patterning. *Cell (Cambridge, Mass.)* **80**, 1–20.

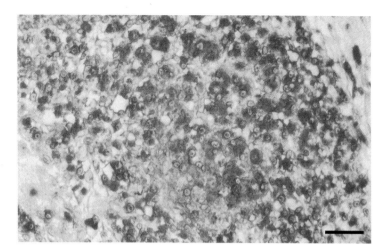

Chapter 2, Fig. 4 Chimeric dorsal muscle obtained by replacing a somite in a 2-day chick embryo with a quail somite. Double staining with monoclonal antibodies 13F4 (detected in blue) specific for the muscle lineage (Rong *et al.*, 1992) and QCPN (detected in brown) specific for quail cells. Quail nuclei are brown and the cytoplasm of muscle cells is blue. Scale bar: 40 μm. Courtesy of M. Coltey.

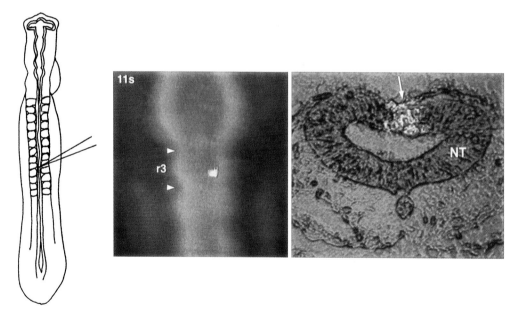

Chapter 3, Fig. 3 DiI injections. (A) Whole neural tube injections of DiI are made by backfilling the micropipette with DiI diluted in isotonic sucrose. The DiI solution is then injected into the lumen of the neural tube, thereby labeling all neural tube cells, including premigratory neural crest cells. (B) Focal injections of DiI are made by injecting a small amount of DiI stock solution into the dorsal neural tube. The embryo received a focal iontophoretic injection of DiI into the dorsal portion of rhombomere 3 (r3) at the 11 somite stage. The arrowheads mark the borders of the rhombomere. (C) A section through the embryo pictured in (B) demonstrates that the DiI labeling was confined to the dorsal portion of the neural tube (NT), with a few ectodermal cells (arrow) also labeled. Modified from Birgbauer *et al.* (1995).

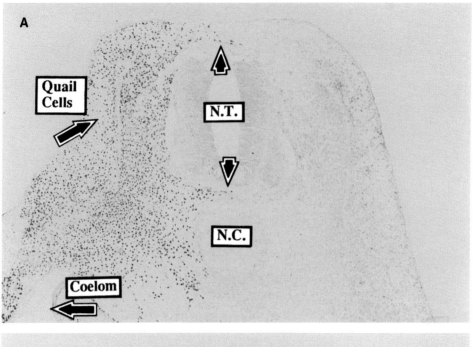

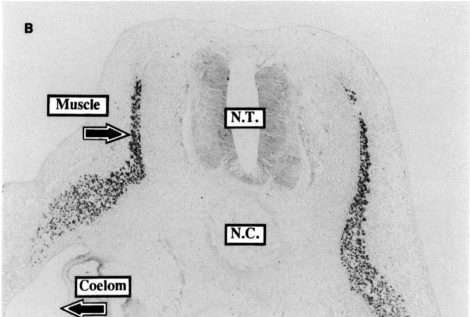

Chapter 4, Fig. 4   A 5-day-old chimeric embryo after a segmental plate graft. (A) Cross section at the thoracic level of a chimeric embryo stained with the anti-quail antibody. The neural tube (N.T.), notochord (N.C.), coelom (arrow), and paraxial mesoderm are visible. Note that in contrast to the Feulgen technique, the antibody technique allows visualization of individual cells at low magnification. (B) Adjacent cross section of the chimeric embryo shown in A, stained with the antimuscle myosin antibody MF20. Skeletal muscle cells (arrow) are stained dark blue and are formed from the grafted quail cells on the operated side of the embryo.

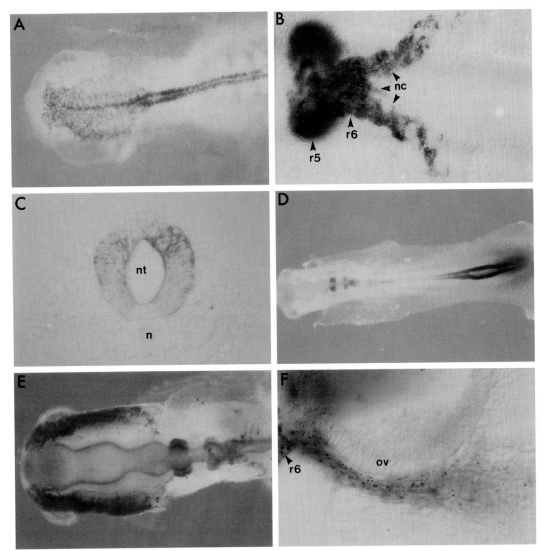

Chapter 11, Fig. 1   (A) Whole mount *in situ* hybridization of a stage 10 chick embryo with probe for *Slug* transcripts. *Slug* expression is detected in the premigratory neural crest at the dorsal midline. In the migratory neural crest, this stage is restricted to the head. From Nieto *et al.* (1994). (B) Flat mount preparation to visualize *Krox-20*-expressing neural crest. Whole mount *in situ* hybridization was carried out to detect *Krox-20* transcripts in a stage 14 chick embryo. The hindbrain was dissected, slit through the ventral midline, and flat mounted. Expression is detected in r3 (not shown), r5, the premigratory neural crest in r6 and caudal r5, and in neural crest cells migrating caudal to the otic vesicle. From Nieto *et al.* (1995). (C) *Krox-20* expression detected in a transverse section of r5. Whole mount *in situ* hybridization was carried out to detect *Krox-20* transcripts. The embryo was fixed, embedded in wax, and sectioned in the transverse plane. From Nieto *et al.* (1995). (D) Double whole mount *in situ* hybridization to detect *Krox-20* transcripts in the hindbrain (NBT/BCIP): blue product) and *Hoxb-9* transcripts in the caudal spinal cord (Vector Laboratories substrate kit II: brown product). (E) Combined whole mount *in situ* hybridization to detect *Krox-20* transcripts (NBT/BCIP: blue product) and immunocytochemistry with HNK-1 antibody and HRP-conjugated secondary antibody to detect neural crest cells (DAB: brown product). (F) Combined DiI labeling and whole mount *in situ* hybridization. DiI was injected into r6, the embryo was incubated until stage 17, and the DiI fluorescence was photoconverted to generate oxidized diaminobenzidine (punctate brown stain). Whole mount *in situ* hybridization was then carried out to detect *Krox-20* transcripts. The r6-derived neural crest expresses *Krox-20*. From Nieto *et al.* (1995). r, rhombomere; nc, neural crest; nt, neural tube; n, notochord; ov, otic vesicle.

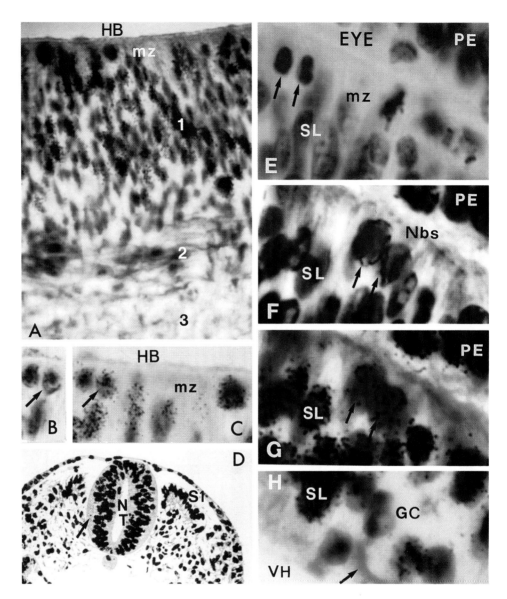

Chapter 16, Fig. 1 Early neurogenesis in the chick brain stem and retina. (A–C) Autoradiographs of two transverse sections of a 3.5-day (HH 21) chick hindbrain (HB) following treatment with [^{3}H]thymidine for 5 hr and stained with the Holmes silver method. More than 50% of the neural epithelial cells of the ventricular zone (1) are labeled whereas neuroblasts and axons of the intermediate (2) and marginal (3) zones are not. (B and C) A pair of apolar daughter cells in the mitotic zone (mz) adjacent to the lumen are both neurofibril positive and labeled (arrows), suggesting a recent cell division. (D) Autoradiograph of a 2-day (HH 12) chick treated with [^{3}H]thymidine for 12 hr between the 9 and the 16 somite stages (ss); nearly all nuclei in the neural tube (NT), somite 1 (S1), and other tissues are heavily blackened (labeled). An unlabeled unipolar neuroblast (arrow) similar to that in Fig. 2C was not labeled. (E–H) Sections of a 3.5-day (HH 21) chick eye show early ganglion cell precursor differentiation. (E) A Feulgen DNA stain shows a daughter cell pair (arrows) in the mitotic zone (mz) of the sensory layer (SL) adjacent to the pigment epithelium (PE). (F and G) Light micrograph and corresponding autoradiograph of the mitotic zone following a 10-hr treatment with [^{3}H]thymidine includes a labeled apolar daughter pair of neuroblasts (arrows) with neurofibril loops. (H) The vitreous humor (VH) side of the same section with several postmitotic ganglion cells (GC) and their axons (arrow). *Note:* A–C and E–H are from double-embedded embryos; D was plastic embedded and prestained with toluidine blue.

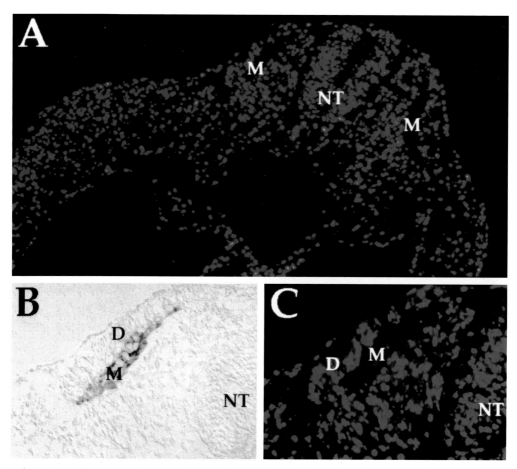

Chapter 16, Fig. 6 The early chick myotome is composed of postmitotic cells. (A–C) Sections through the trunk region of a stage 18 HH chick embryo labeled for 2 hr with BrdU. Cryostat sections were reacted sequentially with the BrdU antibody (A and C) and with the MF20 monoclonal antibody (Hybridoma Study Bank), which recognizes the embryonic form of the myosin heavy chain. While most tissues of the embryo are actively replicative, the myotome (M), recognized by its MF20 labeling, is postmitotic. NT, neural tube; D, dermomyotome.

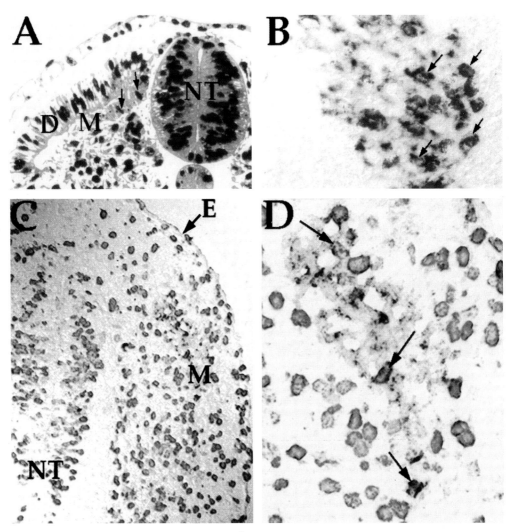

Chapter 16, Fig. 7 (A) Increasing the time of [³H]thymidine exposure of chick embryos to 5 hr leads to the appearance of labeled myogenic cells in the myotome (arrows), indicating that mitotically active myogenic precursors present in the dermomyotome (D) migrate to the myotome in around 5 hr. (B) FREK-expressing cells present in the skeletal muscle masses are replicating. A 6-day-old embryo was exposed for 2 hr to BrdU. Sections at the forelimb level were sequentially hybridized to a FREK nonisotopic RNA probe (in blue) and were reacted with an anti-BrdU monoclonal antibody (in red). In a transverse section through a shoulder muscle, arrows show that FREK expression colocalizes with BrdU-positive nuclei, indicating that FREK-positive cells have undergone DNA synthesis while being exposed to BrdU. (C and D) MyoD-expressing cells are replicating *in vivo*. A stage 23 chick embryo was labeled with BrdU for 2 hr. Transverse sections were then reacted sequentially with a chick MyoD probe (in blue) and an anti-BrdU antibody (in brown). While a majority of MyoD-expressing cells are BrdU negative, we observed colocalization of MyoD and BrdU in a few myotomal cells (arrows). NT, neural tube; M, myotome; E, ectoderm.

CHAPTER 8

Iontophoretic Dye Labeling of Embryonic Cells

Scott E. Fraser

Division of Biology
Beckman Institute
California Institute of Technology
Pasadena, California 91125

I. Introduction
II. Iontophoretic Microinjection of Lineage Tracers
    A. Apparatus for Iontophoretic Dextran Injection
    B. Tools and Tricks
    C. Intracellular Injection Protocol
III. Iontophoretic Application of DiI
    A. Apparatus for DiI Iontophoresis
    B. Iontophoretic Application Protocol
IV. Relative Advantages of Dextran and DiI
    References

I. Introduction

Developmental biology strives to understand the establishment of biological form. In almost every example, embryonic development involves groups of cells that once appeared indistinguishable from one another undergoing morphogenetic movements and phenotypic differentiation, thereby becoming different. Thus, this generation of diversity is in many ways the central task of developmental biology, whether studied at the tissue, cell, or molecular level. Progress at any of these levels requires reliable knowledge of the fate map of the embryo and of the cell lineage of single precursor cells. These are closely related experimental questions. Fate maps are depictions of what cells in various regions of an embryo will become during normal development. Cell lineages identify the range of

Copyright © 1996 by Academic Press, Inc. All rights of reproduction in any form reserved.

phenotypes that arise from single cells. As an example of the importance of this class of data, consider the development of diverse cell types within a single tissue from an apparently homogenous group of precursors. One extreme possibility is that there is an inherent diversity underlying the apparent homogeneity of the cells; the population of precursors is a heterogeneous mixture of unipotent cells, each fated to become a predetermined cell type. Another extreme possibility is that there is a homogeneous set of precursors, able to give rise to many of the different cell types (multipotent or pluripotent) or to all of the cell types (totipotent) in the tissue. In these two scenarios, the environment of the cells would be proposed to play much different roles: in the case of unipotent precursors, it might play no role or it might play a role only in selecting which cell types survive or differentiate; in the case of multipotent or totipotent precursors, it must play a more instructive role. Thus, an important first step in understanding the cell interactions and molecular mechanisms that guide cell phenotype selection must be to test the potency of the precursor cells.

The experimental requirements for cell lineage and fate map studies are very similar. Both require a means of labeling a cell (or distinct group of cells) in a defined region of the embryo, of identifying the progeny of the labeled cell(s) over time, and of scoring the final phenotypes and positions of the progeny. Of course, the ideal label should be indelible so that all descendants of the labeled cell(s) are identified; similarly, it should be unable to pass to neighboring cells. Failure of either of these qualities would result in false negative cases, where true descendants are missed, or false positive cases, where not all of the labeled cells are true descendants. At present, there is no truly ideal approach, but two powerful cell marking techniques have been developed that permit a cell and its progeny to be followed as they move and differentiate: (1) marking the cells with an injectable lineage tracer or (2) marking the cells by infection with a recombinant retrovirus. Intracellular microinjection of the individual cells with fluorescent dextran (Bronner-Fraser and Fraser, 1988; Wetts and Fraser, 1988) or with horseradish peroxidase (HRP) (Holt *et al.,* 1988) can be used to trace lineages because both compounds are large and membrane impermeant. Such tracers are passed from the injected cell solely to its progeny at cell division; thus, all labeled cells must be derived from the injected precursor. In the second approach, precursors are infected with a recombinant retrovirus containing the *lac Z* gene but lacking sequences needed for the infected cell to shed the virus. Therefore, only the descendants of the infected cell will carry the integrated *lac Z* gene (reviews: Cepko 1988; Sanes, 1989). The two techniques have complementary advantages (for a more detailed treatment see Fraser, 1992). The site and timing of the marking are both under experimental control in the tracer injection experiments, but the finite amount of injected compound can be diluted by continued mitotic activity. The retrovirus approach avoids the potential pitfall of dilution, but the identification of any given cell as a member of a clone might rely primarily on statistical arguments.

This chapter presents some of the techniques used for labeling single cells or small groups of cells with fluorescent dyes. Fluorescent dextran labeling of cells offers a direct means to label single cells or small groups of cells, making it appropriate for either fate mapping or cell lineage studies. Lipid-soluble carbocyanine dyes (e.g., DiI and DiA; Honig and Hume, 1984) offer a simpler means to label groups of cells for fate mapping studies; the drawback of the lipid dyes is that it is difficult or impossible to be certain that only a single cell and its progeny were labeled. Although neither of the approaches meets all of the criteria of an ideal cell tracer, each can generate useful and valid data if the potential shortcomings are kept in mind.

II. Iontophoretic Microinjection of Lineage Tracers

A straightforward means to trace cell lineage is to microinject a precursor cell with a macromolecule that is trapped within the cytoplasm; the progenies of the injected cell are recognized by the presence of the tracer within their cytoplasm of the marker which they inherit at mitosis. Such an approach, using the enzyme HRP, was developed for tracing early lineages in the leech embryo (Weisblat *et al.,* 1978) and was first applied in vertebrate embryos to determine the descendants from the blastomeres of early cleavage stage embryos (Hirose and Jacobson, 1979). Because HRP is an enzyme not found in normal animal tissues, sensitive histochemical stains permit the descendants of the injected cell to be identified after considerable development of the embryo. To permit injected cells to be visualized without the need to fix and process the tissue, fluorescent macromolecules, such as fluorescent peptides and fluorescent dextrans (Gimlich and Braun, 1986), were developed for use in cell lineage studies. The dextrans have the added advantage that they are not degraded by the labeled cells, permitting lineages to be assayed after long developmental times. Simple refinements in the injection techniques have permitted the intracellular microinjection of fluorescent dextran (Wetts and Fraser, 1988; Bronner-Fraser and Fraser, 1988) or HRP (Holt *et al.,* 1988) to be applied to the much smaller precursor cells of the vertebrate nervous system. In most settings, the sensitivity of the detection of HRP is outweighed by the ability of fluorescent dextran to be observed in living cells. Because of this advantage and because equivalent results have been obtained with both tracers (Holt *et al.,* 1988; Wetts and Fraser, 1988), only microinjection of fluorescent dextrans will be discussed here.

The microinjection approach can satisfy only some of the criteria for an ideal lineage tracer. Because the microinjection technique is under the control of the experimenter, the position and timing of the labeled cell can be dictated. Of course some cells can be extremely challenging to microinject because of their size or their position. If fluorescent dextran is used, an epifluorescence microscope can be used to validate the presence of only a single labeled cell at the desired location. The dye is not taken up from neighboring cells even when the labeled cell is intentionally killed; instead, it is passed from the injected cell solely to its progeny at cell division. Thus, all labeled cells must be derived from the injected precursor. Fluorescent dextran is not degraded by the labeled cells, making the labeling long lived; however, it is not indelible. Only a fixed amount of the tracer is injected into the precursor, and subsequent growth and division must lead to the dilution of the dye. This dilution can be sufficient to render the dye invisible after several mitoses, although clones as large as 100 to 1000 can be recovered routinely (Bronner-Fraser and Fraser, 1988; Stern *et al.,* 1988). Because the dextran can be fixed in place for histological processing, the fluorescently labeled descendants can be double labeled by a number of immunocytochemical and *in situ* hybridization techniques.

A. Apparatus for Iontophoretic Dextran Injection

The equipment needed for intracellular dye injection is a straightforward application of the technique long used to record intracellularly from cells with sharp micropipettes. The goal is to introduce the tip of the micropipette through the cell membrane, to iontophoretically inject the dye into the cell, and to withdraw the pipette, leaving a labeled, living cell behind in the embryo. The components of the system needed and their role in achieving this goal are outlined below:

1. Pipette

A pipette is a pulled piece of thin-walled glass tubing that must be sharp enough to enter the cell membrane without severely damaging the cell, yet have a large enough lumen to permit dye to quickly flow into the cell. Of course any pipette is a compromise between these two goals, as discussed in the later section on pipette design.

2. Pipette Holder

The holder plays both a mechanical and an electrical role. It mounts the pipette to the micromanipulator and serves as a "half-cell" that connects the liquid inside of the pipette to the input of the current-passing amplifier. The typical holder has a small reservoir that holds a concentrated salt solution and a silver–silver chloride electrode that connects to the amplifier input.

3. Micromanipulator

The manipulator is responsible for moving the pipette into position and holding it stable during the dye microinjection. Among different users, preferences for types of manipulators can approach a religious fervor. Experience shows them all to be correct. Any manipulator that is convenient for the user and that drifts in position less than 1 μm in a few minutes will suffice.

4. Intracellular Amplifier

A current-passing amplifier built for intracellular electrophysiology is needed to record the membrane potential of the impaled cell and to pass current through the pipette tip. The amplifier measures the potential between the inside of the pipette (the inside of the cell when the pipette tip is in a cell) and an indifferent or reference electrode (a silver–silver chloride wire) placed into the egg white through a small hole in the shell. As discussed later, the membrane potential is a useful method for monitoring the successful impalement of the cell and the health of the injected cell, as well as a diagnostic for the pipette slipping into a second cell. A current-passing capability of 10 nA should suffice for most applications.

5. Oscilloscope

An oscilloscope is used for monitoring the potential recorded by the amplifier. A simple oscilloscope will suffice, as the signals are not overly fast (<1 kHz) or small (>10 mV). The most convenient models to use are digital storage oscilloscopes with the ability to perform a "roll" display. Using such an oscilloscope, new data are added to the right side of the screen, pushing old data off of the left side so that the most recent 20–30 sec of data can be observed at a glance.

6. Specimen Holder

A specimen holder is a mount for eggs (or culture dishes) that stabilizes the specimen on the stage of the microscope. It should cover the condenser lens to protect it from the inevitable spills of saline or egg albumen. In the simplest case, the specimen holder can be a large microscope slide held with the conventional slide-holding device of the microscope stage. The egg is stabilized with a ring of modeling clay or a 1-cm segment of foam pipe insulation.

7. Microscope

A fluorescence microscope permits the pipette to be positioned most accurately and allows the quality of an injection to be measured as soon as the injection is completed. The epi-illumination light source should be shuttered and neutral density filters employed to minimize the light exposure to the preparation. This minimizes the bleaching of the dye, hence maximizing the dye signal in the cell and avoiding cell death from the by-products of the dyes being bleached. While some cell types are very resistant to such damage, others can be killed in a few seconds of illumination. Electronic shutters (Uniblitz; Vincent and associates) between the light sources and microscope are best as they permit the light paths to be controlled without directly touching, and hence wiggling, the microscope. To document the dye injection with a minimum of light exposure, a light-intensifying video camera (a SIT or an intensified CCD) can be used to capture images with about 10-fold less light exposure than required for film.

B. Tools and Tricks

1. Pipette Design

The pipette must accomplish two opposed goals: It should have a very small tip, with an outer diameter so small that it can be inserted through the membrane of the targeted cell with little or no damage, and it should have a very large inner diameter so that dye can move quickly into the cell cytoplasm from the pipette lumen, allowing the pipette to be removed from the cell before movement of the embryo or the pipette causes damage to the cell. Finding the appropriate compromise between these two can be a major challenge of the approach and may be different for each cell type, and even each stage of development. The availability of thin-walled aluminosilicate glass tubing has made this task somewhat easier. The glass is somewhat harder than conventional borosilicate glass, requiring a higher heat setting on the pipette puller. When pulled properly, the glass yields micropipettes with a very sharp tip and a large inner diameter. An added benefit is that most cell types seem to seal to the pipette tip more quickly, minimizing the deleterious effects of the impalement. The only drawback to the aluminosilicate glass is that it can be more brittle than conventional glass, requiring some care in tip design. Figure 1 presents the double-pull pipette tips that have been proven the most reliable. The goal is to create a rapidly tapering tip that is sufficiently long to reach conveniently into tissue, yet tapers rapidly enough to have sufficient physical strength and low electrical resistance. The first pull of

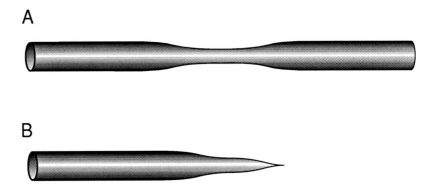

Fig. 1 Pipette tip design. (A) Using the programming feature of the pipette puller to apply a cooling jet of air creates an hourglass shape in the capillary. (B) A second step, in which less cooling and a much greater pull strength is employed, creates a rapid taper tip on the micropipette.

the double-pull design shown in Fig. 1 creates a small-diameter shaft immediately behind the pipette tip, making it easier not only for the pipette to pass through tissue but also to view the preparation as the optical path is less severely distorted by the smaller diameter of the pipette immediately behind the tip. For most preparations, double-pull micropipettes with a resistance of 35–80 MΩ have proved to be the most serviceable.

2. Pipette Filling Solutions

For cell labeling, small fluorescent dextran dyes perform very well. The 3- and 10-kDa dyes are too large to pass from cell to cell through gap junctions, yet they are small enough to rapidly pass from the pipette into the impaled cell. Larger dyes are considerably slower to eject from the pipette tip. The dextran dyes are available commercially (Molecular Probes has the largest variety) or can be synthesized using conventional techniques for labeling antibodies or other proteins.

The dextrans are well tolerated by most cells, although some cell types seem more sensitive; some batches of the dye are toxic for such sensitive cell types. Different lots of the same dye, made by the same recipe or purchased under the same catalog number, can vary wildly in their toxicity. The toxicity of any of the dyes can be minimized by "cleaning" them before use with Micro-Centricon ultrafiltration tubes (Amicon). Make a 100-mg/ml solution of the dye and place it into the Micro-Centricon tubes. The tubes, when spun in a micro-centrifuge, let solutes smaller than their size cutoff (3 kDa) pass through the membrane to the lower chamber. Repeated resuspending of the retained dye in distilled water followed by spinning effectively removes the small by-products that are toxic. After the final spin, resuspend the dye in distilled water to a final volume identical to the starting dye solution. After cleaning, aliquot the dye into 100-μl volumes in sealed tubes and freeze at $-20°C$. Rinsing all lots of dye is recommended as rinsed dyes can be injected to much higher concentrations in the cells.

In contrast to the injection solutions most typically used for pressure injecting substances into cells, which can contain salts and buffers, the best iontophoretic injections are obtained from mixing the dyes in distilled water alone. This is because iontophoresis uses the flow of current to move the dye out of the pipette and into the cell. If the solution contains a significant concentration of salt or buffer, these small, more mobile ions will serve as the major charge carriers, proportionately reducing the expulsion of the dye. With some micropipettes, particularly those with higher tip resistances, the electrical performance of the pipette may be unstable if there are no small salts in the solution. In those cases, add the minimum amount of salt that will stabilize the electrical performance of the micropipettes.

3. Pipette Filling

The dye solutions or other reagents to be iontophoretically injected can be rare or expensive; therefore, a filling technique that minimizes the volume of filling solution is required. A small amount of the dye solution, about 0.25 to 0.5 μl, is drawn into a filling pipette and is deposited inside the aluminosilicate pipette at the taper, as close to the tip as possible. Allow a minute for capillary action to carry the dye into the tip and for any air bubbles to be displaced. The micropipettes with the dye in the tip can be stored in a humidified storage jar for a day. Immediately before the pipette is to be mounted on the manipulator, a second filling pipette is used to back fill the shank of the pipette with electrolyte solution. Dilution of the dye and bubbles will be minimized if the tip of the filling pipette is brought close to, but not into, the dye solution (0.5 mm from the meniscus of the dye). A gentle expulsion of the electrolyte from the filling pipette will "layer" the electrolyte solution on top of the dye solution; 1.2 M LiCl is typically employed as the electrolyte because it is less likely to crystallize in the tip of the filling micropipettes between uses.

For handling and depositing small volumes, a clear filling pipette is best because it permits the solution to be observed and deposited accurately. A homemade filling pipette made from 1-cc disposable plastic tuberculin syringes can be used. Remove the plunger from the syringe body and set it aside. Heat the tip of the syringe body immediately next to the flame (not over) of a microburner until the plastic becomes transparent (not flaming); the tip is then pulled slowly away from the syringe body under visual control. The faster the pull, the smaller diameter the tip. Since the molten plastic provides little resistance, it cannot be pulled by "feel" in the manner typically used for glass tubing. After allowing the plastic to solidify (become translucent), a razor blade is used to cut the tip to length (typically 5 cm). Replace the plunger and press; if air cannot move out of the tip with medium to gentle force on the plunger, the tip is too small in diameter.

4. Iontophoretic Injection

The success of the injections will be maximized by remembering two facts of electrical currents. First, electrical currents only flow in loops. As a result, any break in the pathway from the amplifier, to the electrode holder, through the pipette and preparation, into the indifferent (ground) electrode, and back to the amplifier will be sufficient to prevent the iontophoretic injection. The two most common examples of this problem are air bubbles in the injection pipette or failure to position the indifferent electrode properly. Second, electrical current will take the path of least resistance. Saline or backfilling solution smeared on the outer surface of the injection pipette, on the pipette holder, or near the plug where the pipette holder joins with the amplifier can provide a pathway of much lower resistance than that through the very small opening at the pipette tip. This can short circuit the current flow into the cell, resulting in failed dye injections even though current appears to be flowing.

C. Intracellular Injection Protocol

1. Pull and fill an injection pipette as outlined earlier and mount it into the pipette holder. Make certain that there are no air bubbles in the injection pipette

or in the electrode holder. The electrolyte solution must cover the back opening of the injection pipette to provide a pathway for the current from the amplifier to the injection pipette.

2. Mount the specimen on the stage of the microscope. Insert the indifferent (ground) electrode into the preparation. For *in ovo* injections, the indifferent electrode can be inserted through a needle hole in the end of the chicken egg. Align the specimen so that the targeted region is in the field of view.

3. Turn on the fluorescence epi-illumination and coarsely position the injection pipette so that it is above the preparation, in the beam of exciting light. Under visual control, lower the pipette to the preparation. Contact with the saline can be determined by the motion of the meniscus and by the oscilloscope trace. A stable electrical recording is impossible before the electrical continuity provided by the pipette entering the preparation. Adjust the oscilloscope trace position with the voltage offset controls to position it in the upper half of the oscilloscope screen.

4. Position the pipette with the micromanipulator to directly above the cell to be injected and turn off the epi-illumination source. Lower the electrode slowly, watching the preparation in bright-field and/or the oscilloscope screen. Contact of the pipette tip with the surfacae of the cell typically causes a slight deflection of the oscilloscope trace and an increase in the width (noise) of the trace.

5. "Ring" the pipette tip with the negative capacitance control on the injection amplifier as briefly as possible. This causes a brief electrical oscillation in the amplifier and is thought to facilitate impaling the cell by slightly wiggling the pipette tip and/or destabilizing the membrane structure. Once inside the cell, these currents can kill the cell so make the ring a brief as possible. Some amplifiers have a special control to provide an instantaneous ring. Those using amplifiers without such a circuit develop very quick wrist action on the negative capacitance knob. Some workers prefer to "tap" into a cell. This requires finding a spot on the vibration table, microscope, or manipulator where a small tap causes a small wiggle of the pipette. For injecting chicken eggs this is hard to control, as even small taps can slosh the contents of the opened egg.

6. In an ideal cell penetration (Fig. 2) the potential recorded through the pipette drops precipitously after the "ring" to a new stable value reflecting the cell membrane potential. A sharp transition shows that the cell membranes have quickly sealed to the pipette tip. The value recorded varies with the cell type, stage of the embryo, temperature of the egg, and pipette design, but is typically between 10 and 100 mV. The recorded value is not an accurate measure of the cell membrane potential because the dextran solutions are not ideal electrolytes. However, the cell membrane potential reported can be used to monitor the health of the cell, as well as warn of the pipette moving to another cell. Figure 3 presents the variety of real-world traces that might be obtained on the oscilloscope.

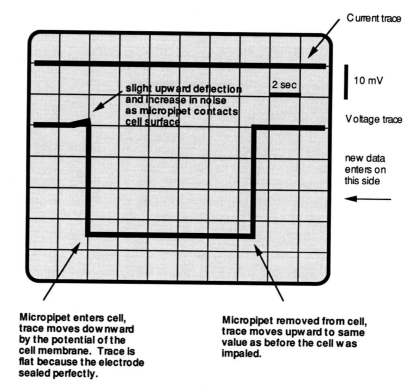

Current trace

10 mV

Voltage trace

new data
enters on
this side

slight upward deflection
and increase in noise
as micropipet contacts
cell surface

2 sec

**Micropipet enters cell,
trace moves downward
by the potential of the
cell membrane. Trace is
flat because the electrode
sealed perfectly.**

**Micropipet removed from cell,
trace moves upward to same
value as before the cell was
impaled.**

Fig. 2 Ideal oscilloscope trace. The sketch shows the appearance of the oscilloscope screen if a digital storage oscilloscope with a roll display is employed. Data continuously enter on the right, pushing previous data toward the left. In an actual injection experiment, pulses of current would interrupt the current and voltage traces; these have been omitted here for clarity.

7. The dye is iontophoresed into the cell with pulses of current, typically positive currents of 2–10 nA at frequencies of 0.5–2 Hz. The periods during the current flow eject the dye, and the periods between pulses can be used to monitor the cell membrane potential. Although some amplifiers are equipped with bridge circuits to permit the potential to be recorded during the pulses, the dextran-filled micropipettes do not perform well in this mode because the dextran is not a well-behaved electrolyte. As a result, the resistance of the pipette tip varies with the flow of current, making it difficult, if not impossible, to properly set the bridge. If better performance is required, some smaller ions must be added to the solution, but this will decrease the iontophoretic injection of the dextran.

The shape of the voltage trace can be used as a method to monitor the electrode tip. If the voltage trace does not return to a somewhat stable value within the first 0.1 sec after a current pulse, the pipette is probably plugging; if it returns immediately, the tip may have broken off.

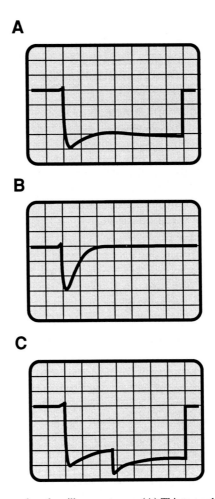

Fig. 3 More realistic examples of oscilloscope traces. (A) This trace shows a nearly ideal injection sequence. The micropipette sealed in rapidly, resulting in only a slight loss of the membrane potential of the cell, followed by a later downward slope of the trace. (B) A stable membrane potential is never recorded in cases where the cell dies or the pipette falls out of the cell before sealing in place. (C) A failed lineage injection is indicated by the sudden change in the potential recorded by the micropipette. When the micropipette drifts between cells in this fashion, at least two labeled cells can be expected.

Some robust cells can be injected quickly with current from continuously "ringing" the pipette with negative capacitance. This should be used with care on small embryonic cells as it kills most of them. Some cell types are too fragile to inject with pulses of current. These are best injected by slowly ramping up the current to 2–4 nA, although it is difficult to measure membrane potential during such injections.

8. The duration of dye iontophoresis varies with a number of factors, including the size of the dextran (smaller = faster), the size of the injection current (larger = faster), and the size of the cells (smaller = faster). For most embryonic cells, 20–30 sec at 4 nA should suffice. Turn off the current and wait for the electrode potential to stabilize.

9. Remove the pipette quickly by turning the knobs of the micromanipulator a predetermined amount. A distance of two to three cell diameters or more, directly along the axis of the pipette, works best. This snaps the pipette free from the cell membrane, allowing it to reseal quickly. Moving the pipette away more carefully and slowly increases the chance of tearing the cell open or of plucking the cell from the tissue by it remaining adhered to the pipette tip. Note the size of the potential change recorded by the pipette on exiting the cell; ideally, it should be close to the transition recorded on entering the cell (see Fig. 2 and 3).

10. Turn on the fluorescence epi-illumination light source and focus on the labeled cell(s) quickly. Score the presence of a single cell and its position. Those embryos with more than one cell cannot be used for cell lineage studies but can be used for fate mapping or cell migration studies.

III. Iontophoretic Application of DiI

Despite the many advantages of iontophoretic injection of fluorescent dextrans, there are several factors that limit its use, ranging from the difficulty of impaling fragile embryonic cells to the considerable expense of the equipment required. Iontophoretic application of the fluorescent lipids DiI and DiO offers a much simpler and less expensive alternative for those experiments in which single-cell lineage data are not required. Iontophoretic application is a refinement of the DiI microinjection techniques covered in other chapters. Although in some settings it has been used to label single cells reliably (Myers and Bastiani, 1993), in the avian embryo, iontophoretic application of DiI is most reliable in labeling from 2 to 30 cells. DiI labels cells brightly and appears to be less phototoxic than fluorescent dextran, making it well suited for time-lapse studies and *in vivo* microscopy. A red-shifted carbocyanine dye, DiI(5) (excited with red light; emits in the infrared) performs very well in this regard. The spectra of DiI(5) are ideally suited to the red excitation line of an Ar–Kr laser on a confocal microscope, and background fluorescence is low at these wavelengths. The dye bleaches very slowly; even prolonged viewing does not seem to cause cell death. The arrival of DiI-CM, a fixable derivative of DiI, solves one of the long-standing limitations of DiI for use with immunocytochemistry or *in situ* hybridization studies.

A. Apparatus for DiI Iontophoresis

The apparatus for DiI iontophoresis can be as complicated as that used for the dextran injections, but excellent results can be obtained with very simple equipment. The injection pipette is not placed intracellularly so there is no need for an oscilloscope or recording amplifier. A simple current source of a 9-V alkaline battery in series with a 100-MΩ resistor suffices; a push button switch or a foot switch can be used to turn the current on and off. Because the dye is being applied to the surface of the cell(s), the pipette can even be held by hand rather than by a micromanipulator.

B. Iontophoretic Application Protocol

1. Pull injection micropipettes in the same fashion as for dextram injections. The ideal tip should be slightly less fine than used for dextran injections (10 MΩ if filled with the dextran solution). Do no break off the tip as typically done for pressure injections.

2. Backfill the tip and about 5 mm of the electrode shank with a 0.5% solution (w/v) of DiI (1,1'-dioctadecyl-3,3,3',3'-tetramethylindocarbocyanine, perchlorate; Molecular Probes, in absolute ethanol). Mount the pipette into a pipette holder with a silver wire that runs down the pipette shank and touches the DiI solution. Unlike for dextran injections, the silver wire does not need to be chloridized.

3. The indifferent (ground) electrode should be inserted into the egg as for dextran injections. The rules of current apply here as well, so apply the same cautions about alternate current paths.

4. Lower the pipette tip into the preparation and close the switch, allowing current to flow for 2–30 sec. Examine the preparation under epi-illumination. Some workers find it convenient to monitor the labeling process continuously with the epifluorescence microscope. In such cases it is important to monitor the preparation for possible phototoxic effects, such as cell blebbing or beading.

5. If no labeled cells result, check for a plugged tip by examining the injection pipette with an epifluorescence microscope. A plugged tip usually has a small crystal of dye fluorescing a different color and brightness. Although it may seem backwards, plugging of the micropipettes is reduced by making the pipette tip sharper and smaller. A larger tip permits the alcohol to leak out of the tip and water to leak in, precipitating the dye.

IV. Relative Advantages of Dextran and DiI

The two dye-labeling approaches share some of the same limitations. For example, both can be diluted to the point that they are no longer detectable by prolonged mitotic activity. The advantages of the dextran technique are that it can reliably label single cells and that the dextran dyes do not transfer from cell to cell. Injecting large amounts of dextran into the extracellular space or intentionally killing a brightly labeled cell does not result in labeled neighbors. The advantages of DiI or related carbocyanine dyes are the ease with which they can be applied and the reduced phototoxicity they exhibit. Perhaps the most reliable way to exploit both sets of advantages is to employ both approaches and compare the results.

References

Bronner-Fraser, M., and Fraser, S. (1988). Cell lineage analysis shows multipotentiality of some avian neural crest cells. *Nature* **335,** 161–164.

Bronner-Fraser, M., and Fraser, S. (1989). Developmental potential of avian trunk neural crest cells *in situ. Neuron* **3,** 755–766.

Cepko, C. (1988). Retrovirus vectors and their applications in neurobiology. *Neuron* **1,** 345–353.

Fraser, S. E. (1992). *In vivo* analysis of cell lineage in vertebrate neurogenesis. *Semin. Neurosci.* **4,** 337–345.

Gimlich, R. L., and Braun, J. (1986). Improved fluorescent compounds for tracing cell lineage. *Dev. Biol.* **109,** 509–514.

Hirose, G., and Jacobson, M. (1979). Clonal organization of the central nervous system of the frog. I. Clones stemming from individual blastomeres of the 16-cell and earlier stages. *Dev. Biol.* **71,** 191–202.

Holt, C. E., Bertsch, T. W., Ellis, H. M., and Harris, W. A. (1988). Cellular determination in the *Xenopus* retina is independent of lineage and birth date. *Neuron* **1,** 15–26.

Honig, M., and Hume, R. I. (1984). Fluorescent carbocyanine dyes allow living neurons of identical origin to be studied in long-term cultures. *J. Cell Biol.* **103,** 171–187.

Myers, P. Z., and Bastiani, M. J. (1993). Growth cone dynamics during the migration of an identified commissural growth cone. *J. Neurosci.* **13,** 127–143.

Sanes, J. R. (1989). Analysing cell lineage with a recombinant retrovirus. *Trends Neurosci.* **12,** 21–28.

Stern, C. D., Fraser, S. E., Keynes, R. J., and Primmett, D. R. (1988). A cell lineage analysis of segmentation in the chick embryo. *Development* **104** (Suppl.) 231–44.

Weisblat, D. A., Harper, G., and Stent, G. S. (1978). Cell lineage analysis by intracellular injection of a tracer enzyme. *Science* **202,** 1295–1298.

Wetts, R., and Fraser, S. E. (1988). Multipotent precursor cells can give rise to all major cell types of the frog retina. *Science* **239,** 1142–1145.

CHAPTER 9

Gene Transfer Using Replication-Defective Retroviral and Adenoviral Vectors

Steven M. Leber,* Masahito Yamagata,† and Joshua R. Sanes‡

* Division of Pediatric Neurology
University of Michigan Medical Center
Ann Arbor, Michigan 48109

† Division of Molecular Neurobiology
National Institute for Basic Biology
Okazaki, Aichi, Japan

‡ Department of Anatomy and Neurobiology
Washington University School of Medicine
St. Louis, Missouri 63110

I. Introduction
II. Retroviral Vectors
    A. Life Cycle of the Retrovirus
    B. Generation of Replication-Defective Retroviral Vectors
    C. Preparation and Storage of Viral Stocks
    D. Titering a Viral Stock
    E. Testing for Replication-Competent Virus
    F. Safety Issues
III. Adenoviral Vectors
    A. Life Cycle of the Adenovirus
    B. Generation of Recombinant Adenoviral Vectors
    C. Preparation and Storage of Viral Stocks
    D. Titering a Viral Stock
    E. Patterns of Expression
    F. Safety Issues
IV. Injection of Virus into Chick Embryos
V. Histology and Histochemistry
    A. Fixation
    B. Histochemical Stain for lacZ

       C. Other Genes and Methods of Detection
       D. Sectioning Tissue
       E. Microscopy and Photography
  VI. Uses of Viral Vectors
       A. Comparison of Gene Transfer Methods
       B. Lineage
       C. Tracing Cell Migration
       D. Inserting Bioactive Genes
    References

I. Introduction

Viruses are obligate intracellular parasites that live by invading a host cell and then using that cell's machinery to replicate their genetic material. As understanding of viral genomes and life-styles increased, it was natural to envision harnessing their skills for the transfer of exogenous genes to vertebrate cells *in vivo,* both for experimental purposes and for gene therapy. Numerous viral vectors have been studied in these contexts, including retrovirus, adenovirus, herpes virus, sindbis virus, vaccinia virus, and adeno-associated virus (Mulligan, 1992; Roth, 1994). For each, enormous effort has been devoted to designing recombinant vectors, attenuating their pathogenicity, and generating high-titer viral stocks. To date, three types of recombinant viral vectors have been used to transfer genes to chick embryos: replication-competent retrovirus, replication-defective retrovirus, and replication-defective adenovirus. The first of these is described in Chapter 10 and the other two are described in this chapter. The chapter begins by describing how the vectors are constructed and how viral stocks are generated (Sections II and III). Methods of introducing the virus into embryos and detecting the gene product, which are nearly identical for the two vectors, are presented thereafter (Sections IV and V). Finally, the advantages and disadvantages of the various methods available for gene transfer are summarized and some recommendations are made about which are best suited for particular experimental purposes (Section VI).

II. Retroviral Vectors

A. Life Cycle of the Retrovirus

Retroviruses consist of an RNA genome encased in a protein core, which in turn is coated by a proteolipid envelope (Fig. 1). The RNA encodes three classes of proteins called pol (for polymerase), gag (for group-associated antigens), and env (for envelope). The pol proteins are tightly associated with the RNA, gag proteins form the core, and env proteins are embedded in the lipid membrane. Numerous retroviral types exist, each with its own peculiar features. However,

PRODUCTION OF RECOMBINANT RETROVIRUS

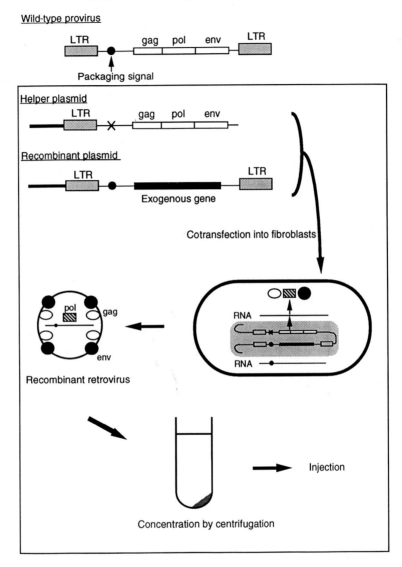

Fig. 1 Replication-incompetent retroviral vectors (see text for details).

the three types that have been used for gene transfer in birds, murine leukemia virus (Galileo *et al.,* 1990), Rous sarcoma virus (Gray *et al.,* 1988), and spleen necrosis virus (Mikawa *et al.,* 1991), all share the features described next.

To initiate an infection, the viral env proteins bind to specific proteins in the host cell membrane. The virion is then internalized by receptor-mediated endocytosis, and its envelope is removed by cellular enzymes. A viral pol protein called reverse transcriptase is then activated and it copies the RNA into DNA. The newly generated DNA moves into the nucleus, where it integrates into a chromosome of the host cell, via the action of an integrase (one of the pol proteins) on long repeated sequences [long terminal repeats (LTRs)] at each end of the viral DNA. Integration occurs when the host cell is in the S phase of its cell cycle. Thereafter, the viral genome, now called a provirus, behaves much like a cellular gene: it is replicated with the chromosome and is transcribed to form RNA from which viral proteins can be translated. Viral pol and gag proteins bind back to specific sequences in the viral RNA (the packaging signals) and assemble new viral cores. The env proteins enter the host cell membrane. Finally, the viral core buds through the host membrane in env-enriched areas, releasing new, infectious particles (Varmus and Brown, 1989; Whitcomb and Hughes, 1992).

B. Generation of Replication-Defective Retroviral Vectors

To generate replication-defective retroviral vectors, it is necessary to remove genes essential for replication and to introduce other genes in their place. The insertion of a reporter gene allows identification of cells carrying the viral genome. Although both steps can be done together, vectors are now available in which viral genes (generally all three) have been removed and replaced by a multiple cloning site. This vector is easily prepared as a plasmid, and straightforward recombinant techniques can be used to introduce sequences that encode a new protein or its antisense copy.

Production of infectious virions from genomes that are missing essential viral genes requires the use of specially constructed packaging cell lines (Fig. 1). These cells are fibroblasts that have been transfected with expression vectors that encode the structural proteins but lack sequences necessary for assembly of the viral RNA into new viral cores (Miller, 1990). The packaging cells thus accumulate the viral structural proteins but cannot make new viruses. To produce replication-defective virions, the helper cells are transfected with a plasmid in which LTRs flank the packaging signals and the exogenous gene. This plasmid directs expression of RNA that can be packaged by the viral structural proteins to form infectious virions.

Virus-producing cell lines can be constructed in any of three ways. Most often, a characterized helper cell line is transfected with plasmids encoding the defective retrovirus and a selectable marker such as neo[R]. These can be on the same or separate plasmids. Stable transfectants are isolated by antibiotic selection and are then subcloned to derive clonal lines. Several lines are tested for viral titer (see below), and the best few are expanded, passaged, or frozen for storage (see, for example, Sanes *et al.*, 1986). As an alternative, fibroblasts can be cotransfected with helper and viral plasmids, and a stable producer line is selected in a single step (see, for example, Gray *et al.*, 1988). Finally, helper cells can be transiently transfected with viral plasmid, and virus is collected from the medium 3–4 days following transfection (see, for example, Galileo *et al.*, 1992). This method avoids the long waiting periods required for selection and subcloning, and thereby permits rapid production of virus. It works best with cell lines that can be transfected with high efficiency, such as QT6 (see below).

The range of host cells susceptible to infection is controlled largely by the env proteins and thus by the *env* gene that the packaging cell harbors. For murine leukemia viruses, some packaging lines produce env proteins that bind to receptors on cells of many species; these generate what are known as "amphotropic" viruses. Other packaging lines generate a different env protein that binds only to rodent cells; it produces a "ecotropic" virus. Of course, amphotropic packaging lines must be used to produce murine viruses that infect chickens. Rous sarcoma and spleen necrosis viruses can both infect avian cells; the terms amphotropic and ecotropic are not applied to them.

C. Preparation and Storage of Viral Stocks

Virus-producing fibroblasts can simply be maintained in serum-containing medium. They can be passaged indefinitely, frozen for long-term storage, and thawed when new virus is needed. They secrete virions into the medium; for infection of cultured cells, the medium can generally be used without further treatment as a source of virus. For most applications *in ovo,* however, the concentration of virus is necessary to bring the titer into an acceptable range. This chapter details protocols for preparing fairly large batches of LZ10 (Gray *et al.*, 1988) and LZ12 (Galileo *et al.*, 1990) viruses. Both vectors have *Escherichia coli* β-galactosidase (*lacZ*) as their exogenous gene and both have been used for lineage tracing in chick embryos (Section VI). LZ10 is derived from a Rous sarcoma virus and is grown in QT6 quail fibroblasts. LZ12 is derived from a Moloney murine leukemia virus and is grown in PA317 mouse fibroblasts, which are themselves derived from 3T3 fibroblasts. Media requirements are slightly different for these two cell types, but the general methods for preparing virus from them are similar.

Virus-producing cells are repeatedly split until forty 10-cm culture plates are confluent. The desired degree of confluency is dependent on cell type: QT6-derived LZ10 producers should be completely confluent for 24–48 hr prior to collection, whereas PA317-derived LZ12 producers should be 90% confluent the day prior to concentration. The medium of the confluent cultures is replaced with 5.5 ml of fresh medium 1 day prior to concentration. On the day of concentration, six 37.5-ml pollyallomer ultracentrifuge tubes are sterilized with 70% ethanol and allowed to dry. The culture medium is then collected in sterile 15- or 50-ml tubes and spun in a tabletop centrifuge at 400–500 g for 10 min to remove debris. The supernatant from these tubes is collected, leaving the bottom 1 ml to avoid transferring cells, and is pipetted into the ultracentrifuge tubes. If necessary, additional medium can be added to fill and balance the tubes. Approximately 2 ml of the viral media can be saved at 4°C to use later for estimating the efficacy of the concentration. The ultracentrifuge tubes are then spun at 40,000 g at 4°C for 1.5 hr (for LZ12) or 2–3 hr (for LZ10). Following centrifugation, most of the supernatant is removed from the tubes; the tubes are tipped to a nearly horizontal position to aspirate all but the last few hundred microliters. The viral concentrate often forms a brown precipitate, but sometimes no precipitate is visible. The virus is removed from the centrifuge tubes by vigorously washing the bottom of the tube approximately 100 times with a sterile 1-ml pipette tip on an ethanol-sterilized 1-ml automatic pipettor set at 200 μl. It is especially important to avoid bubbling during the resuspension. The concentrates from the six tubes are pooled into a sterile 1.5-ml tube. The ultracentrifuge tubes are then washed with 300 μl of supernatant, pipetting approximately 50 times per tube and transferring the same 300 μl from tube to tube. The wash is added to the concentrate, which is then spun for 1–2 min in a microcentrifuge to remove debris that may subsequently clog the injection electrode. Finally, 20- to 40-μl aliquots of the concentrate are placed into 0.5-ml capped microcentrifuge tubes for freezing. One aliquot is saved for titering and the others are transferred immediately to liquid nitrogen or to a −150°C freezer. All of these steps should be done quickly as the virus breaks down at room temperature. Once frozen, the virus lasts for many months; however, the titer drops precipitously if the stock is thawed and refrozen.

If even more concentrated virus is needed, a double concentration can be performed. Instead of leaving only 300 μl per tube at the end of the ultracentrifugation, ~700 μl is left and pooled together into a single, previously sterilized 4-ml polyallomer ultracentrifuge tube, which is then spun at 40,000 g for 2.5 hr. Subsequent resuspension is done as before, except that smaller aliquots are frozen.

Methods for preparing spleen necrosis virus are similar to those outlined above (for details, see Dougherty and Ternin, 1986; Mikawa *et al.*, 1991, 1992).

D. Titering a Viral Stock

Genuine viral titers (numbers of infectious particles per milliliter) are laborious to determine and require the use of special cell lines that lyse when infected (Muenchau *et al.*, 1990). For recombinant retroviral vectors that contain an active *lacZ* gene, however, a simple histochemical method can be used to estimate viral titer. Fibroblasts are plated in a six-well plate on the day prior to titering: 10^5 QT6 or 2×10^4 NIH 3T3 cells/well for LZ12. (Both QT6 and NIH 3T3 cells can be obtained from ATCC. Be sure to use NIH rather than Swiss or Balb/c 3T3 cells; the latter are poorly infected by some viruses.) The next day, the medium is removed from the fibroblasts, and a total of 2 ml of medium plus virus is added to each well. If medium from producer cells is being directly titered, it should first be filtered through a 0.22-μm filter to remove any virus-producing cells which can skew the results even if present only in small numbers. The viral concentrate can be assumed to be cell free and need not be filtered. The producer cell medium is assayed undiluted and is diluted 1:3 and 1:9. For the concentrate, a 40-μl aliquot is mixed with 4 ml of media, and various amounts (e.g., 1.2 ml, 600 μl, 300 μl, 100 μl, 50 μl) are added to fresh medium in a well to a final volume of 2 ml. To enhance the efficacy of infection, polybrene (Sigma; stock solution of 1 mg/ml in water) is added to the medium at a concentration of 6 μl/ml. After 48 hr, the cultures are fixed and stained for lacZ as described in Section V. After incubation overnight, the number of blue cells is counted in 10 to 20 optical fields, using bright-field (not phase-contrast) optics. The number of total blue cells per dish can be calculated from the dish and field sizes. This number should be divided by four to get the approximate number of infectious virions per well since the cells divide approximately every 24 hr. We aim for a titer of approximately 10^3 infectious particles per μl of concentrate (10^6/ml).

E. Testing for Replication–Competent Virus

For many experimental purposes (especially lineage studies), it is imperative to demonstrate that no replication-competent viruses are present in the viral stock. It is strongly recommended that each viral concentrate be screened for a replication-competent virus. This can prevent a great deal of lost time should a wild-type producer appear and spread through the population of producer cells.

A plate of producer cells should be grown to confluency, and a plate of fibroblasts such as QT6 (for LZ10) or NIH3T3 (for LZ12) should be in an active growth phase. The medium is removed from the fibroblasts and is replaced with medium from the producer cells, which should be first filtered through a 0.22-μm sterile filter to exclude live cells. Six microliters of sterile, 1 mg/ml polybrene is added per milliliter of medium. Cultures are incubated for 2–10 days, with the medium replaced as needed. Finally, fresh medium is added, removed 1 day later, filtered through a 0.22-μm filter, and added with polybrene to a new plate of actively growing fibroblasts. After 48–72 hr, this plate is fixed and stained. The presence of any blue cells suggests that a replication-competent virus is present. The longer the wait before the final transfer of medium, the more confident one can be that there are no replication-competent viruses. The initial plate can be fixed and stained to confirm that infection occurred.

F. Safety Issues

Retroviral vectors need to be handled with caution, particularly if they are replication competent. The replication-defective vectors described here are less hazardous because they are less able to produce viremia. Moreover, recombinant vectors do not harbor oncogenes, even though some of their parents (e.g., Rous sarcoma virus) did. Most important, type A Rous sarcoma-based vectors such as as LZ10 infect mammalian cells poorly. (See Chapter 10 for a discussion of the host ranges of Rous viral subgroups A–E).

Nevertheless, it would be a mistake to view the replication-defective vectors as completely innocuous. Even though they do not carry oncogenes, retroviral vectors are mutagens, which can lead to transformation by stable integration of the provirus into a host protooncogenic locus. Moreover, murine leukemia viruses, spleen necrosis viruses, and some Rous subgroups that are used to infect avian cells can also infect human cells. Finally, although the recombinant stocks are nominally helper-free and replication defective, most workers in the field have found that replication-competent recombinants arise on occasion and spread rapidly (Muenchau *et al.,* 1990). For these reasons, care should be taken to avoid viral exposure. Precautions include the use of gloves when handling the viral concentrate, containment of producer cells in laminar-flow hoods, avoidance of aerosols, and disposal in strong bleach containers and glassware that have held virus.

III. Adenoviral Vectors

A. Life Cycle of the Adenovirus

The adenovirus is similar to the retrovirus in some respects. Both bind to cell surface receptors, enter the endosomes, and eventually lose their coat proteins. In both cases, too, the viral genome migrates to the nucleus, where it uses host cell machinery to make new genomes which, in turn, generate new viral proteins. Finally, the viral proteins assemble around the viral genome to form new virions which escape the host cell and spread the infection.

On the other hand, numerous fundamental differences exist between the two viral types, which are crucial to keep in mind when choosing one or the other as platforms for designing recombinant vectors. Some of these differences are: (1) The adenoviral genome is made of DNA instead of RNA. (2) Within the host cell nucleus, adenoviral DNA is maintained episomally in linear form; it does not integrate into the chromosomal DNA. Therefore, the adenovirus does not replicate with the cell and is diluted with cell divisions. On the other hand, it can infect postmitotic cells and it does not cause insertional mutations that are, in rare cases, dominant or carcinogenic. (3) The adenoviral coat is made of protein but contains no lipid. This makes adenoviral particles more stable and easier to concentrate than retroviral particles. (4) The adenovirus lyses its host, whereas the retrovirus does not. Thus, adenovirus-producing cells cannot be maintained in continuous culture.

The adenoviral genome consists of a single, linear piece of double-stranded DNA, approximately 36 kb in length. The genome is complexed with viral proteins to form an icosahedral particle approximately 75 nm in diameter. The genome is organized into early (*E1* through *E4*) and late (*L1* through *L5*) transcriptional regions (Fig. 2). After the virus enters the cells and is uncoated, the early genes are activated and their products trigger DNA replication. Once replication is underway, late genes, including those that encode the viral structural proteins, are expressed. By 48–72 hr after a cell is infected, new virions have formed and cell lysis occurs (Ginsberg, 1984; Becker *et al.,* 1994).

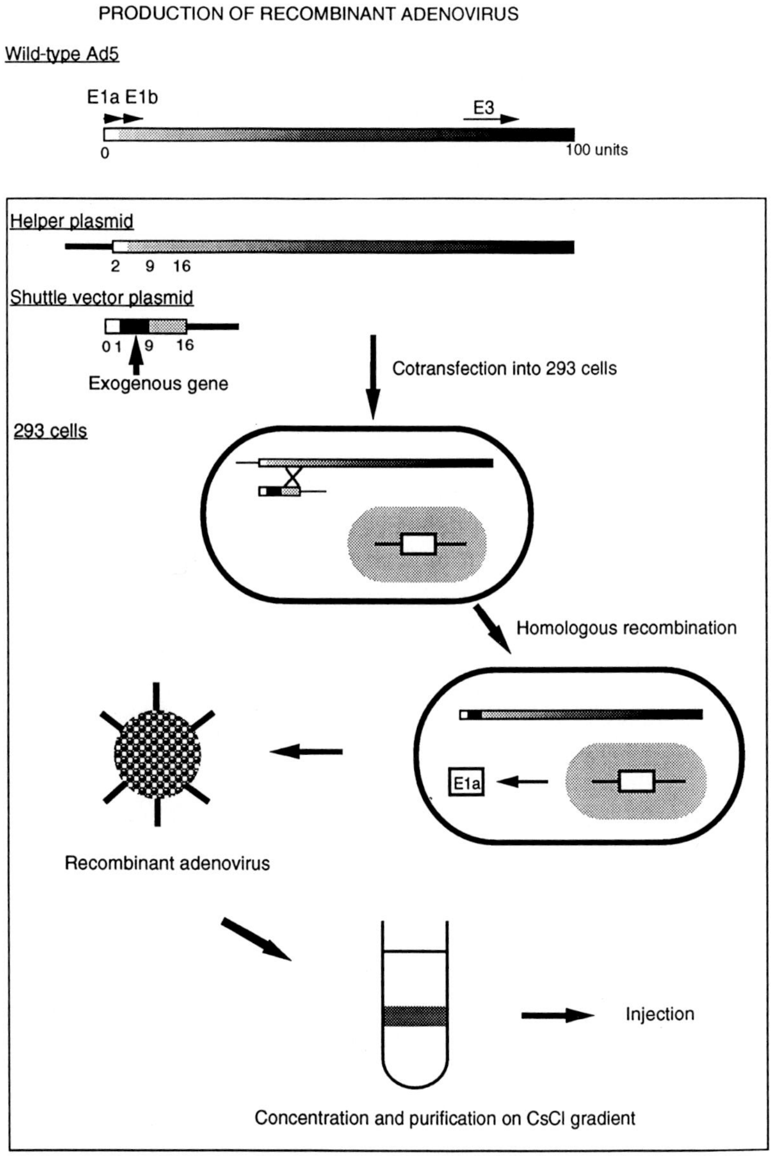

PRODUCTION OF RECOMBINANT ADENOVIRUS

Fig. 2 Replication-incompetent adenoviral vectors (see text for details).

B. Generation of Recombinant Adenoviral Vectors

Although numerous adenoviruses have been characterized, most recombinant vectors are based on human adenovirus serotype 5, which causes respiratory disease in humans (Graham and Prevec, 1991; Berkner, 1992; Grunhaus and

Horwitz, 1992). To render the virus replication defective, essential genes were deleted, including much of the *E1* region. Regions unnecessary for viability, such as *E3,* have also been removed in some cases to decrease the genome size, thereby permitting larger segments of exogenous DNA to be introduced. The important limitation is that only genomes of <105% the size of the wild-type genome (or $1.05 \times 36 = 37.8$ kb) can be packaged (Bett *et al.,* 1993). Thus, in vectors lacking *E1a* and part of *E1b* (2.9 kb), a foreign gene of about 4.7 kb can be inserted ($37.8 - 36 + 2.9 = 4.7$). In a vector that also lack the *E3* region, up to 7.5 kb of the exogenous sequence can be inserted.

To produce replication-defective virions, the widely available human embryonic kidney cell line 293 (sometimes called HEK 293; available from ATCC) is used. These cells were transfected with adenoviral DNA and contain an integrated copy of the *E1* gene (Graham *et al.,* 1977). They can therefore supply the E1 products, much as the retroviral helper lines described earlier supply gag, pol, and env.

In principle, virions can be generated by tranfecting 293 cells with a plasmid that encodes the defective adenovirus. However, the large size of the adenoviral genome makes it difficult to engineer as a single plasmid. A clever alternative that has been adoptive is to use two independent but overlapping genomic fragments that are manipulated separately, then combined by homologous recombination (McGrory *et al.,* 1988). Figure 2 summarizes this approach. The first plasmid (the helper) includes most of the adenoviral genome, but lacks E1a. The second DNA (shuttle vector) contains the exogenous insert plus a short adenoviral sequence that overlaps that of the helper. After cotransfection of these two DNA into 293 cells, this overlap facilitates generation of a linear DNA by homologous recombination. The helper plasmid is too long to be packaged and the shuttle vector lacks packaging signals. In contrast, the properly recombined DNA is shorter than the helper and can be packaged into an adenoviral particle, once the host 293 cells supply the E1a product. Successful recombinants lyse their producers and form plaques on a 293 cell lawn 2–4 weeks after transfection. The supernatant can then be used to infect new 293 cells, as described in the next section. Generally, it is advisable to clone the virus by reinfecting cells at a limiting dilution before going on to prepare large numbers of virions. This procedure ensures that all virions used subsequently will have a common origin and therefore be essentially identical. Detailed protocols for generating adenoviral vectors are presented in another volume in this series (Becker *et al.,* 1994). Moreover, simpler methods for constructing adenoviral rectors are being developed (Miyake *et al.,* in press) and may soon supplant the more cumbersome protocol described here.

C. Preparation and Storage of Viral Stocks

Once a recombinant adenovirus is established, it is relatively easy to propagate by using each stock to reinfect new plates of 293 cells. To optimize production, two factors are crucial. First, 293 cells should be used at the earliest passage available (passage number <25). Once 293 cells are obtained, therefore, they should be expanded and frozen so that new vials can be thawed frequently and old stocks discarded after several passages. Second, the multiplicity of infection (number of virions per 293 cells) needs to be regulated; in our experience, a multiplicity of 0.01 is best.

To obtain a viral stock, virions are added to a 70–80% confluent culture of 293 cells. Over the next 2–3 days, the infected cells will start to round up. Eventually, the media will turn acidic and cells will begin to detach from the dish. The progress of the infection should be monitored daily, and the cells should be taken as this stage. The medium contains some virions and can be used for some purposes. Generally, however, many more virions are trapped within the cells than released into the medium. The cells can be harvested with the medium simply by pipetting them off the plate; neither scraping nor trypsinization is required. Luckily, the virions are quite stable so they can be released with a minimal loss of activity by either freezing and thawing this suspension or by collecting the cells in a small volume of saline by centrifugation, then freezing and thawing them a few times. Typically, stocks of 10^5–10^8 active virions per ml can be prepared by this method.

To obtain higher titer stocks, virions can be concentrated from the lysate. A commonly used method is polyethylene glycol precipitation. However, this crude concentration is not suitable for microinjection because a precipitate forms that clogs the tips of glass pipettes. A density-gradient technique should be used instead, which yields highly concentrated and purified single particles (Precious and Russell, 1985). Briefly, the cleared lysate is applied to a stepwise gradient of CsCl (0.8 ml of $\rho = 1.45$ and 1.5 ml of $\rho = 1.33$ in a 13×15-mm tube). The tube is centrifuged at 90,000 g for 90 min in a swinging bucket rotor. The white band that appears at the middle of the gradient is collected and dialyzed against phosphate-buffered saline (PBS). In this way, more than 10^{10} viruses/ml of solution can be obtained.

Viral supernatants in serum-containing medium can be stored at −20°C and are relatively resistant to freeze–thawing. In contrast, the CsCl-purified concentrate is labile. However, the purified particles can be stabilized by adding 10% glycerol. The concentrate can be stored at 4°C for a few days without a significant decrease in the titer, but it should be aliquoted and frozen at −70°C for long-term storage.

D. Titering a Viral Stock

The viral titer is most simply determined with plaque-forming or end-point dilution assays, using 293 cells as indicators (Precious and Russell, 1985). In the plaque-forming assay, lysed cells form clear plaques in a lawn of cells, much as what happens following the transfection of cells during the initial generation of the virus. In the end-point dilution assay, serial dilutions are applied to 293 cells in microwells, and the titer is calculated from the greatest dilution that still leads to cell lysis. As an alternative, the titer of lacZ-containing adenoviral vectors can be estimated by infection of cells that cannot produce virus, followed by staining for lacZ, as detailed in the next section. To assess the ability of a virus to infect avian cells, the QT6 quail fibroblast line and chick embryonic fibroblasts (easily prepared from embryonic day 10 embryos) are useful.

Plaque-forming and end-point assays determine actual viral titer, but are relatively laborious. Assays based on an activity of the exogenous gene are inherently less accurate since they reflect levels of expression as well as actual titer. However, such assays are not only simpler and faster than genuine titration, but also provide the investigator with information about expression that may be useful in designing experiments *in ovo*.

E. Patterns of Expression

Over a dozen studies have been published in which replication-defective retroviral vectors have been used to transfer genes to chick embryos (Section VI). In contrast, the application of recombinant adenoviral vectors to chickens is recent and limited (Yamagata *et al.,* 1994). Therefore, it is too early to know how widely applicable the adenoviral method will be. In our study, an adenovirus was used in which the expression of lacZ was directed by a cytomegalovirus (CMV) late promoter/enhancer. Infection led to the expression of lacZ in cells in many embryonic chick tissues, including somite, notochord, dorsal root ganglion, optic tectum, spinal cord, muscle, cartilage, fat, skin, lens, lung, and heart (Yamagata *et al.,* 1994). There were, however, some tissues in which little expression was observed. More recently, we have constructed and tested an adenovirus with a Rous sarcoma virus enhancer/promoter and found better expression in the central nervous system (M. Yamagata and J. R. Sanes, unpublished). These results suggest that an appropriate choice of regulatory elements will permit use of the adenoviral vector for gene transfer to many, if not most, parts of the chick embryo.

F. Safety Issues

Adenoviral vectors are considered to be quite safe (Crystal *et al.,* 1994). Because adenoviral genomes are episomal (they do not integrate into the genome), they do not cause insertional mutations like retroviruses. Even wild-type, replication-competent adenoviruses cause only mild syndromes such as colds in humans. Furthermore, most adults are immune to the serotype 5 adenovirus. The recombinant vectors used in birds are replication defective and are missing genes such as *E1a* whose products are potentially harmful. However, there is a risk that the replication-defective vectors could recombine with endogenous viral genomes to produce replication-competent viruses, and studies in rodents have revealed some pathogenicity associated with the injection of high-titer viral stocks. Thus, standard virological precautions should be observed when handling adenoviral vectors: use gloves and safety hoods, avoid aerosols, and autoclave or bleach used glassware.

IV. Injection of Virus into Chick Embryos

Because surgical methods for introducing retrovirus and adenovirus are so similar, they are described together here. Virus is thawed, then kept on ice until it is used. The virus is mixed with 4% (v/v) fast green and, if necessary, diluted with culture medium. For retrovirus, 10% (v/v) 1 mg/ml polybrene is also added. Electrodes are pulled from 1.0-mm-outer-diameter × 0.5-mm-inner-diameter, non-omega glass capillary tubing, using an electrode puller. Almost any electrophysiology-type puller will suffice; we use an old one that was made by World Precision Instruments and is no longer adequate for electrophysiology. After pulling, the tip is broken, either by pinching it with forceps or by pushing it against a piece of soft rubber with a razor blade. The latter method may produce a sharper edge and more of a bevel. An opening that is just barely large enough to see under the highest power of a dissecting microscope, around 10–30 μm in diameter, is best. The electrode can be marked every 5 mm with a sharp-pointed felt-tip pen, starting from the end of the shank, to facilitate the estimation of injection volumes.

The electrode is filled by attaching the open end of the electrode to a vacuum and inserting the tip of the electrode into the viral mixture. Care must be taken not to allow the tip to come out of the solution or the viral mixture will be sucked out the back of the electrode into the tubing. Clogging of the electrode during filling is frequent. This can usually be overcome by turning off the vacuum and applying a strong positive pressure to push the debris out of the electrode. When this fails, it is necessary to break the electrode back a short distance to increase the size of the opening. Alternatively, the virus suspension can be sonicated briefly to break up any clumps. With a proper-sized opening, filling is slow and may take a minute or more.

Eggs can be opened in numerous ways. Placing the eggs on their sides in the incubator is effective. At the time of injection, they are "candled" on the end of a fiber optic light source to visualize the positions of the embryo and air cavity. Injections are performed under a stereo dissecting scope with illumination from a fiber optic light source. The egg is wiped with 95% ethanol, and a thumbtack is inserted through the shell into the air cavity and again, very gently, at the position overlying the embryo. A rubber pipette bulb is then squeezed and placed over the hole in the air sac, and the air is gently sucked out. A new air bubble can then be seen overlying the embryo when the egg is recandled. Clear cellophane tape placed over both holes prevents the yolk from leaking out and minimizes the amount of broken shell that falls onto the embryo. Using fine scissors previously cleaned with alcohol, an opening is cut in the shell overlying the embryo. Depending on the electrode size and the tissue to be injected, it may be necessary to deflect some of the extraembryonic membranes. This can be done with a pair of sharpened, alcohol-sterilized forceps. Failure to remove the membranes may cause the electrode to dent the membranes and then advance suddenly to puncture the embryo when the membrane finally breaks.

The electrode is attached to a PicoPump (World Precision Instruments), an Eppendorf microinjector, or a similar pressurized ejector. If the virus is to be injected into a very precisely defined or small space (e.g., the spinal canal), the electrode should be held by a micromanipulator. If the injection is into a large space such as the ventricles of the brain, it is easier to inject freehand, gripping the electrode holder and resting the side of the hand on a hard surface. The duration of ejection is controlled by a foot pedal connected to a solenoid that controls the air supply (a pedal is supplied with the PicoPump). We use a series of short pulses and monitor the injection visually, using the fast green in the viral stock.

The best diameter for an electrode tip varies with the application. Small-tipped electrodes clog easily. On the other hand, broad, blunt tips have difficulty penetrating the tissue, resulting in tissue damage and leakage of the virus. The leakage may be deleterious to the experiment. In general, it is easier to inject into a fluid-filled cavity than into tissue, but both can be done.

Following injection, electrode is withdrawn and a drop of ~50 μl of ampicillin (50 mg/ml) is placed onto the membranes near the embryo. The hole overlying the embryo is then sealed tightly with clear cellophane tape and the egg is returned to the incubator on its side. Some expression of lacZ has been found within 24 hr of injection, but levels seem variable for the first 48 hr after infection. We therefore wait at least 2 days before analyzing the embryos.

We have occasionally encountered difficulty in infecting certain batches of chick embryos with retroviral vectors. This has been particularly true when the eggs come from flocks of older hens. Changing suppliers or having the supplier use a new batch of younger hens has alleviated the problem.

V. Histology and Histochemistry

A. Fixation

For lacZ staining, embryos are fixed in 2% formaldehyde (made from either formalin or paraformaldehyde) and 0.4% glutaraldehyde in PBS, pH 7.2–7.4. Fixation can be done either by perfusion followed by immersion or by immersion alone. It is necessary to limit the total time of fixation to approximately 1 hr as overfixation can decrease the activity of the lacZ. Organic fixatives, such as alcohols, destroy lacZ activity and are useful primarily if the virally introduced gene is detected immunohistochemically.

Cultured cells can be fixed in the same solution as embryos, but the fixation time should be limited to 5 min.

B. Histochemical Stain for lacZ

The staining solution for demonstrating lacZ activity is as follows (Sanes *et al.*, 1986):

Final concentration	Volume stock solution/ml
1 mg/ml X-Gal	25 μl of 40 mg/ml stock in DMSO
4–16 mM potassium ferrocyanide	20–80 μl of 200 mM stock
4–16 mM potassium ferricyanide	20–80 μl of 200 mM stock
2 mM MgCl$_2$	2 μl of 1 M stock
PBS, pH 7.2–7.3	Dilute total volume to 1 ml

The lower concentrations of potassium ferri- and ferrocyanide result in maximum sensitivity in culture, but permit diffusion of the reaction product. As a result, the higher concentrations are better in tissue because the diffusion out of X-Gal-positive cells is less. When preparing the incubation mixture, bring the PBS to room temperature before adding X-Gal because crystals may form. Cells or tissue are incubated overnight in the dark at room temperature. Incubation at 30°C results in better staining but also may increase background. After staining overnight, the culture or tissue should be rinsed several times in PBS, then stored in 2% formaldehyde, 2% glutaraldehyde, and PBS at 4°C.

Certain tissues have light background staining with X-Gal; this staining increases during the time of the rinse. Leave the tissue in PBS for several hours before transferring it into the secondary fixative (2% formaldehyde/2% glutaraldehyde). Because the background staining varies reproducibly among tissues and brain laminae, it may be useful if it is very light.

C. Other Genes and Methods of Detection

Instead of using a histochemical reaction for lacZ, commercially anti-lacZ antibodies can be applied. Several antisera are available commercially, and we have deposited a monoclonal antibody to lacZ, 40-1, in the Developmental Studies Hybridoma Bank (maintained by NIH at the University of Iowa). If immunofluorescence is used, it is important to minimize the amount of glutaraldehyde in the primary fixation. This approach will allow the use of specific cell markers along with the retroviral labeling, but often precludes the use of whole mounts. Moreover, if the lacZ-positive clones are rare, prohibitively large volumes of antibodies may be necessary to stain a few clones.

Not all viruses use *lacZ* as a reporter gene. The RCASBP(A) virus, described in Chapter 10, for example, uses alkaline phosphatase instead. Refer to Chapter 10 for a description of alkaline phosphatase histochemistry.

D. Sectioning Tissue

Histochemically stained cells can be examined in whole mounts or in thick or thin sections prepared in any of several ways. Sectioned material allows excellent cellular resolution but obscures the relationship between populations of stained cells. In contrast, whole mounts allow a direct visualization of stained cells from many angles. The ideal strategy, when feasible, is to stain and examine whole mounts, then cut sections for a more detailed study of regions of interest. The steps used to analyze lacZ-positive cells in spinal cord are summarized next (Leber *et al.*, 1990; Leber and Sanes, 1995).

First, the entire spinal cord was dissected from the animal after fixation, the tissue was rinsed in PBS, and then the tissue was immersed in X-Gal solution. Following this incubation, the tissue was rinsed again in PBS and was progressively cleared in graded glycerol to reveal cells buried deep in the tissue. Slabs (200–400 μm) of spinal cord containing stained clones were then cut by hand using a fine razor blade, and the slabs were examined in whole mount from various directions under a dissection microscope to determine the relationship between the stained cells. For a more detailed analysis, the glycerol was gradually washed out with saline, and the tissue was dehydrated and embedded in Epon. Care was taken to avoid using propylene oxide because the X-Gal reaction product is soluble in this solvent. The plastic-embedded spinal cords were cut on a microtome at a section thickness of 20 μm, using disposable metal blades. The sections generally had a great deal of surface chatter, but this was hidden by using immersion oil as the mounting medium. When necessary, basic fuchsin was very effective as a counterstain for the blue-stained cells. Subsequently, some 20-μm plastic sections were removed from the slides, remounted, and sectioned at 1 μm. The semithin sections could be stained with toluidine blue to demonstrate Nissl substance. Alternatively, thin sections were taken for electron microscopy.

Similar whole mount staining can be done in brain until about E10, at which time the brain becomes too thick to allow adequate penetration of the X-Gal solution. At older ages or for thick tissues, another approach is to fix the tissue as described earlier, rinse it in PBS, and then take Vibratome sections of the tissue. Sections (200 μm) are picked up and put into X-Gal in 96-well plates. These are stained overnight at room temperature, then rinsed as described earlier. After rinsing, the sections are fixed in 2% formaldehyde, 2% glutaraldehyde in PBS, rinsed again, and mounted on slides. This method allows excellent visualization of the relationship between cells and tissue and lamina boundaries, but bending and folding of the Vibratome sections can make the reconstruction of serial sections difficult.

An alternative method is to freeze fixed and rinsed tissue, take serial cryostat sections, and stain all the sections for lacZ. This approach allows observation of the relationship between stained cells and tissue/lamina boundaries quite well without much distortion of tissue, but the dispersal of clones of cells across many sections necessitates the use of complex reconstruction methods.

It is also possible to stain whole mount tissue for lacZ followed by paraffin embedding and sectioning. However, the X-Gal reaction product is soluble in organic solutions and is extracted unless dehydration and clearing are rapid. One solution to this problem is to use Bluogal (BRL Life Technologies, Gathersburg,

MD), which is structurally similar to X-Gal but much less soluble in organic solvents. The Bluogal reaction product is somewhat grayer than that of X-Gal, which can decrease contrast in thick sections. On the other hand, the Bluogal product is more suitable for electron microscopy than that of X-Gal because it forms a darker and finer electron-dense precipitate (Weis *et al.*, 1991).

E. Microscopy and Photography

Whole mounts are best viewed with a dissecting microscope. They should be submerged in saline for photography to avoid glare. Sections are best viewed with bright-field optics on an upright microscope. Faintly stained cells can be seen better if a red filter is used. Nomarski or phase-contrast optics are useful in defining tissue and laminar locations in uncounterstained tissue, but can obscure faintly X-Gal-positive cells. Sections can be photographed, although the dispersal of cells throughout the depth of the section usually makes it hard to focus on more than a small area of the clone. The arrangement of X-Gal-positive cells in a thick section is often best documented using a drawing tube. Computerized reconstruction that allows rotation of the clones through space is ideal, but is unnecessary in most cases.

VI. Uses of Viral Vectors

A. Comparison of Gene Transfer Methods

Two vectors for transferring genes to avian cells *in vivo* have been described: replication-defective retrovirus and replication-defective adenovirus. A third vector type, the replication-competent retrovirus, is discussed in Chapter 10. A fourth method, direct microinjection of plasmid, is clearly feasible, based on success with tracer injection (Chapter 8) and preliminary results with plasmids (S. Fraser, unpublished). A final set of methods, transfection of cells with lipid-coated (Holt *et al.*, 1990) or polyion-conjugated (Curiel, 1993) DNA, holds great promise, but has been little applied to avian embryos so far (Demeneix *et al.*, 1994). Table I summarizes the advantages and disadvantages of the first four of these methods (there are insufficient data to evaluate the fifth). The following paragraphs annotate the table, and subsequent subsections focus on particular applications.

Retroviruses offer the best means for stable introduction of foreign genes into cells. They are generally nonpathogenic, and the genes they transfer become permanent elements of the host cell genome and are thereby transferred to that cell's progeny without dilution. Limitations are that (1) infection is restricted to mitotically active target cells; (2) specific cells cannot be targeted for infection; and (3) the expression of inserted genes can be affected by the insertion site of the provirus in the host chromosome and by interference between viral and internal promoters.

Table I
Comparison of Methods for Transferring Genes to Avian Cells
In Ovo

Agent for transfer	Microinjection	Replication-competent retrovirus	Replication-defective retrovirus	Replication-defective adenovirus
Innocuous to recipient cell	−	+++	+++	+
Ability to transfer vector to numerous cells	−	+++	+	++
Ability to transfer genes to postmitotic cells	+++	−	−	+++
Ability to target vector to specified cells	+++	−	+	+
Capacity to transfer large genes	+++	+	++	+/++
Stable integration	−	+++	+++	−
Safe to investigator	+++	−	+	++

In essence, the replication-defective retroviruses are suitable when it is important to infect only a few cells whereas the replication-competent retroviruses are best used when it is important to infect many or most of the cells in a tissue. Limitations of the replication-competent vectors are (1) they can spread uncontrollably through the embryo, making it difficult to limit gene transfer to a specific tissue unless technically arduous interstrain transplantation methods are used (Chapter 10); (2) they pose more serious safety issues than methods based on replication-defective vectors; and (3) they can only package exogenous genes of ≤2 kb.

Adenoviral DNA does not integrate into the genome, so expression of its genes is transient. For studies in avian embryos, however, this is not much of a problem: adenovirally introduced genes are generally expressed for at least a few weeks, which is longer than most experiments run. The great advantages of adenoviral over retroviral vectors are (1) the high titers that can be obtained; and (2) their ability to infect postmitotic cells (Stratford-Perricaudet *et al.*, 1992; Breakefield, 1993). (3) In addition, expression of the reporter gene is relatively insensitive to interference from viral sequences (because nearby viral promoters have been excised) or site-specific host genomic influences (because the virus remains episomal), favoring the use of adenoviral vectors for testing tissue-specific promoters *in vivo* (Friedman *et al.*, 1986; Bessereau *et al.*, 1994). In addition to the instability of expression discussed earlier, disadvantages include the potential for toxic and immune response to adenoviral proteins encoded by genes that have not been excised from the recombinant vectors.

B. Lineage

Replication-incompetent retroviruses have been used for studies of cell lineage in rodent since the mid-1980s (Sanes *et al.*, 1986; Price *et al.*, 1987) and they remain the only viral vector suitable for this purpose. In the chick, these retroviruses have been used to elucidate the lineage of neurons and glia in spinal cord, dorsal root ganglion, enteric ganglia, retina, and optic tectum, as well as in a variety of nonneural tissues (e.g., Gray *et al.*, 1988; Galileo *et al.*, 1990; Frank and Sanes, 1991; Leber *et al.*, 1990; Mikawa *et al.*, 1992). Their particular advantage lies in the fact that their label is stably expressed and allows progeny to be traced throughout development. In addition, the injection of virus is quite simple and cells can be labeled even if they are relatively inaccessible or too small to be labeled with an intracellular dye or tracer. Because replication-competent retroviral vectors spread and adenoviral vectors do not integrate, they are both unsuitable for lineage analysis. Direct injection of tracers has provided an excellent alternative to lineage tracing (see Chapter 8) and permits labeling of a single identified progenitor; however, injection methods suffer from the dilution of injected label as cells divide. For a comparison of the advantages and disadvantages of microinjected tracers and retroviral genes as lineage tracers, see Frank and Sanes (1991). An ideal method would involve microinjection of a plasmid capable of integrating into the genome. Methods for accomplishing this goal are under development, but have not been perfected yet.

The primary disadvantage of the retroviral method lies in the impossibility of directing label to a single cell. The ideal situation is one in which clones of cells appear as isolated clusters. This can occur when clonally related cells do not migrate away from their siblings. Careful choice of a viral dose can then provide a reasonable sample size without obscuring clonal boundaries. Even in an ideal situation, however, the number of clones per animal may vary considerably and infections may cluster spatially. Two approaches can be used to test the interpretation that isolated clusters represent clones. First, a quantitative analysis can be done. If the number of viruses injected is decreased 10-fold, for example, the number of clones should also decrease 10-fold but the number of cells per clones should be unchanged (see, for example, Gray *et al.*, 1988). If, on the other hand, some clusters are polyclones, then dilution should increase their average size as well their number. The second approach is to inject a mixture of viruses that contain different exogenous genes and then to demonstrate that the cells in each cluster express only one type of label. For example, viruses bearing an ordinary *lacZ* gene can be mixed viruses encoding a fusion protein that targets *lacZ* to the nucleus (see, for example, Galileo *et al.*, 1990). If clusters are clones, each should contain only cytoplasmically stained or only nuclear-stained cells. A technically arduous but more comprehensive approach uses mixtures of hundreds of individual viruses, each identifiable by a single-cell PCR assay (Walsh and Cepko, 1992). Despite these measures, however, an element of doubt always remains as to the identity of clones marked by retrovirus-mediated gene transfer.

C. Tracing Cell Migration

Since the early days of the field, embryologists have tracked the migratory paths of cells by labeling them with a dye or by transplanting them from one animal to another. In the course of lineage-tracing experiments with replication-defective retroviruses, it became apparent that these vectors could also be used to study cell migration in the nervous system (Gray *et al.*, 1988). Since clonally related cells have a common site of origin at the ventricular surface and since cells migrate out of the ventricular zone asynchronously, the distribution of cells at intermediate stages of development reflects their migratory pathway. In addition, the spread of cells within the ventricular zone is an indication of how much mixing occurs within the neuroepithelium. This method has been used to map migratory paths in the laminated optic tectum and the nonlaminated spinal cord. In both structures, mixing in the ventricular zone is progressively restricted as development proceeds, radial migration is prominent, and tangential migration (parallel to the surface of the brain) along axonal pathways occurs as well (Gray and Sanes, 1991; Leber and Sanes, 1995).

Adenoviral vectors also hold promise for tracing cell migrations. One potential advantage is that they can be introduced into postmotitic cells, such as neurons, to trace migrations that occur following the completion of neurogenesis. Another advantage is the high titer of adenoviral stocks. For example, we have been able to inject enough adenoviral particles into the lumen of a single somite to label a dozen or more cells, which were then viewed as they migrated toward the limb (Yamagata *et al.*, 1994). Such an experiment would have been impossible with retroviral vectors because a lumen full of retroviral inoculate would contain at most a few active virions.

D. Inserting Bioactive Genes

All three of the viral vectors described in this chapter can be used to transfer bioactive genes or their antisense copies to avian cells, to perturb cellular differentiation, and thereby learn about the function of the gene. Each vector has its own advantages. The replication-competent viruses can transform an entire tissue, as detailed in Chapter 10. In contrast, replication-defective viruses provide a means of generating small groups of transgenic cells in a wild-type environment. This strategy has two main advantages: it favors the detection of cell autonomous and direct effects of the transgene, and it permits testing of genes that would be generally deleterious or lethal if expressed in a whole animal. For example, Galileo *et al.* (1992) infected tectal cells with a retrovirus bearing an antisense copy of the integrin $\beta 1$ subunit, which serves as a cellular receptor for numerous membrane- and matrix-bound ligands. Cells expressing the antisense construct were often unable to move from the ventricular zone to the tectal plate, thus demonstrating a role for integrins in neuroblast migration. The important point is that this result could not have been obtained by the overall attenuation of integrin levels: integrin "knockout" mice are early embryonic lethals (Yang *et al.,* 1993), and general interference with integrin function in avian embryos would surely be lethal as well.

A problem that arises in transferring bioactive genes with replication-defective retroviruses is detection of the infected cells. To circumvent this problem, vectors have been designed that contain a bioactive gene plus *lacZ*. Thus, the infected cell's progeny can be identified histochemically and, in many cases, the abnormality can be assessed from the distribution, shape, and size of the lacZ-positive cells. Particularly useful in such vectors has been the use of ribosome-binding sequences from a picornavirus (Ghattas *et al.,* 1991). The insertion of this so-called "IRES" permits translation of two genes from a single transcript, thereby avoiding the problems frequently encountered when two separate promoters are linked to generate two separate transcripts, each encoding a single gene.

Finally, no studies of adenovirally transferred bioactive genes in birds have yet appeared, but we see great promise for these vectors in light of their successful use for gene therapy in mammals, including humans (Kozarsky and Wilson, 1993; Crystal *et al.,* 1994). They should see many uses in the nervous system, where transfer to postmitotic cells is frequently essential. Moreover, their combination of high titer and replication incompetence should make them ideal for transferring genes to a significant fraction of the cells in a tissue without risking uncontrolled spread and viremia.

References

Becker, T. C., Noel, R. J., Coats, W. S., Gómez-Foix, A. M., Alam, T., Gerard, R. D., and Newgard, C. B. (1994). Use of recombinant adenovirus for metabolic engineering of mammalian cells. *Methods Cell Biol.* **43,** 161–189.

Berkner, K. L. (1992). Expression of heterologous sequences in adenoviral vectors. *Curr. Top. Microbiol. Immunol.* **158,** 39–66.

Bessereau, J. L., Stratford-Perricaudet, L. D., Piette, J., Le Poupon, C., and Changeux, J. P. (1994). *In vivo* and *in vitro* analysis of electrical activity-dependent expression of muscle acetylcholine receptor genes using adenovirus. *Proc. Natl. Acad. Sci. U.S.A.* **91,** 1304–1308.

Bett, A. J., Prevec, L., and Graham, F. L. (1993). Packaging capacity and stability of human adenovirus type 5 vectors. *J. Virol.* **67,** 5911–5921.

Breakefield, X. O. (1993). Gene delivery into the brain using virus vectors. *Nat. Genet.* **3,** 187–189.

Crystal, R. G., McElvaney, N. G., Rosenfeld, M. A., Chu, C.-S., Mastrangeli, A., Hay, J. G., Brody, S. L., Jaffe, H. A., Eissa, N. T., and Danel, C. (1994). Administration of an adenovirus containing the human CFTR cDNA to the respiratory tract of individuals with cystic fibrosis. *Nat. Genet.* **8,** 42–51.

Curiel, D. T. (1993). Adenovirus facilitation of molecular conjugate-mediated gene transfer. *Prog. Med. Virol.* **40,** 1–18.

Demeneix, B. A., Abdel-Taweb, H., Benoist, C., Seugnet, I., and Behr, J. P. (1994). Temporal and spatial expression of lipospermine-compacted genes transferred in chick embryos *in vivo*. *BioTechniques* **16,** 496–501.

Dougherty, J. P., and Temin, H. M. (1986). High mutation rate of a spleen necrosis virus-based retrovirus vector. *Mol. Cell. Biol.* **7**, 4387–4395.

Frank, E., and Sanes, J. R. (1991). Lineage of neurons and glia in chick dorsal root ganglia: Analysis *in vivo* with a recombinant retrovirus. *Development (Cambridge, UK)* **111**, 895–908.

Friedman, J. M., Babiss, L. E., Clayton, D. F., and Darnell, J. E. J. (1986). Cellular promoters incorporated into the adenovirus genome: Cell specificity of albumin and immunoglobulin expression. *Mol. Cell. Biol.* **6**, 3791–3797.

Galileo, D. S., Gray, G. E., Owens, G. C., Majors, J., and Sanes, J. R. (1990). Neurons and glia arise from a common progenitor in chick optic tectum: Demonstration with two retroviruses and cell type-specific antibodies. *Proc. Natl. Acad. Sci. U.S.A.* **87**, 458–462.

Galileo, D. S., Majors, J., Horwitz, A. F., and Sanes, J. R. (1992). Retrovirally-introduced antisense integrin RNA inhibits neuroblast migration *in vivo*. *Neuron* **9**, 1117–1131.

Ghattas, I. R., Sanes, J. R., and Majors, J. E. (1991). The encephalomyocarditis virus internal ribosome entry site allows efficient coexpression of two genes from a recombinant provirus in cultured cells and in embryos. *Mol. Cell. Biol.* **11**, 5848–5859.

Ginsberg, H. S. (1984). "The Adenoviruses." Plenum, New York.

Graham, F. L., and Prevec, L. (1991). Manipulation of adenoviral vectors. *In* "Methods in Molecular Biology" (E. J. Murray, ed.), pp. 109–128. Humana Press, Clifton, NJ.

Graham, F. L., Smiley, J., Russell, W. C., and Nairn, R. (1977). Characteristics of a human cell line transformed by DNA from human adenovirus type 5. *J. Gen. Virol.* **36**, 59–74.

Gray, G. E., and Sanes, J. R. (1991). Migratory paths and phenotypic choices of clonally related cells in the avian optic tectum. *Neuron* **6**, 211–225.

Gray, G. E., Glover, J. C., Majors, J., and Sanes, J. R. (1988). Radial arrangement of clonally related cells in the chicken optic tectum: Lineage analysis with a recombinant retrovirus. *Proc. Natl. Acad. Sci. U.S.A.* **85**, 7356–7360.

Grunhaus, A., and Horwitz, M. S. (1992). Adenoviruses as cloning vectors. *Semin. Virol.* **3**, 237–252.

Holt, C. E., Garlick, N., and Cornel, E. (1990). Lipofection of cDNAs in the embryonic vertebrate central nervous system. *Neuron* **4**, 203–214.

Kozarsky, K. F., and Wilson, J. M. (1993). Gene therapy: Adenovirus vectors. *Curr. Opin. Genet. Dev.* **3**, 499–503.

Leber, S. M., and Sanes, J. R. (1995). Migratory paths of neurons and glia in the embryonic chick spinal cord. *J. Neurosci.* **15**, 1236–1248.

Leber, S. M., Breedlove, S. M., and Sanes, J. R. (1990). Lineage, arrangement and death of clonally related neurons in chick spinal cord. *J. Neurosci.* **10**, 2451–2462.

McGrory, W. J., Bautista, D. S., and Graham, F. L. (1988). A simple technique for the rescue of early region 1 mutation into infectious human adenovirus type 5. *Virology* **163**, 614–617.

Mikawa, T., Fischman, D. A., Dougherty, J. P., and Brown, A. M. C. (1991). *In vivo* analysis of a new LacZ retrovirus vector suitable for cell lineage marking in avian and other species. *Exp. Cell Res.* **195**, 516–523.

Mikawa, T., Cohen-Gould, L., and Fischman, D. A. (1992). Clonal analysis of cardiac morphogenesis in the chicken embryo using a replication-defective retrovirus. III: Polyclonal origin of adjacent ventricular myocytes. *Dev. Dyn.* **195**, 133–141.

Miller, A. D. (1990). Retrovirus packaging cells. *Hum. Gene Ther.* **1**, 5–14.

Miyake, S., Makimura, M., Kanegae, Y., Harada, S., Sato, Y., Takamori, K., Tokuda, C., and Saito, I. (1996). Efficient generation of recombinant adenoviruses using adenovirus DNA-terminal protein complex and a cosmid bearing the full-length virus genome. *Proc. Natl. Acad. Sci. U.S.A.*, in press.

Muenchau, D. D., Freeman, S. M., Cornetta, K., Zwiebel, J. A., and Anderson, W. F. (1990). Analysis of retroviral packaging lines for generation of replication-competent virus. *Virology* **176**, 262–265.

Mulligan, R. C. (1992). The basic science of gene therapy. *Science* **260**, 926–932.

Precious, B., and Russell, W. C. (1985). Growth, purification and titration of adenoviruses. *In* "Virology: A Practical Approach" (B. W. J. Mahy and W. J. Brian, eds.), pp. 193–205. IRL Press, Oxford.

Price, J., Turner, D., and Cepko, C. (1987). Lineage analysis in the vertebrate nervous system by retrovirus-mediated gene transfer. *Proc. Natl. Acad. Sci. U.S.A.* **84,** 156–160.

Roth, M. G., ed. (1994). "Protein Expression in Animal Cells" Methods Cell Biol., Vol. 43. Academic Press, San Diego, CA.

Sanes, J. R., Rubenstein, J. L. R., and Nicolas, J.-F. (1986). Use of a recombinant retrovirus to study post-implantation cell lineage in mouse embryos. *EMBO J.* **5,** 3133–3142.

Stratford-Perricaudet, L. D., Makeh, I., Perricaudet, M., and Briand, P. (1992). Widespread long-term gene transfer to mouse skeletal muscles and heart. *J. Clin. Invest.* **90,** 626–630.

Varmus, H., and Brown, P. (1989). Retroviruses. *In* "Mobile DNA" (D. E. Berg and M. M. Howe, eds.), pp. 53–108. Am. Soc. Microbiol., Washington, DC.

Walsh, C., and Cepko, C. L. (1992). Widespread dispersion of neuronal clones across functional regions of the cerebral cortex. *Science* **255,** 434–440.

Weis, J., Fine, S. M., David, C., Savarirayan, S., and Sanes, J. R. (1991). Integration site-dependent expression of a transgene reveals specialized features of cells associated with neuromuscular junctions. *J. Cell Biol.* **113,** 1385–1397.

Whitcomb, J. M., and Hughes, S. H. (1992). Retroviral reverse transcription and integration: Progress and problems. *Annu. Rev. Cell Biol.* **8,** 255–306.

Yamagata, M., Jaye, D. L., and Sanes, J. R. (1994). Gene transfer into avian embryos with a recombinant adenovirus. *Dev. Biol.* **166,** 355–359.

Yang, J. T., Rayburn, H., and Hynes, R. O. (1993). Embryonic mesodermal defects in α_5 integrin-deficient mice. *Development (Cambridge, UK)* **119,** 1093–1105.

CHAPTER 10

Manipulating Gene Expression with Replication-Competent Retroviruses

Bruce A. Morgan* and Donna M. Fekete†

* Cutaneous Biology Research Center
Harvard Medical School and Massachusetts General Hospital
Charlestown, Massachusetts 02129

† Department of Biology
Boston College
Chestnut Hill, Massachusetts 02167

I. Introduction
    A. Advantages of Virus-Mediated Alteration of Gene Expression in Chick Embryos
    B. Replication-Competent vs. Replication-Defective Vectors
    C. General Virology
    D. Optimizing Retrovirus-Mediated Expression in Chick Embryos
II. Materials
    A. Plasmids
    B. PCR Primers
    C. Equipment and Supplies
III. Methods
    A. Virus Construction
    B. Virus Production
    C. General Preparation
    D. Prototype Injection Protocols for Solid Tissue
    E. Prototype Injection Protocols for Lumenal Spaces
    F. Developing a Novel Infection Protocol
IV. Results and Discussion
    A. Correlating Infection with Resulting Phenotype
    B. Further Restriction of Gene Expression
    C. Alternative Infection Protocols
V. Conclusions and Perspectives
    References

Copyright © 1996 by Academic Press, Inc. All rights of reproduction in any form reserved.

I. Introduction

A. Advantages of Virus-Mediated Alteration of Gene Expression in Chick Embryos

The obvious advantages of the chick for embryological studies have been tempered by the difficulties of genetic analyses in this organism. The ability to manipulate gene expression in the mouse embryo has rendered it the organism of choice for genetic studies, but the difficulty of physically manipulating the mammalian embryo limits the combination of these approaches to study development. Although transgenic approaches may ultimately become routine in the chick, the long reproductive cycle and culture requirements will limit their general utility. The use of retroviral vectors to alter gene expression has proven a valuable alternative to transgenic approaches. Many of the genetic manipulations that have proven so powerful in the mouse can be mimicked with retroviral vectors. To date, the gain of function experiments has been the most successful. The potential role of a protein is assayed by expressing it in places or times at which it would not normally be found (Morgan *et al.*, 1992; Riddle *et al.*, 1993). This approach can also be used to free the expression of a gene from the requirement of interaction with inducing factors, thereby allowing the separation of coinduced genetic pathways to study their respective functions in isolation (Laufer *et al.*, 1994). The comlimentary approach of inactivating gene expression is in theory also possible by several methods. The most promising involves the expression of dominant negative proteins which interfere with the wild-type protein. The high levels of expression achieved with retroviral vectors should be sufficient to achieve the required stoichiometry for successful interference. The high efficiency of the viral promoter has also encouraged attempts at gene inactivation by antisense RNA expression. To date, these attempts have been less successful, but they may ultimately prove effective.

The use of retroviruses to alter gene expression has several advantages stemming from the comparative ease with which different expression patterns may be generated with the same virus. Many genes are reused in different tissues and at different times to mediate development. By varying the infection protocol, a single high titer virus stock may be used to address the role of a gene in many different developmental decisions. The low cost, quick turn around time, and technical simplicity of these experiments also allow the simultaneous generation of a number of alternative (e.g., mutant) constructs in parallel.

B. Replication-Competent vs. Replication-Defective Vectors

All avian retroviral vectors currently in use for gene transfer were initially derived from naturally occurring proviruses. A provirus is a double-stranded DNA form of a retrovirus that resides in the chromosome of a host cell. The provirus is generated by reverse transcription of single-stranded viral genomic RNA. Two identical strands of genomic RNA are surrounded by a protein core in an infectious virus, and the protein core is in turn enveloped by a membranous coat embedded with surface proteins. The core proteins, three enzymes (reverse transcriptase, integrase, and protease), and surface proteins are encoded by the viral structural genes *gag, pol,* and *env* respectively. A virus that has a complete genome is replication competent. That is, it can infect a host cell, generate and integrate a new provirus, transcribe and translate the viral structural genes, and assemble and bud off new infectious particles (Fig. 1). Viruses that are missing portions of the genome will be referred to as replication defective.

Both replication-competent and replication-defective retroviral vectors are available for mediating gene transfer into avian host cells. They are constructed and amplified as bacterial plasmids to generate large quantities of proviral DNA. This DNA is then transfected into the appropriate host "producer" cells *in vitro.* Following transfection, the producer cells generate large quantities of infectious virions and release these into the media. This supernatant is collected, concentrated, and used to infect embryos or tissue culture cells. An alternative procedure using infected cells instead of culture supernatant to infect embryos is also possible. In this chapter, detailed protocols for all of these steps are provided for replication-competent vectors. Similar protocols for replication-defective viruses are presented elsewhere in this volume.

In the case of replication-defective retroviral vectors, significant deletions exist in the structural genes to make room for the insertion of exogenous sequences. The result is that a host cell infected with a replication-defective virus can permanently carry and express one or more retrovirus-mediated transgenes, but the cell itself will not generate new infectious virions.

In the case of replication-competent retroviral vectors, such as those designed by S. H. Hughes and colleagues (Hughes and Kosik, 1984; Petropoulos and Hughes, 1991; Boerkoel *et al.,* 1993; Hughes *et al.,* 1987; Greenhouse *et al.,* 1988), the viral structural genes and other important regulatory sequences are intact. The source virus from which these were derived is the avian oncogenic virus. Rous sarcoma virus (RSV) RSV is a member of a larger group of related retroviruses, collectively called avian sarcoma and leukemia viruses (ASLVs), that share a great deal of sequence homology. RSV is unusual among ASLVs in that in addition to *gag, pol,* and *env,* it also carries a host-derived oncogene, *src,* which is about 2 kb in length. The Hughes group removed *src* and some surrounding sequences and replaced them with a convenient *Cla*I restriction site. It is at this site that a transgene can be easily inserted (gene X in Fig. 1). A series of such vectors has been generated, with small sequence differences that affect splicing of the transgene, host tropism (as described later), and strength of the promoter in the long terminal repeat (LTR). As a prototype of this series of vectors, this chapter focuses on the replication-competent, avian leukemia virus LTR, splice acceptor, Bryan high titer polymerase, A-envelope subgroup RCASBP(A). These distinctions will be discussed briefly later. It has been empirically determined that the vectors of this series can carry up to 2.4 kb in additional sequence, although the precise upper limit has not been determined. Like wild-type viruses, replication-competent avian vectors are able to carry out all aspects of the viral

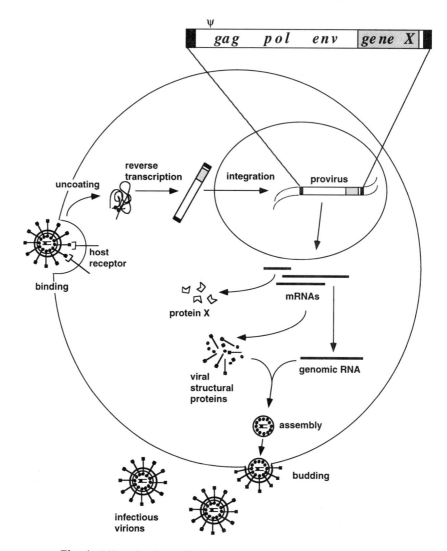

Fig. 1 Life cycle of a replication-competent retrovirus vector (see text).

life cycle, as well as encode an additional transgene (Fig. 1). Thus, the transgene can be spread from cell to cell, making experiments much less dependent on initial titers for widespread infection of a host embryo.

The choice of whether to use replication-defective or replication-competent vectors depends on the specific requirements of the experiment, taking into account the advantages and disadvantages of each. Some of these are listed in Table I. One of the most significant differences is that it is considerably easier to make viral stocks using replication-competent vectors as they are not depen-

Table I
Advantages and Disadvantages of Replication-Defective versus Replication-Competent Retroviral Vectors for Gene Transfer into Embryos

	Replication defective	Replication competent
Ease of making viral stocks	Harder, need packaging cells	Easy
Titer of unconcentrated virus	2×10^4–5×10^5/ml	2×10^5–5×10^6/ml
Limit on size of exogenous gene(s)	Approximately 10 kb	2.0–2.4 kb
Can encode multiple transgenes	Yes	Not practical
Envelope subgroups available	A, B	A, B, D, E
Widespread infection	Limited by initial titer	Yes, but can be limited by injection parameters or by transplantation protocols

dent on the use of specialized packaging cells. A second major advantage is that the overall extent of infection is much greater with replication-competent vectors because of their ability to spread beyond the initial population of infected cells. Obviously, though, this could be a detriment in certain experimental situations, where widespread gene transfer could prove lethal to embryos. Later in this chapter we provide methods to combine the use of viral infection of donor tissue with transplantation into resistant hosts, which can circumvent some of the potential drawbacks of global infection in embryos.

C. General Virology

1. Life Cycle of the Retrovirus

There are several aspects of the avian retroviral life cycle that are important to keep in mind when using these as tools for gene transfer into animals since retroviral infection involves an intimate relationship between the retrovirus and the infected host cells (Table II). The first point concerns the ability of the retrovirus to recognize the target cell. This binding and subsequent internalization of the retrovirus depends on both the specific envelope protein on the surface of the virion and the specific viral receptor on the surface of the host cell. Both features are, to some extent, under the control of the experimenter and may need to be optimized for the particular target tissue type as described later.

The second point is that the virus can only integrate into dividing cells during the mitotic (M) phase of the cell cycle as described for murine leukemia virus (Roe *et al.*, 1993). This aspect of the viral life cycle may place a limitation on the time during which a cell population is accessible to retrovirus-mediated gene transfer *in vivo*, if the target cells (such as neurons) do not remain mitotic throughout the life of the animal.

Table II
Relationship between Host Cell and Virus in the Retrovirus Life Cycle

Components of retroviral life cycle	Requirement	Viral genome
Binding to host cell	Envelope proteins and cell receptor on host cell	*env*
Internalization and uncoating of genomic RNA		?
Reverse transcription of genomic RNA into double-stranded DNA	Reverse transcriptase Viral LTRs, tRNA primer	*pol*
Integration into host cell genome	Integrase activity M phase of cycling host cell	*pol*, LTR
Transcription and RNA processing	Intact retroviral promoter; host cell transcriptional machinery;	LTR
	splicing from splice donor site (six amino acids into *gag* coding sequence) to splice acceptor sites in *env* and *src* (or transgene)	SD and SAs
Translation and post-translational processing	Host cell translational machinery, post-translational processing (e.g., glycosylation); proteolytic cleavage of precursor proteins	*gag* (PR)
Assembly of viral core	gag polypeptides	*gag*
Packaging of viral genomic RNA	Packaging sequences dispersed through the genome	
Budding off host cell	Envelope proteins	*env*

The third point concerns the splicing patterns of mRNAs utilized by ASLVs. Two or three distinct alternative mRNAs are generated for ASLVs or RSV, receptively. For RSV and RSV-derived vectors (such as RCASBP), the three alternative splice variants are shown schematically in Fig. 2. The full-length RNA can be packaged into new virions as genomic RNA or it can be used as the mRNA for the viral core proteins (MA, p10, CA, NC, PR), all encoded by *gag*. A translational frame shift of the same mRNA produces the enzymes reverse transcriptase (RT) and integrase (IN). A shorter transcript generated by alternative splicing is used for translating the viral envelope proteins, SU and TM. Finally, the shortest splice variant is used for the translation of the exogenous transgene (or *src* in the case of RSV). In most cases, this short transcript makes up about 20–30% of the virally encoded RNAs and so is fairly abundant. This alternative splice places a practical upper limit on the level of expression achieved. Alteration of the splice acceptor site or the 5′-untranslated sequences can be used to reduce expression below this amount.

The fourth point is that, once in the cell, both transcription and splicing of viral sequences are not discernibly cell-type specific. Thus tissue specificity of expression is controlled largely by regulating the scope of infection, as detailed later.

RCASBP/ X

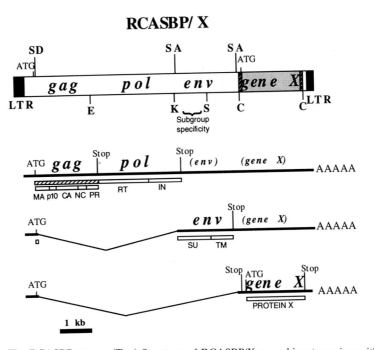

Fig. 2 The RCASBP vector. (Top) Structure of RCASBP/X recombinant provirus with the sequence of gene X inserted at the *Cla*I site. Polylinker sequences (not to scale) are indicated as hatched bars on either side of gene X. Key restriction sites in the generation of the vector are indicated: E, *Eco*RI; K, *Kpn*I; S, *Sal*I; C, *Cla*I. The E–K fragment was used to insert the Bryan high titer polymerase gene, whereas the K–S fragment was used to insert envelope genes of different subgroups. LTR, long terminal repeat; SA, splice acceptor; SD, slice donor. (Bottom) Solid lines: three resulting RNA variants, with the splicing indicated. Stop refers to the presence of a stop codon. Open bars beneath each mRNA indicate the precursor proteins encoded by each and the final protein products generated by proteolytic cleavage. CA, capsid; IN, integrase; MA, matrix; NC, nucleoprotein; PR, protease; RT, reverse transcriptase; SU, surface (receptor-binding); TM, transmembrane. Nomenclature according to Leis *et al.* (1988).

The fifth point to note is that many hours may be required for the series of steps initiated by binding of the virus to the host cell, culminating in physiological levels of protein expression. In a developing organism, this can be an important and perhaps limiting variable. We have empirically determined that the MA (matrix) core protein is detectable by immunohistochemistry within 18 hr of injection into the neural tube cavity of embryos, while no protein is detectable at 10 hr. During the first several days of embryonic development, 10–18 hr is considerable, and this should be taken into account when designing experiments.

2. Envelope Subgroups

The viral surface protein, or SU, is a glycosylated protein that is tethered to the cell surface by a transmembrane protein, TM. Sequence variability within

SU defines five major subgroups of ASLVs, designated envelope subgroups A,B,C,D, and E. These distinctions are based on which receptors they interact with on host cells (i.e., tropism) and their ability to block each other from superinfecting a host cell (i.e., interference). Several small regions of the viral *env* gene are responsible for these differences in envelope subgroups (Dorner *et al.*, 1985). The variable regions are included within a 1.1-kb *Kpn*I–*Cla*I fragment; this fragment has been swapped in order to make vectors of different subgroups (see Fig. 2). To date, RCASBP is available in subgroups A, B, D, and E. RCANBP, a vector that is similar to RCASBP but has no splice acceptor, is available in subgroups A, B and D. It is important to note that the infection efficiency of all subgroups, with the exception of A, is improved by the presence of polybrene (see Section III).

Often viral constructs differing in their envelope subgroup may be under construction simultaneously in the laboratory, raising the potential of cross-contamination. PCR primers have been designed to distinguish between envelope subgroups A, B, and E (D. J. Goff, D. M. Fekete, and C. L. Cepko, unpublished) by choosing sequences in the hypervariable regions (Dorner *et al.*, 1985). We routinely use these to verify that plasmid DNA used for transfections to generate viral stocks is subgroup specific. They can also be used on DNA prepared from producer cells to detect the presence of contaminating provirus. The primers are listed in Section II,B.

3. Host Cell Receptor Types

The lack of cross interference between the different envelope subgroups suggests that each viral subgroup interacts with a distinct receptor protein. Among ASLV receptors, only the A subgroup receptor has been identified (Young *et al.*, 1993). When this receptor is compared with the few other retroviral receptors that have been cloned, no clear relationship is evident; that is, they do not all form members of a family (Odorizzi and Trowbridge, 1994). Because of the importance of cellular receptor proteins in mediating viral infection, it should be emphasized that they can, in theory, pose a significant limitation on the ability of the virus to infect a target population of cells. However, since the receptors for the B, D, and E envelope subgroups have not yet been identified, very little is known about the distribution of specific viral receptors on different cells and tissues during embryogenesis. Empirical data concerning this issue are described in Section III,C.

4. Chicken Strains

Related to the issue of viral tropism is the existence of strains of chickens that differ in their susceptibility or resistance to different envelope subgroups. Viral resistance to ASLV subgroups is denoted by a standard nomenclature, e.g., C/E chickens (or cells) are resistant to the E envelope subgroup, C/A,B are resistant to A and B envelope subgroups, and C/O are not resistant to any of the five subgroups. Variability among chickens has practical considerations for retrovirus-mediated gene transfer.

First, standard chicken strains that are purchased through commercial vendors are typically C/E, although this need not be true for every bird in the flock. For most chicken strains, multiple loci exist that contain E subgroup sequences; these are referred to as endogenous viruses (Crittenden, 1991). Despite these endogenous viral sequences, such birds are adequate for most experiments in which A, B, or D subgroup viruses are used. A strain of chickens susceptible to the E subgroup virus does exist, called line $15b_1$ (C/O).

Second, line 0 chicken cells (C/E) are desirable for growing viral stocks as they do not contain any of the known ASLV endogenous viruses. This minimizes the chance of recombination beween the exogenous virus being introduced into the cells and cryptic endogenous viruses. Third, if multiple replication-competent plasmid constructs and viral stocks are being generated in the laboratory simultaneously, the possibility exists of getting cross-contamination in the stocks. It was mentioned previously that envelop-specific PCR primers can be used to verify the subgroup specificity of the plasmid DNA or the proviruses in the producer cells. As an alternative, cells derived from different strains of chickens can be used to test the subgroup specificity of the stocks. Table IV lists several strains that are available (at least part of the year) from the USDA Poultry Research Laboratory.

Finally, the availability of both resistant and sensitive strains has been used to advantage for gene transfer. It is possible to create chimeras consisting of a resistant embryo that has received an implant or transplant derived from a sensitive strain (Riddle et al., 1993; Fekete and Cepko, 1993b). Viral infection and transgene expression in such chimeras are then limited to the transplanted cells or tissues as detailed in Section IV,B,1.

D. Optimizing Retrovirus-Mediated Expression in Chick Embryos

It is imperative that pilot studies be conducted in order to optimize infection of the tissue or cell type of choice for the requirements of the experiment. These requirements vary widely and focus on considerations of the size of the infection domain required at a given time of development, the percentage of the cells in this domain that must be infected, and the degree to which the infection must be constrained to that domain over the course of the experiment. The nature of the transduced protein and its role in development will define these requirements. For a secreted signaling molecule, incomplete infection of a region may be sufficient and small regions of infection may suffice to mimic naturally occurring sources of the protein. For a transcription factor involved in regulating the interactions of cells in a development field, it may be necessary to infect every cell within a large developmental primordium such as that of a rhombomere or even a limb bud. The degree to which infection must be restricted to an initial target region will also vary with the insert. Many genes have discrete developmental windows within which they may exert their activity. Spread outside the target region subsequent to this developmental window may be irrelevant. Other genes may have profound effects outside the target region and may require more rigorous restriction.

Four basic aspects of virus biology impinge on the process of determining the site, timing, and extent of initial infection that will result in the appropriate viral spread. The first is that virus uptake is receptor mediated. To achieve infection or spread, the cell must express the appropriate receptor for the virus subtype. This is particularly important for initial infection where receptor density may normally limit the apparent titer of a viral inoculum. Most studies addressing the tissue tropism of RSV vectors *in vivo* suffer from bias inherent in the infection protocol, and it is advisable to test this directly for the different virus subgroups. Particularly at early stages of development, different results may be achieved with different subgroups (see Section III,E,5).

The second aspect of virology is that *in vivo,* the virus spreads largely from cell to adjacent cell in solid tissues, even when those tissues border on a luminal space (e.g., the neural tube). This makes the spread of infection predictable within the other constraints described.

The third aspect of virus biology is the fact that the virus can only integrate into the genome of replicating cells. Therefore, quiescent cells are resistant to initial infection and serve as barriers to viral spread. Furthermore, the spread of virus is more rapid in tissues containing rapidly dividing cells, thereby exaggerating both the clonal expansion effect of rapid proliferation as well as the inhibitory effects on the spread into adjacent tissues which divide at a slower rate.

Finally, basement membranes surrounding endothelia and epithelia appear to serve as effective barriers to viral spread, at least over short developmental periods (unpublished observations).

Given these observations, the design of an infection protocol must consider the number, position, and density of initial infection foci which can be generated by injection and the manner in which those foci will spread as developmental proceeds. In a practical sense, there are two basic types of injections: injections into solid tissue and injections into confined cavities. In luminal injections, sufficient virus may be delivered to infect every cell lining the lumen, provided that they have receptors and are dividing. As such, these injection protocols are much less dependent on viral spread to achieve large domains of infection. In contrast, very few viral particles may be delivered to a solid tissue by injection. Therefore, the subsequent spread of isolated foci of infection is more important in these protocols. Specific protocols for each type will be described later, but two general considerations apply to most experiments.

The first is that most experimental designs will call for injection of as little as $0.01–1.0$ μl of concentrated virus per embryo. As a result, perhaps the single most important factor in optimizing infection is the generation of a virus stock with high titer (expressed as IU/ml, infectious units/ml). Viral titers of greater than 10^6 IU/ml before concentration and greater than 10^8 IU/ml after concentration are routinely obtained using procedures outlined below, and titers over 10^9 are achievable. In our hands, a viral stock of less than 5×10^7 IU/ml would not be considered useful for high efficiency infection of either the limb bud or the neural tube.

The second observation is that there is a lag between the binding of the virus to the cell and expression of the transduced gene which may be as much as 12-18 hr and must be accounted for in designing an infection protocol. Although infection earlier in development may circumvent this problem, there appears to be some constraint on infection prior to stage 8. The difficulty in achieving infection at early stages may vary with viral subtype and/or tissue type, and should be investigated for the tissue of interest.

II. Materials

A. Plasmids

RCASBP(A), RCASBP(B), RCASBP(D)

RCANBP(A), RCANBP(B) (contact S. Hughes; National Cancer Institute, Frederick, MD)

RCASBP/AP(A), RCASBP/AP(B), RCASBP/AP(E), RCASBP(E) CLA 12, SLAX 12, pRD-4 (contact the authors)

B. PCR Primers

rcas-5′	ACGCTTTTGTCTGTGTGCTGC (does not bind RCANBP)
DMF04	ATCTCTGCAATGCGGAATTCAGTG
SX12	ACGTGGGACGTGCAGCCG
Aenv3′	CAGCGGTACTGCTGCCCCACC
Aenv5′	CTCCTTAGACGCCCCCTCTTTC
Benv3′	ATCCTTTTGACCGACCCAG
Benv5′	CCCCACACATCCTGACAAAT
Eenv3′	TCTGCACATCTCCACAGGTGTAAA
Eenv5′	CTTGATCGCCCCGTGGGTCAATCC

C. Equipment and Supplies

3C2 hybridoma supernatant (Potts *et al.*, 1987) (Developmental Studies Hybridoma Bank, Department of Biology, University of Iowa)

Eggs: SPAFAS, Inc. for SPF-11 (usually C/E) fertilized eggs; see Table III for other strains

Wooden, rotating egg incubator from Petersime (Gettysburg, OH)

Benchtop metal egg incubator from Kuhl (Flemington, NJ)

Stoelting microsyringe pump (catalog No. 51219) with standard gears

Stoelting 55023 Prior tilt arm micromanipulator with 55038 post stand magnetic base

Hamilton No. 1507 gas-tight 100- and 50µl Luer-lock syringes

Microcapillaries: 100 mm o.d. × 0.75 mm i.d. × 100 mm Omega Dot (FHA Brunswick ME)

18.5-gauge syringe needle (Luer mount)

Tygon B44-4X tubing

Egg holders: 0.5-in. rings cut from 1.5-in. diameter plastic pipe and notched on opposing sides

Dolan Jenner A3200 fiber optic illuminator fitted with IR and daylight conversion filters

Daylight conversion filter for stereoscope objective (Tiffen A80).

III. Methods

A. Virus Construction

1. Insert Design

The first step in virus construction is the generation of an appropriate insert. Total insert size should be less than 2.4 kb and no minimum size is required; smaller inserts may be favored. Sequences that interfere with full-length transcription of the virus or normal spicing of the viral transcripts are not tolerated. The minimal requirements beyond the coding sequence include *Cla*I ends. Since translation of the inserted coding region involves translation termination and reinitiation, extensive sequences 5' to the initiation codon of the inserted sequences may decrease translation. The *Cla* 12 adapter plasmid has a convenient polylinker between two *Cla*I sites and may be used to generate *Cla*I ends (Fig. 3) (Hughes *et al.*, 1987). Subcloning into this vector can prove an efficient way to generate an insert which may be excised by *Cla*I digestion and inserted into the RCASBP and RCANBP vectors.

When high levels of expressed protein are required, it is desirable to append the 5'-untranslated region of *src* to the coding region. This has been found to confer efficient expression on heterologous coding sequences (S. H. Hughes, personal communication; B. A. Morgan, unpublished). The *Cla* 12 NCO adapter plasmid was designed to add the 5'-untranslated region of the *src* gene to the sequences that are to be expressed (Hughes *et al.*, 1987). SLAX 12 was constructed by transferring the *Cla*I to *Cla*I fragment of this adapter plasmid to a pBluescript (Stratagene) derivative to add the copy number advantages and t3 and t7 primer-binding sites of the Bluescript backbone to the *Cla* 12 NCO polylinker (Fig. 3). To avoid altering the N terminus of the encoded protein, the coding sequences must be fused in frame with the ATG of the SLAX 12 *Nco*I site. The sequence

Cla 12

ATC GAT AAG CTC GGA ATT CGA GCT CGC CCG GGG ATC CTC TAG AGT CGA CCT GCA GCC
Cla 1   Eco R1 Sac 1 Sma 1Bam H1 Xba 1 Sal 1 Pst 1

CAA GCT TAT CGA T
Hind III Cla 1

SLAX 12 NCO

ATT AAC CCT CAC TAA AGG GAA CAA AAG CTG GAG CTC ATC GAT TCT AGA CCA CTG TGG
        T3 Primer   Cla1

CCA GGC GGT ACG TGG GAC GTG CAG CCG ACC ACC ATG GCC ATG ATT ACG AAT TCG AGC
            SX12 Primer   Nco1   Eco R1

TCG CCC GGG GAT CCT CTA GAG TCG ACC TGC AGC CCA AGC TTA TCG ATA CCG TCG ACC
    Sma 1Bam H1   Pst1   Hind III Cla1

TCG AGG GGG GGC CCG GTA CCC AAT TCG CCC TAT AGT GAG TCG TAT T
Xho 1   Apa 1   Kpn 1   T7 Primer

Fig. 3 Adapter plasmids. The polylinker regions of the adapter plasmids *Cla* 12 (top) (Hughes *et al.*, 1987) and SLAX 12 NCO (bottom). The 5′ to 3′ strand is shown. The T3, T7, and SX12 primer-binding sites are shown as arrows below the sequence which indicate the orientation of the primer (arrowhead 3′). SLAX 12 NCO was constructed by inserting a *Cla*I linker adjacent to the *Sac*I site in pBluescript II SK+ (Stratagene) and replacing the *Cla*I to *Cla*I fragment of the resulting plasmid with the *Cla*I to *Cla*I interval of *Cla* 12 NCO (Hughes *et al.*, 1987).

surrounding the initiator codon of the insert dictates which of the three methods are used to insert the coding region in SLAX 12. When the initiator codon of the protein is embedded in an *Nco*I site (CCATGG), direct cloning into this plasmid is straightforward. When the nucleotides directly upstream of the initiator ATG are not a pair of cytidines, but the second codon begins with a guanine (+4 nucleotide), mutagenesis of the insert sequence to an *Nco*I site will not affect the coding regions and may be followed by cloning into the SLAX 12 vector. This involves a two-step approach in which mutagenesis is performed on a short stretch between the region upstream of the ATG of the insert and some unique downstream site which is also found in the SLAX 12 polylinker. This segment may be cloned into SLAX 12 and sequenced with the t3 and t7 primers, which flank the polylinker. The remaining coding sequences can then be added, thereby avoiding inadvertent mutagenesis of the downstream sequences during PCR amplification of the full-length gene.

When the +4 nucleotide is not a guanidine, a third strategy must be employed to generate an *Nco*I compatible 5′ overhang (5′-C-A-T-G). This can be achieved by PCR with a primer that adds a 5′ cytosine to the coding sequences, followed by digestion with exonuclease III to generate single-stranded 5′ overhangs (Fig.

198   Bruce A. Morgan and Donna M. Fekete

4). When convenient unique sites occur in the coding sequence to be mutagenized, it is preferable to amplify a relatively small piece to avoid inadvertent mutagenesis. This piece may then be easily sequenced before the remaining downstream

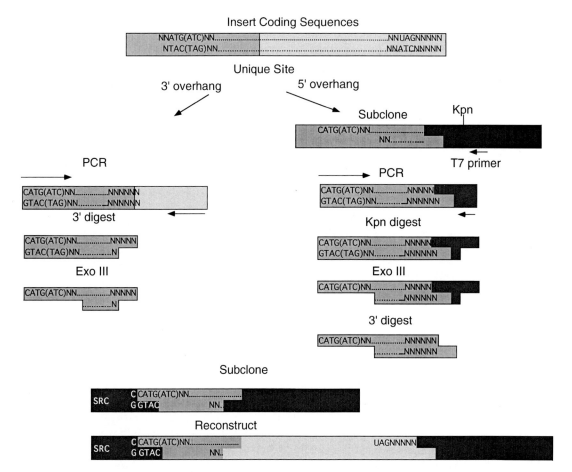

Fig. 4 NCO mutagenesis. Strategy for generating an *Nco*I compatible 5′ overhang without altering the coding sequences. (Left) Strategy when a unique restriction site which generates a 3′ overhang upon digestion is present in the insert sequences. (Right) Strategy when the only unique sites generate 5′ overhangs upon digestion. In this case, the fragment is subcloned into pBluescript II SK. A site in the vector is then used as the unique 3′ overhang (shown as *Kpn*I). PCR is then performed between a primer with the sequence CATG N$_{15}$ (where ATG N15 is the 5′ end of the coding sequences to be inserted) and a 3′ primer from the coding sequence (left) or the plasmid backbone (shown as T7 primer at right). Digestion of the 3′ end with the appropriate restriction enzyme results in the generation of an exonuclease III-resistant 3′ overhang. Brief exonuclease III digestion then converts the 5′ blunt end to a 5′ overhang. This fragment is then cloned into SLAX 12 NCO at the *Nco*I site. The 3′ coding sequences from the original insert are then inserted into this plasmid to reconstruct the insert with the *src*-untranslated region appended to the 5′ end.

sequence is appended to it by a subsequent ligation. A restriction site that occurs once in the insert and generates a 3′ overhang upon digestion is preferable for the 3′ end of the amplified product since such sites are resistant to exonuclease III digestion (Fig. 4). If such a site is not available, it may be preferable to subclone the fragment to be amplified into pBluescript II SK which contains an ample polylinker flanked by 3′ overhang sites. In this case, the t3 or t7 primer may be used for the 3′ PCR primer. If subcloning is omitted, the 3′ primer shoud be synthesized from a sequence downstream of the unique site used for the construction.

1. Primers:

    5′: CATGN$_{15}$ where N15 is the coding sequence from +4 to +18.
    3′: 19 nt of coding sequence running 3′-5′ and downstream of the restriction site used for construction. Alternatively, a primer binding the flanking plasmid may be used.

2. PCR: PCR in a 50-μl reaction using a 100-ng template, 100 pmol each primer (5′ primer should be phosphorylated) for 15 cycles.
3. Phenol extract and ethanol precipitate the product.
4. Generate blunt ends by polishing with 1 unit of T4 DNA polymerase in the presence of 100 μM dNTPS at 37°C for 15 min.
5. Phenol extract and ethanol precipitate.
6. Cleave the 3′ restriction site with the appropriate enzyme, then heat inactivate and ethanol precipitate.
7. Resuspend in 50 μl of Exo III buffer. Remove 5 μl and reserve for gel analysis. Add 100 units of Exo III and incubate at room temperature for 3 min. Phenol extract and purify on a low melt agarose gel. The band should be fuzzy when compared with the undigested control and shifted to a slightly lower molecular weight.
8. Ligate to appropriate digested and gel-purified SLAX 12 vector. After sequence analysis has confirmed the integrity of the mutagenized insert, the 3′ coding sequences should be appended by digesting this plasmid with the unique 3′ restriction site and some site in the 3′ polylinker to accept an appropriate fragment from the original coding sequence plasmid.

2. Virus Assembly

The choice of vector subtypes is dictated by considerations described earlier. It is advisable to clone the insert into both RCASBP and RCANBP of the corresponding envelope subgroup. RCANBP differs from RCASBP by lack of the splice acceptor upstream of the *Cla*I insertion site (Fig. 2). This virus serves as a control for nonspecific effects of infection with a virus of a similar genomic structure since the inserted coding sequences will not be translated in the host cell. The vectors are digested with *Cla*I, dephosphorylated with alkaline phosphatase, gel purified, and ligated to the *Cla*I insert generated earlier. The resultant plasmid is quite large and only moderate in copy number. The colonies resulting from transformation with this plasmid are often discernibly smaller than colonies derived from transformation with a contaminating vector in the insert preparation.

Orientation of the insert is conveniently determined by PCR using a primer that binds in the insert and primers binding adjacent to the insertion site in the RCASBP vector (Fig. 5). If SLAX 12 is routinely used, the SX12 primer from the *src*-untranslated sequence may be used in lieu of a specific primer from the inserted coding sequence (primer X in Fig. 5). Parallel reactions with the internal primer and either rcas5′ or rcas3′ are performed. This reaction consists of 100 ng of template plasmid, 50 pmol of each primer, 100 μM dNTPS, $1 \times Taq$ buffer containing 2 mM MgCl$_2$, and 0.5 units of *Taq* polymerase for 20 cycles of {93°C (45 sec); 52°C (45 sec); 72°C (1 hr 45 sec)}. Both flanking primers are within 50 nt of the *Cla*I insertion site. Amplified product with the DMF-04 primer but not with the rcas5′ primer in conjunction with a 5′ to 3′ internal primer is indicative of appropriate orientation for insert expression. The opposite result indicates that the virus will encode an antisense transcript. Orientation of the insert can also be determined by sequencing the plasmid with the rcas5′ primer which hydridizes just upstream of the insertion site.

B. Virus Production

1. CEF Production and Culture

Primary cultures of chicken embryo fibroblasts (CEFs) must be produced from a strain compatible with the virus subtype to be used (see Table IV). The QT6 quail cell line is not recommended for growing virus stocks: although QT6 cells

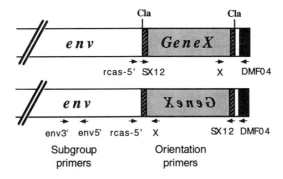

Fig. 5 Primers for PCR amplification for determining subgroup specificity of the virus and orientation of the insert (see text).

can be infected as efficiently as CEFs (and thus used for titering, see later) they grow RCOS, RCAS, and RCASBP very poorly when compared to CEFs (S. H. Hughes, personal communication). Line 0 is used for all subgroups except E. This procedure describes a technique for pooling four to six embryos to generate CEFs. An alternative approach, which may yield healthier cultures, is to prepare CEFs separately from each of six embryos, grow for several days, and choose the line that is growing the fastest (S. H. Hughes, personal communication). CEF cultures produced in this manner will survive for 4 to 6 weeks in culture.

Reagents

Ethanol-sterilized surgical instruments (forceps, razor blade)

Stir bar, autoclaved

125- or 250-ml Erlenmeyer flask, autoclaved

One dozen eggs, incubated for 10 days

Fetal calf serum (FCS)

0.25% trypsin–1 mM EDTA (GIBCO)

Dimethyl sulfoxide (DMSO)

Dulbecco's modified Eagle's medium (DMEM; high glucose, glutamine, sodium pyruvate)

1. Wear gloves (ethanol-sterilized). Place the embryo in a petri dish. Cut off limbs and head with the razor blade and remove viscera with forceps.
2. Collect four or five embryos in a 10-cm petri dish and mince well with a razor blade.
3. Transfer tissue with a 5-ml wide-mouth pipette into an Erlenmeyer flask with 10 ml of 37°C trypsin solution. Digestion with dispase and collagenase may yield healthier cultures (S. H. Hughes, personal communications). Add stir bar and mix at low speed for 15 min. Small pieces of tissue should begin to dissolve.
4. Allow big chunks to settle for about 5 min and transfer supernatant to sterile 50-ml plastic centrifuge tube.
5. Add an equal volume of 100% FCS. Invert to mix. Repeat step 4.
6. Spin at 1000 rpm with a clinical centrifuge for 5 min at room temperature. Save pellet.
7. Resuspend pellet in 10 ml of 100% FCS and spin again.
8. Resuspend pellet in chick culture media (10% FCS, 2% chicken serum in DMEM).
9. Plate cells into multiple 10-cm tissue culture plates at three different concentrations: 10^7, 10^6, or 3×10^5 cells/plate.
10. Check the cells and change the media daily. Expect to see many floating and dead cells in the first few days. In a few days, surviving cells begin to grow very quickly. Choose the fastest growing dishes with the fewest dead

cells to freeze. When the cells are confluent, trypsinize and split 1:4. One to 2 days later when the cells reach 80% confluence, collect by trypsinization, resuspend in 3 ml of 10% FCS, 12% DMSO in DMEM, and freeze in 1-ml aliquots. Upon thawing each 1-ml aliquot, plate the cells into two 6-cm plates. One plate can be used as the stock by passaging every other day at 1:4 and 1:8 dilutions.

2. Transfection and Amplification of Producer Populations

Since the entire process of generating a producer stock takes 7–12 days, a recent thaw of CEFs derived from a strain permissive for the vector class should be employed. Allow these cells to recover from thawing for several days. When they are growing rapidly, proceed with transfection. Because the virus will spread, almost any transfection protocol will suffice. The following protocol works well. Other protocols may be substituted, but DEAE dextran is toxic to CEFs and should not be used (S. H. Hughes, personal communication).

Reagents
2× HEPES-buffered saline (280 mm NaCl, 50 mM HEPES, 105 mM Na$_2$HPO$_4$, pH 7.05)
15% glycerol in phosphate-buffered saline (PBS)
250 mM CaCl$_2$
PBS
8 mg/ml polybrene in H$_2$O, stored at $-20°C$ in 1-ml aliquots

1. Split a densely confluent 6-cm plate 1:6 and incubate overnight.
2. Generate a DNA precipitate by dissolving 6 μg of super-coiled plasmid in 500 μl of 250 mM CaCl$_2$ and then adding 500 μl of 2X HEBS dropwise with rapid agitation. Allow the DNA suspension stand at room temperature for 15 min until a fine-grained precipitate forms.
3. Remove media from the plate and add 1 ml media and the DNA precipitate.
4. Incubate for 10 min at 37°C and then add an additional 8 ml of media.
5. Incubate for 4 hr at 37°C.
6. Remove the media and add 2 ml 15% glycerol. Incubate for 90 sec and then add 10 ml PBS. Aspirate the PBS and wash two more times with PBS. Add media and incubate at 37°C. Note that all viral subgroups except A should be grown in the presence of 8 μg per ml polybrene added to the media from a 1000× stock solution.
7. Cells should be passaged for a week or more to ensure that the virus spreads through the culture. Splitting the cells 1:4 at confluence keeps them growing rapidly. The culture should be amplified to five 15-cm plates during this period. At the last split (to 15-cm dishes), an aliquot of the cells should be plated on a chamber slide or a 24-well culture dish to assess the extent

of infection by staining with an antibody to the viral MA protein (see Section III,B,5).

3. Virus Harvest

When cells are first confluent after the last split, replace media with a minimal volume (12 ml) of low serum media [either 2% FCS, 0.2% chick serum in DMEM or 10% NuSerum V (Collaborative Biomedical Products, Bedford, MA) in DMEM]. The lower serum content of the media makes it easier to resuspend the concentrated virus and does not affect the titer for most preparations. After 24 hr, remove media and filter through a 0.45-μm cellulose acetate filter with a glass fiber prefilter (Costar). Collect the filtrate and save two small aliquots for titration. The remainder may be aliquoted for use as an unconcentrated stock, concentrated directly, or, in most cases, frozen for subsequent concentration. Add fresh media and repeat the harvest over the next 2 days. Following the last virus collection, rinse one plate with PBS, scrape the cells into a centrifuge tube, pellet, and freeze for subsequent analysis if necessary (see later). Depending on the virus and confluence of the cells, the titers of the unconcentrated viral stocks should vary between 5×10^5 and 10^7 IU/ml. Since there may be variations between the different collections, they should be processed separately to achieve the highest titer possible. Although many viruses survive repeated freeze/thawing with only a mild loss of titer (twofold), others are more sensitive to freeze/thawing.

4. Virus Concentration and Storage

To concentrate the virus, centrifuge for 3 hr at 22,000 rpm in a Beckman SW 28 rotor at 4°C. Aspirate the supernatant, leaving a small volume (100–200 μl) over the pellet (which may not be visible). Shake gently on a rotating platform for 15 min on ice to resuspend the pellet. Resuspend by repeated gentle pipetting with a pipetteman, pool identical samples, and divide into 20-μl aliquots. Surprisingly, the yield may vary from 30 to 300%, and titers of 10^9 IU/ml may be achieved.

In general, virus stocks are frozen in liquid nitrogen and stored at −80°C. However, the stability of the virus may be affected by the inserted sequences. Aliquots smaller than 20 μl may lose titer upon prolonged storage in liquid nitrogen. Stable viruses maintain titer for months or years at −80°C.

5. Virus Titration

Approximate titer of the concentrated or unconcentrated virus stock can be determined by infection of CEFs or the quail cell line QT6 (see Table III). This is accomplished by serial dilutions of the virus and staining infected cultures 48 hr after infection. After this brief incubation, secondary spread of the virus does not result in darkly staining cells, and the progeny of a single infected cell can

Table III
Some Useful Strains of Chickens or Quails

Chicken strain	Susceptibility to viral infection		
	A subgroup	B subgroup	E subgroup
SPF-11[a]	+	+	−
Line 15b$_1$ (C/O)[b]	+	+	+
Line 0 (C/E)[b]	+	+	−
Line alv6 (C/A,E)[c]	−	+	−
Line C (C/A)[b]	−	+	+
QT6 cells (C/B)[d]	+	−	(+)
Line 7$_2$ (C/A,B,E)[b]	−	−	−

[a] The SPF-11 chickens currently sold by SPAFAS behave as C/E, although they are bred by crossing a C/O with a C/E strain, so the genotype can vary.

[b] Available from the USDA Poultry Research Laboratory, East Lansing, Michigan.

[c] Line alv6 is a transgenic chicken constituitively expressing A subgroup envelope protein (Federspiel et al., 1991).

[d] QT6 is a chemically induced fibroblast cell line derived from Japanese quail (Moscovici et al., 1977).

usually be identified. In practice, unconcentrated viruses with stable inserts usually have a titer of 10^5 to 10^7 IU/ml whereas concentrated viruses range from mid 10^6 to 10^9 IU/ml. To titer, plate CEFs at 20% of confluence in 6- or 24-well dishes and incubate overnight. Dilute virus stocks through 10^{-6} in tissue culture media. Aspirate media from successive wells and replace with 0.5 ml fresh media with 1 μl of a 10^{-6}, 10^{-5}, and 10^{-4} dilution of virus (concentrated) or a 10^{-4}, 10^{-3}, and 10^{-2} dilution (unconcentrated). Incubate for 48 hr, remove media, and fix for 15 min in 4% paraformaldehyde in PBS. Wash three times (5 min each) with PBS. Block with PBST (10% serum, 0.1% Triton X-100 in PBS) (10 min). Stain for 30 min with a 1:5 dilution of 3c2 monoclonal anti-MA in PBST. Wash three times with PBST. Detect with a Vecta Stain secondary detection kit (Vector Labs) as recommended by the manufacturer.

Failure to generate a high titer viral stock may make it difficult to achieve adequate infection. More importantly, it may indicate that the insert is either deleterious to the viral life cycle or deleterious to the producer cells. If this is the case, mutation or deletion of the offensive sequences are selected for during the multiple rounds of replication of the virus which occur in prep production and after injection into the embryo. The stability of the inserted sequence and expression level of the inserted protein should be confirmed for all viral stocks, particularly those which are difficult to generate at high titer.

6. Assaying Insert Stability and Expression

Where possible, the expression of the protein should be assayed by Western blotting of the protein from the producer cultures or assayed by some functional criteria. When an antibody to the encoded protein is not available, epitope tagging of the inserted sequences is advised if this addition does not affect protein function. A SLAXMYC vector encoding a myc epitope tag 3′ of the insertion site may be used to facilitate this process (U. Hofer and P. Goetinck, personal communication).

A comparison of the titer of RCASBP and RCANBP virus derivatives with the identical insert determines the source of any difficulty in generating a high titer stock. If the RCANBP virus reaches high titer in the normal time period but the RCASBP virus does not, this indicates that the encoded protein is interfering with the production of the virus or the proliferation of the cell. If both viruses grow slowly, this indicates that the DNA sequences themselves are interfering with virus propagation. Since illegitimate recombination is comparatively frequent during virus reproduction, deleterious sequences may be removed from the insert by deletion. The resulting virus will have a competitive advantage in subsequent rounds of replication both during prep production and after injection *in ovo.*

Deletions in the virus may be detected by amplification of the insert region of the provirus population in the producer culture. Cells frozen at the end of harvest may be used to determine if the insert remains in the majority of the proviruses. PCR between a primer 5′ to the insertion site (rcas5′) and a primer in the 3′ LTR (DMF-04) can be performed on genomic DNA from the producer cell population and amplification products can be compared to those generated by PCR on the starting plasmid construct. The presence of aberrant-sized bands suggest selection for deleted viruses.

It is possible to circumvent these problems by altering offensive sequences and minimizing the number of rounds of replication that occur both during the production of a viral stock and in the embryo after injection. However, where possible, the use of replication-incompetent vectors should be considered when these problems arise. The opportunity for selection for mutant viruses is thereby greatly reduced.

C. General Preparation

1. Lowering and Windowing Eggs

If the incubator used does not shift the eggs periodically, the embryo may stick to the egg shell which makes subsequent manipulations difficult. For injections after stage 12 or so, this can be avoided by removing 1 to 3 ml of albumin from the egg after a day of incubation. This protocol differs slightly from conventional approaches but is preferable for some of the specialized chick strains used. Place the eggs on their sides in a plastic egg tray. Squirt with 70% ethanol and air dry for 5–10 min. Using a 21-gauge needle attached to a 5-ml syringe, poke two holes in the egg—one at the upper (i.e., side) surface and one at the pointed end of the egg. Withdraw 1.5 ml of albumin from the pointed end. Cover both holes with clear tape. Using small curved scissors, pierce the tape on the upper surface and cut a hole in the shell about 0.5 in. in diameter. Peer in, locate the embryo, and enlarge the hole in a direction sufficient to expose the embryo.

Stage the embryo and then inject or return to the incubator for later use. If the yolk is damaged in this procedure (albumin is difficult to draw up or is cloudy and yellow), throw the egg away.

2. Needle Preparation

Injection needles are prepared by pulling glass capillaries on a pipette puller. Omega dot capillary pipettes (No. 30-30-0 1.0 mm o.d.; 0.75 mm i.d.; 100 mm long; FHC, Brunswick, ME) are pulled on a Flaming/Brown micropipette puller (Sutter) set to generate moderately tapered needles. Using a fine forceps, break the tip of the capillary to generate a tip with an outer diameter of approximately 10–15 μm. Pipettes that are fortuitously broken at an oblique angle tend to penetrate the tissue more easily than blunt tips. A supply of pulled capillaries should be prepared prior to injection.

3. Injection Setup

The injection syringe and a tube of mineral oil should be placed under vacuum to degas for 15 min. Fill the injection syringe with mineral oil, being sure to avoid bubbles. This may require removing the plunger and allowing the oil to flow through the barrel. Insert the plunger and expel all but enough oil to fill the injection capillary (usually about 25 μl). Attach the capillary to the syringe tubing and slowly fill with oil. Add 1/40 volume filter-sterilized Fast Green (1% in H_2O) and centrifuge for 30 sec at 6000 g to pellet the particulates. Place a drop (10 μl) of virus on a piece of Parafilm in a sterile plastic dish, lower the needle tip into the drop, and slowly backfill the syringe. The viscosity of the viral inoculum is considerable and it may take several minutes to fill the syringe. Be sure to adjust the plunger to generate slight positive pressure while observing the meniscus between inoculum and oil prior to removing the tip from the drop. After withdrawal the plunger should be adjusted to a slight positive pressure that is insufficient for forward flow while the needle tip is in the air. If injections are interrupted, the needle tip should be lowered into a bath of PBS to prevent clogging. Any leftover virus can be stored on ice for subsequent use if the needle fails.

The eggs are stabilized for all injections using homemade egg holders composed of hollow $\frac{1}{4}$ in. Plexiglas tubes, 1.5 in. in diameter, 0.5 in. high, with two opposing indentations designed to hold the eggs on their sides (see Fig. 6).

D. Prototype Injection Protocols for Solid Tissue

When designing an infection into solid tissue, the limiting factor is usually adequate infection. The volume of virus that is effectively delivered to a solid tissue is less than 0.01 μl. Hence viral titers in excess of 5×10^7 IU per ml are required for the reproducible infection of small clusters of cells at the injection

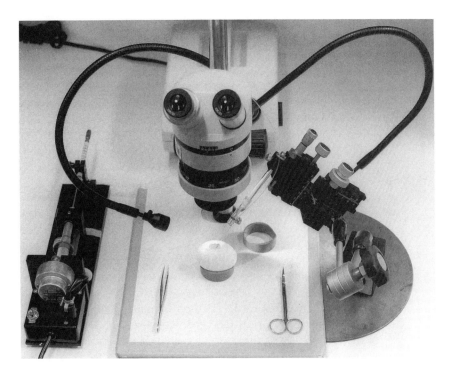

Fig. 6 Injection apparatus. A typical injection setup, including micromanipulator, microinjector, dissection microscope, fiber optics, and egg holder.

site. Broad patches of infection cannot be generated at the time of injection Instead, multiple independent foci of infection are generated by separate injections. Broad domains of infection are then generated by the subsequent spread and coalescence of the initial infections. Hence injection protocol strategies are dominated by considerations of infection spread and clonal expansion. The pattern of cell division in a tissue can be used to modulate the spread of the virus from the initial infection. In regions of rapid cell division, the virus spreads more efficiently to adjacent cells, compounding the clonal expansion of the infected cells. In regions of slower cell division, both viral spread and clonal expansion are decreased. Basement membranes or barriers of quiescent cells prevent viral spread.

The limb bud provides an excellent example of the use of growth characteristics of a tissue to modulate infection. The limb arises from the proliferation of lateral plate mesenchyme at stage 17. The nascent bud induces a specialized structure in the ectoderm along the distal tip of the limb, the apical ectodermal ridge (AER). The remarkable growth of the limb requires rapid cell division throughout the limb. However, the distal outgrowth of the limb is dependent on the hyperproliferation of the cells immediately adjacent to the AER in the so-called progress zone resulting in elongation by the preferential addition of cells at the distal margin. A cell infected in the progress zone will give rise to a clone of cells arranged in a wedge that extends distally from the position of the cell at the time of injection. Spread of the infection of this clone occurs most rapidly in the hyperproliferative progress zone, leading to the exaggeration of the wedge shape of the domain of infection. Proximal spread of the infection is comparatively minimal.

In contrast, injection of the virus into more proximomedial regions away from the progress zone does not result in a clear bias between proximal and distal spread of infection and can result in localized patches of infection. Thus, sectors starting at almost any level along the proximal/distal (P/D) axis and extending distally may be generated by varying the time at which cells beneath the AER are infected. Local infections along the P/D axis may be generated only after this region of the bud has been displaced from the progress zone. Examples generated at a specific stage in limb development are diagrammed in Fig. 7A. Saunders' (1948) AER extirpation experiments provide an accurate map of the time at which various regions along the P/D axis of the limb are displaced from the progress zone.

For many experiments, limited regions of altered gene expression within the limb may be preferred. The protocols listed in Section III,D,1 for injection onto the limb bud will achieve this result. The stage of the embryo at infection and the position of the injection will determine the resulting domain of infection. Multiple injections into a single limb bud may be employed to achieve larger infection domains. In principle, complete infection of the limb bud may be achieved by multiple injections in the progress zone of a very young limb bud. However, it is much more practical to generate a few foci of infection early in development in the lateral plate mesenchyme that includes the limb bud precursors. These foci spread to encompass much of the presumptive limb mesenchyme by stage 19, including the progress zone. From this point on, the progressively added distal cells will be infected. Natural boundaries restrict further viral spread. The margins of the limb serve as one limit to infection spread while the lower proliferative rate of the flank mesenchyme inhibits spread along the body axis and the neural tube basement membrane inhibits the spread of infection across the midline. It has been empirically determined that microinjection of the lateral plate mesenchyme of a stage 10 embryo achieves this result. Injection protocols for complete infection of the limb bud are described in Section III,D,2.

1. Limb Bud Injection Protocol

1. If albumin has not been removed previously, do so prior to windowing the egg (see Section III,C,1).
2. Cut a small window in the dorsal surface of the egg with a curved iris scissors.
3. To inject the subridge mesenchyme, orient the AER in the region to be injected parallel to the long axis of the injection capillary under 20–40×

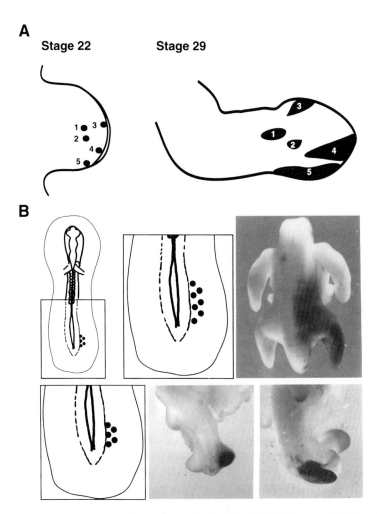

Fig. 7 Limb infections. (A) Focal infection of the limb bud. (Left) A stage 22 right wing bud. Numbered dots represent points of injection of a 1×10^8 IU/ml virus stock. (Right) The resulting domains of infection in a stage 29 wing 2.5 days later. Note that injections dorsal and proximal to the progress zone (1,2) lead to isolated patches of infection in the limb mesenchyme. In contrast, injection into the progress zone at various points along the A/P axis (3,4,5) lead to sectors of infection extending from within the manus to the distal tip of the limb. (B) Infection of the limb bud precursors. (Left) A late stage 10 embryo. The area in the box is magnified to show the array of injections used to infect the limb bud primordia. (Right) An array of seven injection sites used to completely infect the limb bud and surrounding flank. (Far right) The infection resulting from this infection protocol detected as the dark alkaline phosphatase precipitation product generated by whole mount *in situ* hybridization with a probe to the viral RNA. Although infection extends into the anterior flank, it is still restricted to the right side of the embryo and does not include the wing bud or the tail. The array of five injection sites shown below results in infection restricted to the limb bud. (Left) Infected embryos at stage 21 and 24. The viral message has been detected by whole mount *in situ* hybridization with a probe to the inserted cDNA and is detected as a dark alkaline phosphatase precipitation product. Note that the infection encompasses the entire limb bud and is largely restricted to the limb bud at these stages. Lighter staining in the other limb buds of the embryo at the far right reflects expression of the endogenous gene and is not a result of infection.

magnification. The amnion should be removed from the area above the limb in embryos beyond stage 20. Injection at an approximately 45° angle with the plane of the AER is effective. The virus must be delivered within 1–200 μm of the AER to ensure infection in the progress zone. A very fine needle with a tip diameter under 10 μm should be used to facilitate penetration of the tissue. For injections outside the progress zone, the injection needle can be oriented facing proximally along the proximal distal axis of the limb.

4. Cover the window with transparent cellophane tape and incubate in stationary racks.

2. Infection of Limb Bud Precursors

1. Prepare the embryo as described earlier. When incubated at 99.7°F, SPAFAS SPF eggs will reach stage 10 after approximately 36 hr of incubation. Precise staging is crucial for reproducible infections.

2. Orient the axis of the embryo perpendicular to the micropipette with the tail closest to you under 10–20× magnification. The embryo has very little contrast at this stage and is more easily viewed if both the illumination source and the microscope objective are fitted with blue (daylight correction) filters. Slight positive pressure on the injection syringe should be set to flow slowly when the tip is immersed in an embryo but not flow when in the tip is in air. Pressure may be adjusted by gently tapping the plunger.

3. Bring the tip of the needle to the surface of the embryo and orient the tip over the lateral plate by moving the embryo. Extend the needle into the embryo. If the embryo is substantially distorted by this process, the needle is too blunt and a finer needle should be tried. Insert the needle into the embryo. If the tip of the needle is in the subembryonic space, the inoculum will appear fuzzy and diffuse rapidly. Slowly withdraw the needle tip until it is in the mesenchyme. At this point, flow from the needle will slow and be focused in a sharp dot and will not appear diffuse. Withdraw the needle slowly, shift the embryo, and repeat the injection. A closely spaced array of three to five injections is sufficient to completely infect the limb bud (see Fig. 7B). A larger number of injections leads to a high percentage of completely infected limb buds early in development, but the adjacent flank may also be infected. The smaller number of injections results in more restricted infection, but the limb bud may be only partially infected in some embryos. If it is necessary to avoid ectodermal infection, withdraw the needle quickly to avoid injection of the virus on the ectodermal surface. The total volume of injected material in the mesenchyme is very small (0.01 μl). Injection of additional virus does not appear to be productive as it merely leaks into the yolk or supra ectodermal space and does not contribute to productive mesenchymal infection. Injection of additional virus on the dorsal surface can lead to scattered ectodermal infections.

4. Cover the window with transparent tape and incubate. Over the ensuing several days, a mortality of 5–10% is not uncommon, primarily due to the stress of injection rather than the resulting infection. Higher mortality rates may indicate toxic effects of viral infection.

E. Prototype Injection Protocols for Lumenal Spaces

What follows are general protocols that have been developed for the infection of ectodermally derived tissues, including the neural tube (and/or neural crest prior to emigration), the otocyst, the subretinal space, or the surface ectoderm (with an emphasis on infection of the otic placode). Embryo and needle setup are as described earlier. However, for reproducibility of lumenal injections it may be desirable to precisely control the volume of inoculate injected and a slightly different apparatus is used.

1. Injection Setup

A mechanical (motorized) microinjector is often used to deliver precise volumes to the neural tube when trying to optimize other variables (such as envelope subgroup, presence or absence of polybrene, time of injection). We use a Stoelting microsyringe pump (catalog No. 51219) with standard gears and a 100-μl Luer-lock Hamilton syringe. This apparatus delivers 1 μl of virus in 53 sec. Other gears are available from the manufacturer which will vary the rate of injection. Degas heavy mineral oil before using it to fill the tubing of the injector apparatus. Secure the tubing to the pipette slot of the micromanipulator. Since this tubing is rather inflexible, a 0.5 in. long piece of flexible Tygon tubing (B44-4X) is used to bridge the gap to the back end of the injection capillary. Push oil out to the tip of the pipette. Place a drop of virus on a piece of parafilm (not sterile) placed in a petri dish. Backfill the pipette with 4–5 μl of virus by manually pulling back the plunger of the microinjector syringe. Apply positive pressure before removing the pipette tip from the drop of virus.

2. Injection Protocol

In general, luminal spaces are relatively easy to target with the assistance of a micromanipulator. The key to observing structures prior to the development of the vasculature is to set the fiber optic to illuminate the embryo at a very oblique angle. This is easiest when the embryos are not very low in the egg (hence the removal of only 1.5 ml of albumen). Up until embryonic day 3 it is usually possible to insert the injection pipette directly through the amnionic membrane with a slight rapid advance of the micromanipulator. Pipettes that have difficulty penetrating the amnion or the tissue are best replaced immediately. After embryonic day 3, it is often helpful to use fine (No. 5) dissection forceps to tear a small hole in the amniotic membrane before lowering the pipette. The structure of interest can usually be injected by a novice within a single practice session.

3. Variation in Time of Injection into the Neural Tube

Although it might seem intuitively obvious that earlier injections will lead to more widespread infection in embryos, this has not been our experience at early stages of development (Fekete and Cepko, 1993a). At least two drawbacks are associated with injections on the first day *in ovo* [i.e., prior to stage 8 of Hamburger and Hamilton (1951)]. First, the survival rate following viral injection decreases from 80–90% at stage 10 to 20% at stage 4/5 to 0% at stage 3. Second, even embryos that survive injections prior to stage 8 typically exhibit much lower levels of virus-mediated gene expression 48 hr later when compared to embryos injected after stage 8, at least with respect to infection of the neural tube (S. A. Homburger and D. M. Fekete, unpublished observations).

4. Variation in the Envelope Subgroup of the Virus

We had previously reported no differences between A and E subgroup viruses in their ability to infect the neural tube and/or neural crest (Fekete and Cepko, 1993a) using RCASBP vectors encoding alkaline phosphatase. For both A and E subgroups, the central nervous system was well infected 48 hr after injections into the neural tube at stage 13 and was rather poorly infected following injections at stages 8–10. By comparison, the neural crest was relatively well infected by injections at these earlier stages. This analysis has been extended to include the B subgroup and to include vectors either with or without alkaline phosphatase. The presence of the B subgroup virus, either alone or in the presence of the A subgroup, yields significant improvement (about threefold) in virus expression in the central nervous system or otic placode (Kiernan *et al.,* 1994). For example, 48 hr after injections of A+B vectors into the neural tube at stages 8–11, 36–93% of the tissue in the forebrain, hindbrain, retina, or inner ear was expressing the marker gene (alkaline phosphatase). The values increased to 78–98% for B subgroup vectors that did not encode alkaline phosphatase (and that were approximately fivefold higher titer). These results suggest that in the early neural tube, the receptor for the B subgroup is present at higher levels, is more accessible to the inoculum, and/or is more efficiently used for viral entry than the A subgroup receptor. These results also raise the exciting possibility that widespread infection of the central nervous system during the stages of compartmentalization is feasible with this technique.

We have also found that both B and E subgroups yield higher infectivity *in vivo* in the presence of polybrene (Fekete and Cepko, 1993a; S. A. Homburger and D. M. Fekete, unpublished), confirming reports for *in vitro* infections (Toyoshima and Vogt, 1969). *In vivo* there was very little difference in infectivity of subgroup E using polybrene concentrations of 800 and 80 μg/ml; both concentrations were better than 8 μg/ml which was optimal for *in vitro* experiments). More precise titering of polybrene concentrations in the inoculum has not been attempted. An 80-μg/ml final concentration of polybrene in the inoculum is routinely used; it is added to the virus immediately after thawing from a 8-mg/ml stock solution (stored frozen).

5. Infection Efficiency

As a general note of caution, despite efforts to control precisely the site and stage of injection, and the exact volume of virus injected, there can still be an unsettling degree of variability in the percentage of expressing tissue when assayed 48 hr later. This is particularly true for injections into the neural tube prior to its closure and probably reflects the fact that it is impossible to contain the inoculum at the precise site of injection. The anterior neuropore and posterior neuropore both remain open up to stage 11. Beyond this stage the anterior neuropore is still a "weak link" and is often forced open if excess virus is injected into the neural tube. More consistent results are obtained when injecting into an enclosed space; this is recommended if earlier expression is not essential to the experimental design.

F. Developing a Novel Infection Protocol

In general, the infection protocol is a compromise between two conflicting goals. The first is to achieve complete and reproducible infection of a target tissue at a defined developmental stage. The second is to restrict infection to that tissue. When morphological assays of phenotypic effects are employed, there is frequently a span of several days between the time of injection and the assessment of effects. It is therefore necessary to characterize the reproducibility of both the initial infection process and the subsequent spread of the infection. Since the virus may continue to spread between the time it exerts its effects and the time they are assayed, phenotypic effects may only be correlated with the probability that a given region was infected at a particular time in development. The greater the time between the infection and harvest, the greater the variability.

To simplify the process of studying the infection resulting from an injection protocol, we and others have inserted the human placental alkaline phosphatase gene (AP) into RCASBP (A), (B), and (E) subtype vectors (Fekete and Cepko, 1993a). This allows the detection of virus-infected cells in large numbers of embryos by a simple whole mount histochemical procedure. This approach assumes that the AP gene product does not affect the infected cells and thereby influences virus spread, cell survival, or differentiation. This assumption has been confirmed in lateral plate mesenchyme and limb mesenchyme for days 1.5 to 5 of development by comparing infections resulting from RCASBP/AP injection with those from injection of other RCASBP-derived viruses. It may not be true for the neural tube where infection and/or expression of the viral gene products appears to be decreased in the presence of AP. In any event the infection resulting from injection of an experimental virus may differ from an "innocuous virus" and should be independently assessed. This may be done by detecting viral message by whole mount *in situ* hybridization with a probe to the viral RNA (see Chapter 11). The pRD-4 plasmids containing the *Kpn*I to *Cla*I fragment of RCASBP may be used to generate a convenient probe for whole mount detection (B. A. Morgan, unpublished).

1. Whole Mount Human Placental Alkaline Phosphatase Detection

1. Fix in 4% paraformaldehyde in PBS (2 hr to overnight).
2. Wash well in PBS (five times for 1 hr or overnight).
3. Incubate at 65°C for 30 min in PBS to inactivate endogenous alkaline phosphatase.
4. Incubate in detection buffer 3 (30 min).
5. Incubate in detection solution (signal may increase for several hours).
6. Wash in TE (10 mM Tris, pH 7.5, 10 mM EDTA) for 10 min.
7. Wash in PBS three times (10 min each).
8. Postfix in 4% paraformaldehyde for 1 hr at room temperature.

Detection buffer 3	Detection solution
100 mM Tris, pH 9.5	100 μl 50× NBT
100 mM NaCl	50 μl 100X X-Phos
50 mM MgCl$_2$	5 ml detection buffer 3

100× BCIP: 5-bromo-4-chloro-3-indolyl phosphate (10 mg/ml in H$_2$O)

50X NBT: nitro blue tetrazolium chloride (50 mg/ml in 70% dimethyl formamide/30% H$_2$O)

IV. Results and Discussion

A. Correlating Infection with Resulting Phenotype

The power of this approach lies in the ease with which gene expression may be altered in specific areas of the embryo at different times in development. The major difficulty in interpreting the effects of altering gene expression with replication-competent vectors arises because the virus may spread between the time of injection and the time of assay. When the period between injection and assay is short (a few days), it is relatively easy to predict the course of infection from its extent at harvest. Hence the dissection of molecular pathways, which frequently involves short-term assays, is well suited to this approach. However, when morphological assays are employed, several weeks may intervene between injection and assay. Therein lies the advantage of complete infection of a developmental field; viral spread is no longer an issue when infection is complete. The variability then arises in the time between injection and complete infection. This may be very short for lumenal injections, but may be several days for injections into solid tissue. Precise staging of infected embryos and positioning of injections are crucial to reducing variability. Nevertheless, the initial infections and the time required for the infection to spread sufficiently to encompass the entire developmental field will not be identical. This drawback can be turned to an advantage. The penetrance of a phenotype may be used to infer the developmental time at which a gene exerts specific effects. In practice, a percentage of the injected embryos must be harvested at intermediate stages of development to assess the course of infection in the population. The penetrance of a given phenotype can then be correlated with the probability that a tissue was infected at a given stage in development.

In the limb bud infection protocol described earlier, infection is performed at day 1.5. Effects of distal skeletal elements cannot be reliably assayed before day 11, making it impossible to directly relate the degree of infection at an early stage with a particular phenotype in an affected embryo. Complete infection of the limb bud, and therefore an end to effective spread of the virus, is achieved between stages 19 and 24. A population approach may be employed to correlate the degree of infection of early harvested specimens with the range of phenotypes later in development (Morgan *et al.,* 1992; Morgan and Tabin, 1994). The continuous spread of the virus during the course of incubation increases the penetrance of phenotypes which result from transduced gene activity later in development. Because there is a proximal to distal progression of differentiation in the limb, this will be observed in two ways. The effects of altered gene expression on a given developmental process (e.g., cartilage condensation) will be evident more frequently in distal structures where this process occurs later, allowing more time for viral spread. Furthermore, at a given level along the proximal distal axis, phenotypes resulting from influences on later developmental events will also be observed more frequently than those reflecting earlier activity.

B. Further Restriction of Gene Expression

1. Restriction of Viral Spread by Generating Chimeric Embryos

Situations may exist in which the spread of virus beyond the specific target cells will compromise the experiment, either because of extraneous or indirect effects on other cells or because of lethality. In such cases, it may be preferable to use replication-defective viruses if sufficient infection can be achieved with these vectors. If not, replication-competent vectors can be used in combination with a grafting technique to limit spread. The graft consists of infection-sensitive target tissue in the form of dissectable chunks or pelleted cells, and the host is an embryo from an infection-resistant strain (Fekete and Cepko, 1993b; Riddle *et al.,* 1993). We have experience with two distinct combinations of sensitive donor and resistant host strains of chickens (Table IV). Although the B subgroup viruses (with or without intermixed A subtypes) were found to yield optimal infection (see Section III,E,4), the host embryos (line 7_2 c/A,B,E) needed for this grafting paradigm had lower fertility and lower survival rates following surgical manipulation than the other strains. Thus we prefer to use the E subgroup combinations when this subgroup can sufficiently infect the target population.

2. Tissue-Specific Expression of Viral Inserts

An alternative approach to restricting gene expression to a target population involves restricting insert expression without restricting viral spread. Such approaches employ related vectors, RCANBP (N=No splice acceptor) or RCONBP (O=RAV-0 LTR, weaker viral promoter), which lack the splice acceptor upstream of the insertion site. In theory, insert expression may be restricted by inclusion of either a tissue-specific splice acceptor or a tissue-specific promoter in the inserted sequences. This strategy has been used successfully with a muscle-specific promoter (Petropoulos *et al.,* 1991). The same constraints on size and content of the inserted sequences apply to these replication-competent viruses and may limit the general utility of this approach, but it has clear advantages in some instances.

C. Alternative Infection Protocols

Some workers prefer to implant infected cells into the embryo to initiate infection (Petropoulos and Hughes, 1991). For most infections, the injection of a high titer virus stock is preferable. However, infection at very early stages has proven difficult and may be limited by receptor availability. The persistent source of concentrated virus created by implanted cells may generate more consistent infection at these stages.

V. Conclusions and Perspectives

To date, replication-competent retrovirus-mediated gene expression has been used to address the role of several gene families in different developing tissues.

Table IV
Donor and Host Embryo Combinations for Grafting Retrovirus-Infected Tissue

Virus strain	Donor line (sensitive)	Host line (resistant)
A and/or B envelope subgroup	Line 0 (C/E)	Line 7_2 (C/A,B,E)
E envelope subgroup	Line 15b$_1$ (C/O)	Line 0 (C/E)
		SPAFAS SPF-11 (C/E)[a]

[a] Not all SPF-11 embryos will be C/E (see Table III).

Many of the genes in these families are active in the formation of several tissues, and the ability to restrict infection and thereby limit genetic perturbation to a specific region of the embryo has been essential for ruling out possible indirect effects on morphogenesis. This approach has been used to mimic normal expression domains that vary from a few hundred cells to broad developmental fields. Short-term assays have been instrumental in dissecting complex genetic pathways and longer term assays have helped to discern the role these pathways play in morphogenesis. Different infection protocols have allowed the use of the same virus to test the role of a gene in different tissues. As infection protocols for other tissues are developed, the power of this approach will continue to increase.

Acknowledgments

We thank Stephen Hughes for critical reading of the manuscript and helpful advice. B.A.M. is supported by a grant from the Shisheido Corporation. D.M.F. is supported by a Clare Boothe Luce Professorship, the National Science Foundation, the March of Dimes Foundation, and the Deafness Research Foundation.

References

Boerkoel, C. F., Federspiel, M. J., Salter, D. W., Payne, W., Crittenden, L. B., Kung, S.-J., and Hughes, S. H. (1993). A new defective retroviral vector system based on the Bryan strain of Rous Sarcoma Virus. *Virology* **195,** 669–679.

Crittenden, L. B. (1991). Retroviral elements in the genome of the chicken: Implications for poultry genetics and breeding. *Crit. Rev. Poul. Biol.* **3,** 73–109.

Dorner, A. J., Stoye, J. P., and Coffin, J. M. (1985). Molecular basis of host range variation in avian retroviruses. *J. Virol.* **53,** 32–39.

Federspiel, M. J., Crittenden, L. B., Provencher, L. P., and Hughes, S. H. (1991). Experimentally introduced defective endogenous proviruses are highly expressed in chickens. *J. Virol.* **65,** 313–319.

Fekete, D. M., and Cepko, C. L. (1993a). Replication-competent retroviral vectors encoding alkaline phosphatase reveal spatial restriction of viral gene expression/transduction in the chick embryo. *Mol. Cell. Biol.* **13,** 2604–2613.

Fekete, D. M., and Cepko, C. L. (1993b). Retroviral infection coupled with tissue transplantation limits gene transfer in the chicken embryo. *Proc. Natl. Acad. Sci. U.S.A.* **90,** 2350–2354.

Greenhouse, J. J., Petropoulos, C. J., Crittenden, L. B., and Hughes, S. H. (1988). Helper-independent retrovirus vectors with Rous-associated virus type O long terminal repeats. *J. Virol.* **62,** 4809–4812.

Hamburger, V., and Hamilton, H. L. (1951). A series of normal stages in the development of the chick embryo. *J. Morphol.* **88,** 49–91.

Hughes, S. H., and Kosik, E. (1984). Mutagenesis of the region between *env* and *src* of the SR-A strain of Rous sarcoma virus for the purpose of constructing helper-independent vectors. *Virology* **136,** 89–99.

Hughes, S. H., Greenhouse, J. J., Petropoulos, C. J., and Sutrave, P. (1987). Adaptor plasmids simplify the insertion of foreign DNA into herlper-independent retroviral vectors. *J. Virol.* **61,** 3004–3012.

Kiernan, A. E., Homburger, S. A., and Fekete, D. M. (1994). Optimization of retroviral gene transfer into the embryonic nervous system of chicks. *Neurosci. Abstr.* **20,** 255 (abstr.).

Laufer, E., Nelson, C., Johnson, R., and Morgan, B. A. (1994). Sonic hedgehog and fgf-4 act through a signalling cascade and feedback loop to integrate growth and patterning of the developing limb bud. *Cell* **93,** 993–1003.

Leis, J., Baltimore, D., Bishop, J. M., Coffin, J., Fleissner, E., Goff, S. P., Oroszlan, S., Robinson, H., Skalka, A. M., Temin, H. M., and Vogt, V. (1988). Standardized and simplified nomenclature for proteins common to all retroviruses. *J. Virol.* **62,** 1808–1809.

Morgan, B. A., and Tabin, C. J. (1994). Hox genes and growth: Early and late effects on limb bud morphogenesis. *Development (Cambridge, UK)*, *Suppl.*, 181–186.

Morgan, B. A., Izpisùa-Belmonte, J., Douboule, D., and Tabin, C. (1992). Targeted misexpression of Hox-4.6 in the avian limb bud causes apparent homeotic transformations. *Nature (London)* **358,** 236–239.

Moscovici, C., Moscovici, M. G., Jimenez, H., Lai, M. M. C., Hayman, M. J., and Vogt, P. K. (1977). Continuous tissue culture cell lines derived from chemically induced tumors of Japanese quail. *Cell (Cambridge, Mass.)* **11,** 95–103.

Odorizzi, G., and Trowbridge, I. (1994). Recombinant Rous sarcoma virus vectors for avian cells. *Methods Cell Biol.* (in press).

Petropoulos, C. J., and Hughes, S. H. (1991). Replication-competent retrovirus vectors for the transfer and expression of gene cassettes in avian cells. *J. Virol.* **65,** 3728–3737.

Petropoulos, C. J., Payne, W., Salter, D. W., and Hughes, S. H. (1991). Appropriate in vivo expression of a muscle-specific promoter by using avian retroviral vectors for gene transfer. *J. Virol.* **66,** 3391–3397.

Potts, W. M., Olsen, M., Boettiger, D., and Vogt, V. M. (1987). Epitope mapping of monoclonal antibodies to gag protein p19 of avian sarcoma and leukaemia viruses. *J. Gen. Virol.* **68,** 3177–3182.

Riddle, R. D., Johnson, R. L., Laufer, E., and Tabin, C. (1993). Sonic hedgehog mediates the polarizing activity of the ZPA. *Cell (Cambridge, Mass.)* **75,** 1401–1416.

Roe, T. Y., Reynolds, T. C., Yu, G., and Brown, P. O. (1993). Integration of murine leukemia virus DNA depends on mitosis. *EMBO J.* **12,** 2099–2109.

Saunders, J. W. (1948). The proximo-distal sequence of origin of the parts of the chick wing and the role of the ectoderm. *J. Exp. Biol.* **108,** 363–402.

Toyoshima, K., and Vogt, P. K. (1969). Enhancement and inhibition of avian sarcoma viruses by polycations and polyanions. *Virology* **38,** 414–426.

Young, J. A. T., Bates, P., and Varmus, H. E. (1993). Isolation of a chicken gene that confers susceptibility to infection by subgroup A avian leukosis and sarcoma viruses. *J. Virol.* **67,** 1811–1816.

CHAPTER 11

In Situ Hybridization Analysis of Chick Embryos in Whole Mount and Tissue Sections

M. Angela Nieto,★ Ketan Patel,† and David G. Wilkinson†

★ Instituto Cajal
28002 Madrid, Spain

†Laboratory of Developmental Neurobiology
National Institute for Medical Research
Mill Hill, London NW7 1AA
United Kingdom

I. Introduction
II. When to Hybridize to Sections or Whole Mounts
III. Solutions
IV. Whole Mount *in Situ* Hybridization
    A. General Precautions
    B. Preparation of Labeled RNA Probe
    C. Fixation and Pretreatment of Embryos
    D. Hybridization, Posthybridization Washing, and Immunocytochemical Detection of Probe
    E. Photography and Sectioning
V. Double Detection of Two RNAs
VI. Double Detection of RNA and Protein
VII. Combined DiI Labeling and *in Situ* Hybridization
VIII. *In Situ* Hybridization to Tissue Sections
    A. General Precautions
    B. Preparation of Tissue Sections and Subbed Slides
    C. Prehybridization Treatments
    D. Posthybridization Washing and Immunocytochemical Detection
IX. Troubleshooting Guide
References

METHODS IN CELL BIOLOGY, VOL. 51
Copyright © 1996 by Academic Press, Inc. All rights of reproduction in any form reserved.

I. Introduction

The *in situ* analysis of the temporal and spatial regulation of gene expression in embryos is critical for elucidating the developmental functions of genes and for unraveling the cellular interactions that regulate tissue patterning and differentiation. Patterns of gene expression can be visualized either by detecting mRNA using *in situ* hybridization or by detecting the encoded protein product by immunocytochemistry. Since RNA and protein expression do not always correlate, the detection of protein has the advantage of being a more accurate guide to sites of gene action, but the production of specific antibodies can be difficult and time-consuming. In contrast, specific probes for *in situ* hybridization to mRNA are readily produced from cloned DNA or by the synthesis of oligonucleotides.

The method of *in situ* hybridization to RNA involves a series of procedures: (a) synthesis of a labeled nucleic acid probe complementary to the target mRNA, (b) fixation and permeabilization of tissue, (c) hybridization of the probe to the tissue and washing to remove unhybridized probe, and (d) detection of the probe.

Many alternatives exist for the type of probe and for the methods of labeling and visualization. Single-stranded RNA probes labeled with ^{35}S have been the most widely used for the hybridization of tissue sections because of their high sensitivity, but have several drawbacks. The main problem is that the signal is not at a single cell resolution. Methods with a similar sensitivity have been developed using RNA probes labeled with a nonradioactive hapten (Harland, 1991; Wilkinson, 1992; Conlon and Herrmann, 1993). Following hybridization and washing, the location of the probe is detected with a hapten-binding protein conjugated to an enzyme. This latter enzyme catalyzes the conversion of a chromogenic substrate to an insoluble, colored product, thus producing a signal at the sites of the target mRNA. In addition to greater speed and safety, nonradioactive methods have the major advantages of giving a single cell resolution and allowing *in situ* hybridization not only of tissue sections, but also of whole embryos. This whole mount *in situ* hybridization gives a direct visualization of the spatial pattern of RNA expression (Figs. 1A and 1B, see color insert) and can easily be carried out simultaneously on many embryos, thus facilitating a complete time course analysis.

A number of haptens and enzyme conjugates of hapten-binding proteins are available. The haptens digoxigenin (DIG), fluorescein, and biotin can be detected with commercially available antibodies or, for the latter, with streptavidin. Enzymes include alkaline phosphatase (AP), β-galactosidase, and horseradish peroxidase (HRP). For each of these enzymes, a variety of chromogenic substrates can be used that yield different colored products. Currently, the reagents that have found widespread favor due to their high sensitivity and low backgrounds are DIG-labeled probes detected with an AP-conjugated anti-DIG antibody and the chromogenic substrate mixture of 5-bromo-4-chloro-3-indolylphosphate

(BCIP) plus 4-nitro blue tetrazolium chloride (NBT). Fluorescein-labeled probes detected with an AP-conjugated antifluorescein antibody and BCIP/NBT give similar results.

This chapter describes methods for nonradioactive *in situ* hybridization in whole mount and tissue sections, for the double detection of two RNAs, and for combining *in situ* hybridization with immunocytochemistry or with lineage tracing.

II. When to Hybridize to Sections or Whole Mounts

For many purposes, the *in situ* hybridization of whole embryos is the method of choice as it is easier and often provides more information than the hybridization of sections. If sections are required, it is much less work to section embryos after whole mount hybridization and signal detection (Fig. 1D) than it is to prepare sections and then hybridize (Fig. 1E). However, whole mount hybridization does have several limitations that can be overcome by the hybridization of tissue sections:

1. The extent of penetration of reagents into tissues limits the size of embryos that can be used for whole mount *in situ* hybridization. Although low backgrounds have been obtained with chick embryos up to stage 25, much stronger signals are obtained when the tissue is at the surface than when it is internal, and thus some sites of expression could be missed. This problem can be alleviated to some extent by longer hybridization and washing steps. In addition, access of the reagents can be increased by bisecting embryos or by dissecting out the tissue of interest prior to hybridization.

2. Comparison of the expression of two genes in the same embryo can be achieved by the detection of two mRNAs in whole mount, but with the color reagents currently available, it may be difficult to detect overlaps in expression. It is currently not possible to analyze the expression of three or more genes in whole mount, but the hybridization of adjacent tissue sections allows the spatial domains of a number of genes to be compared in the same embryo. However, unless very thin sections are cut, it cannot be ascertained whether individual cells are coexpressing different mRNAs.

III. Solutions

TE buffer: 10 mM Tris–HCl, 0.1 mM EDTA, pH 8.0

5× transcription buffer: 200 mM Tris–HCl, pH 7.9, 30 mM MgCl$_2$, 10 mM spermidine, 50 mM NaCl

Nucleotide mix: 10 mM GTP, 10 mM ATP, 10 mM CTP, 6.5 mM UTP, 3.5 mM digoxigenin-UTP or fluorescein-UTP, pH 7.5 (Boehringer)

Phosphate-buffered saline (PBS): prepare using Dulbecco "A" tablets (Oxoid)

PBT: PBS, 0.1% Triton X-100

Proteinase K: 10 mg/ml stock in sterile H_2O

Paraformaldehyde fixative: 4% paraformaldehyde in PBS. Heat at 65°C with occasional agitation until dissolved, cool, and then filter. Use on the day of preparation. *Note:* take precautions with paraformaldehyde fumes which are toxic.

Glutaraldehyde: 25% stock solution (Sigma)

Prehybridization solution: 50% formamide, 5× SSC, 2% blocking powder (Boehringer, Cat. No. 1096176; dissolve directly in this mix), 0.1% Triton X-100, 0.1% CHAPS (Sigma), 1 mg/ml tRNA, 5 mM EDTA, 50 μg/ml heparin

20× SSC stock solution: 3 M NaCl, 0.3 M sodium citrate, pH 7.0

KTBT: 50 mM Tris–HCl, pH 7.5, 150 mM NaCl, 10 mM KCl, 1% Triton X-100

NTMT: 100 mM Tris–HCl, pH 9.5, 50 mM $MgCl_2$, 100 mM NaCl, 0.1% Triton X-100

NBT stock solution: 75 mg/ml NBT (Boehringer) in 70% dimethylformamide

BCIP stock solution: 50 mg/ml BCIP (Boehringer) in dimethylformamide

IV. Whole Mount *in Situ* Hybridization

A. General Precautions

It is important that solutions used for processing the embryos prior to hybridization are free of ribonuclease to avoid the degradation of the cellular RNAs. We find it sufficient to autoclave the PBS used for making fixative and pretreatment solutions and to use disposable plastic tubes. In order to obtain low backgrounds it is important that the washes are thorough, but do not damage the embryo. We use a variable speed rocking platform (Denley Reciprocal Mixer) adjusted such that the embryos are gently agitated during prehybridization, hybridization, and washing steps; this is easier to achieve if the container is not completely full. For the high temperature incubations, microtubes are placed in a heater block (Techne Dri-Block DB-1) turned on its side on a rocking platform. Alternatively, an incubator containing a rocking platform can be used. When changing solutions, allow the embryos to settle to the bottom of the container and leave some liquid above them so that surface tension does not flatten them. A variety of different containers can be used, partly depending on the equipment available. We use 7-ml flat-bottomed tubes (Bijoux tubes, Sterilin) for the fixation and pretreatment of embryos, and 2-ml microtubes (Eppendorf) for hybridization, washing, and immunodetection.

B. Preparation of Labeled RNA Probe

The probe is synthesized by the *in vitro* transcription of the DNA template in the presence of ribonucleotides, one of which is hapten conjugated (e.g., with DIG or fluorescein), such that labeled RNA that is complementary, or "antisense," to the target mRNA is produced. The DNA template can then be degraded, but this step is optional. The RNA probe is purified away from unincorporated nucleotides, which can give high backgrounds, by ethanol precipitation in the presence of ammonium acetate or lithium chloride. Since the signal strength is related to the sequence complexity of the probe, it is recommended that, whenever possible, long probes (~0.5–3 kb) be generated. However, because long probes penetrate less efficiently into the tissue, they are size reduced by limited alkaline hydrolysis to obtain optimal signals. As a rule of thumb, probes of >1 kb are degraded to an average of ~500 bases whereas probes of <1 kb are not degraded, but the optimal conditions have not been systematically investigated and presumably depend on the extent of tissue crosslinking.

The most common method used to generate a probe is by cloning cDNA sequences into a vector containing T7, T3, or SP6 RNA polymerase initiation sites, such as the pGEM (Promega) or Bluescript (Stratagene) plasmid vectors. Preparations of the plasmid construct are generated by standard protocols, such as the alkaline lysis method. It it not necessary to use highly pure DNA and even small-scale minipreps can be used; however, if the plasmid prep contains ribonuclease A (to degrade bacterial RNA), this should be removed by several phenol/chloroform extractions. Probes including plasmid sequences can yield high backgrounds, so to ensure that only cDNA sequences are transcribed the construct is linearized at a restriction site at the 5' end of the cDNA. Because aberrant transcripts are produced from DNA with a 3' overhang, this linearization should be carried out with restriction enzymes that generate either a 5' overhang or a blunt end. After checking that linearization is complete, the DNA is phenol/chloroform extracted, ethanol precipitated, and redissolved at 1 $\mu g/\mu l$ in TE buffer. The transcription reaction is carried out as follows.

1. Mix these reagents in the following order at room temperature:
   8.5 μl sterile distilled water
   4 μl 5× transcription buffer
   2 μl 0.1 *M* dithiothreitol
   2 μl nucleotide mix
   1.5 μl linearized plasmid (1 $\mu g/\mu l$)
   0.5 μl placental ribonuclease inhibitor (100 U/μl)
   1.5 μl SP6, T7, or T3 RNA polymerase (10 U/μl)
2. Incubate at 37°C for 2 hr.
3. Remove a 1-μl aliquot and run on an agarose gel containing 0.5 μg/ml ethidium bromide to estimate the amount synthesized. This gel must be ribonuclease free, but does not need to be denaturing (e.g., containing formaldehyde). An RNA band ~10-fold more intense than the plasmid band should be seen, indicating that ~15-μg probe has been synthesized.

4. Add 2 μl ribonuclease-free DNase I (1 U/μl) and incubate at 37°C for 15 min. This step is optional.

5. If the transcript is 1 kb or greater in length, reduce the average size to ~500 bases. Add an equal volume of 80 mM NaHCO$_3$, 120 mM Na$_2$CO$_3$ and heat at 60°C for a period of time (minutes) given by time (min) = (L-0.5)/(0.055L), where L is the starting length of the transcript. It is advisable to check on an agarose gel the size of the product compared with a ~500-base transcript since overdegraded probes can give low signals and high backgrounds.

6. Add 130 μl distilled H$_2$O, 50 μl 10 M ammonium acetate, and 400 μl ethanol, mix, and incubate at −20°C for 30 min. Do not incubate at a lower temperature as this may precipitate unincorporated nucleotides.

7. Spin for 10 min in a microfuge, wash pellet with 70% ethanol, and air dry the pellet.

8. Redissolve in 150 μl ice-cold distilled H$_2$O, add 50 μl 10 M ammonium acetate and 400 μl ethanol, incubate at −20°C for 10–20 min, and repeat step 7.

9. Redissolve in ice-cold TE at ~0.1 μg/μl and store at −70°C. Use 1–5 μl for each milliliter of hybridization mix.

C. Fixation and Pretreatment of Embryos

Before hybridization, embryos are fixed and subjected to several pretreatments. The conditions used are a compromise between, on the one hand, fixing RNAs *in situ* and preserving morphology and, on the other, permeabilizing the tissue such that the probe can access target RNA. This is achieved using a crosslinking fixative, paraformaldehyde, then partially digesting cellular proteins with proteinase K, followed by refixation. Prior to hybridization, the embryos are incubated with hybridization mix lacking the probe in order to block nonspecific-binding sites.

A common problem with whole mount hybridization is the trapping of reagents in enclosed cavities, such as the neural tube, leading to high backgrounds. For this reason, it is important to dissect open any such cavities, e.g., by tearing a hole in the dorsal hindbrain. A fixation time of 2 hr is adequate for chick embryos up to stage 17, but overnight fixation gives the same results and can be more convenient. The optimal proteinase K treatment varies according to the stage of embryo since surface tissues will be digested more rapidly than deeper tissues; we digest embryos at stages 3–6 for 5 min, stages 6–12 for 10 min, and stages 12–25 for 20 min. If excessive tissue disintegration occurs during *in situ* hybridization or if poor signals are obtained, it is advisable to optimize the period of digestion with the batch of proteinase K being used.

In the following protocol, the incubations are at room temperature unless otherwise indicated. The embryos are gently agitated during steps 3–9 and 11.

1. Dissect embryos in PBS, removing as much extraneous tissue as possible.

2. Incubate in paraformaldehyde fixative at 4°C for 2 hr to overnight.

3. Rinse the embryos with PBT twice for 5 min.

4. Dehydrate the embryos by washing for 10 min each in a graded methanol series diluted in PBT (25% methanol, 50% methanol, 75% methanol) and then twice with 100% methanol. The embryos can now be stored at −20°C for several months and are stable for several days at room temperature.

5. Rehydrate the embryos by washing for 10 min in the graded methanol series in PBT (75% methanol, 50% methanol, 25% methanol) and then twice in PBT.

6. Treat the embryos with 20 μg/ml proteinase K in PBT for 5–20 min at room temperature.

7. Rinse the embryos with PBT for 5 min.

8. Refix the embryos with fresh 0.2% glutaraldehyde/4% paraformaldehyde in PBT for 20 min.

9. Rinse the embryos with PBT twice for 5 min.

10. Remove most of the liquid, add 1 ml prehybridization solution, and allow the embryos to sink.

11. Replace with fresh 1 ml prehybridization solution and incubate at 55–65°C for 2 hr to overnight. The embryos can be stored at −20°C at this point for several months.

D. Hybridization, Posthybridization Washing, and Immunocytochemical Detection of Probe

Embryos are incubated with a hapten-labeled probe, the unhybridized probe is removed by washing at moderate stringency, and nonspecific binding sites are blocked with sheep serum. The bound probe is detected with an AP-conjugated anti-hapten antibody, washed, and incubated with a chromogenic substrate for alkaline phosphatase. This produces a colored precipitate at the site of the target RNA. The protocol described here has been simplified from an earlier version (Wilkinson, 1992) by eliminating the ribonuclease treatment of the embryos following hybridization. This latter step is intended to remove the unhybridized probe, but also decreases the specific signal, and omission gives a major increase in sensitivity. We have also found that preabsorption of antibody with embryo powder can be omitted, but as this could depend on the antibody preparation it is advisable to test this.

For hybridization, the probe is used at 0.1–0.5 μg (equivalent to 1–5 μl of purified probe) per ml of hybridization mix, but if high backgrounds are obtained it may be beneficial to decrease the probe concentration. Hybridization and washing can be carried out between 55° and 65°C, and the washing solutions should be prewarmed. For many probes, 55°C is best since stronger signals are obtained, and this can be especially important for probes that are short (~200 bp) or AT rich, but if the probe gives a background problem, a higher temperature should be tested. In addition, in cases where the probe might hybridize to transcripts of related genes, then this can be avoided by higher stringency hybridization or washing. It is especially important that the embryos are agitated sufficiently to ensure thorough washing after hybridization and incubation with antibody, and it may be beneficial to increase the number and/or length of washes, especially for later stage embryos.

1. Incubate embryos with hybridization mix containing the probe overnight at 55–65°C. Incubations of up to 3 days can be used without detriment and may enable penetration of the probe into large embryos.
2. Wash with 2× SSC, 0.1% CHAPS, three times for 20 min at 55–65°C.
3. Wash with 0.2× SSC, 0.1% CHAPS, three times for 20 min at 55–65°C.
4. Rinse with KTBT, twice for 10 min at room temperature.
5. Preblock the embryos with 20% sheep serum in KTBT for 2–3 hr or longer at 4°C.
6. Incubate with 1/2000 dilution of anti-DIG or anti-fluorescein antibody (Boehringer) in 20% sheep serum in KTBT and rock overnight at 4°C. The antibody can be preabsorbed for 1 hr with embryo powder as described later, but this step may not be needed.
7. Wash the embryos with KTBT at room temperature for 1 hr, five or more times, then overnight at 4°C. The overnight wash is optional, but gives lower backgrounds, and it is more convenient to monitor a slow color reaction if it is started on the following morning.
8. Wash twice in NTMT for 15 min and transfer to a glass embryo dish for easier observation; crystals can form if plastic petri dishes are used. The NTMT can contain 1 mM levamisol, which inhibits many endogenous alkaline phosphatases, but we have not found this to be needed.
9. Incubate in the dark with NTMT containing 3 μg/ml NBT stock solution, 2.3 μl/ml BCIP stock solution. Periodically monitor the reaction and when a strong signal is produced and/or any background is observed, stop by washing several times with KTBT, and store in PBS. If the embryos are overstained, it is possible to partially destain them in PBS containing 1% Triton X-100 or in methanol, but care has to be taken that the latter does not remove too much signal. Sometimes the color reaction yields a brown product. The reason for this has not been identified, but it is possible to convert the product to a blue color by washing in PBT or by brief incubation in methanol.

The following steps are used to preabsorb the antibody. For a 2-ml final solution, place ~3 mg embryo powder (prepared as described below) in a microtube and add 0.5 ml 20% sheep serum in KTBT and 1 μl antibody. Shake gently at 4°C for several hours or overnight. Spin for 1 min in a microfuge, remove the supernatant, and dilute it to 2 ml.

Embryo powder is prepared as follows:

1. Homogenize stage 15–17 chick embryos in a minimum volume of PBS.
2. Add 4 volumes of ice-cold acetone, mix, and incubate on ice for 30 min.
3. Spin at 10,000 *g* for 10 min and remove supernatant. Wash pellet with ice-cold acetone and spin again.
4. Spread the pellet out and grind it into a fine powder on a sheet of filter paper and allow it to air dry. Store in an air-tight tube at 4°C.

E. Photography and Sectioning

Photography of whole embryos can be carried out using a dissection microscope fitted with a camera. If required, the embryos can be orientated as follows. Pour a ~2- to 3-mm layer of 1% agarose into a petri dish, allow it to set, and then with a hot glass capillary melt troughs that can accommodate the embryos. Overlay with PBS and orientate the embryos in the troughs as required. Higher power photographs can be shot by mounting the embryos under a coverslip. An easy way to achieve this is to place two blobs of petroleum jelly about 1 cm apart on a microscope slide, pipette the embryo between and orientate as desired, and then lower a coverslip on top, gently pushing it down as required. Depending on the site of expression, it can be very useful to partially dissect the embryo in order that the tissue can be flattened during mounting such that expressing cells are in the same plane of focus. For example, the hindbrain can be dissected free of underlying tissues, slit along the ventral midline, and mounted as a "kipper" preparation to visualize the neural crest (Fig. 1B). In order to visualize nonexpressing tissues, a light counterstaining with eosin can be used, but since this can obscure the signal we instead routinely use differential interference contrast (Nomarski) optics.

A color reversal film such as Kodak EPY64T can be used directly for slides or for preparing prints. Typically, an exposure equivalent to ASA 32 (e.g., ASA64 + 1 stop) gives the best results with this film, but it may be necessary to try several different exposures. Alternatively, color negative film can be used, which has the virtue of being cheaper to print from, though it can be difficult to achieve a consistent color balance if using commercial printers. For black and white photography, a film such as Kodak TMax 100 is suitable.

It can be very informative to observe gene expression in sectioned tissue, e.g., to visualize dorsoventrally restricted expression in transverse sections. This can be achieved by carrying out *in situ* hybridization on tissues sections as described next, but it can be more convenient to section whole mount hybridized embryos (Fig. 1C). Signals can be detected in sectioned material if they are strong in the whole mount, but it can be difficult for weak signals, for which it is advisable to cut thick sections. Sections can be prepared for cryostat sectioning as follows.

1. Fix the stained embryos overnight in 4% paraformaldehyde in PBS.
2. Wash several times in PBS and equilibrate overnight with 30% sucrose.
3. Mount on a cryostat chuck with OCT compound (BDH) and freeze on dry ice.
4. Cut 10- to 15-μm sections on a cryostat.

Alternatively, embryos can be embedded in wax and sections cut on a microtome, as follows.

1. Fix the embryos in 4% paraformaldehyde in PBS overnight at 4°C. This step is especially important for wax embedding because the NBT/BCIP reaction product will dissolve in the solvents used.
2. Wash the embryos twice for 10 min with PBS and then replace the solution with methanol for 5 min, with isopropanol for 10 min, with tetrahydronaph-thalene (Aldrich) for 15 min, and then with fresh tetrahydronaphthalene. This must be carried out in a fume hood.
3. Add an equal volume of paraffin wax at 60°C and incubate for 20 min with occasional shaking to mix, then replace this with paraffin wax, three times for 20 min each, all at 60°C.
4. Transfer to an embryo dish at 60°C, place at room temperature, orientate using a warmed needle (if necessary, observing with a dissection micro-scope), and let the wax set.
5. Cut sections (e.g., 10 μm), mount on subbed slides, and dry at 37°C over-night.
6. Dewax for 2–5 min with Histoclear (National Diagnostics).
7. While the slide is still wet, mount the sections under a coverslip using Permount (Sigma) mounting agent.

V. Double Detection of Two RNAs

It can be very useful to detect the products of two genes simultaneously, e.g., to map how the expression domain of one gene relates to that of another or to analyze the effects of an experimental manipulation on several molecular mark-ers. This can be achieved by taking advantage of multiple labeling and detection systems to detect two RNAs in the same embryo. In the method described here, both of the probes labeled with different haptens are detected with AP-coupled antibodies, and this necessitates sequential incubations with antibody, each fol-lowed by a color reaction. A quicker alternative is to simultaneously incubate with antibodies coupled to different enzymes, such as AP and HRP, and then to carry out sequential color reactions. However, because of the lower stability of HRP, this method is much less sensitive and can only be used to detect abundant RNAs. A limitation to the currently available substrates is that it is difficult to unambiguously detect cells expressing two different transcripts, so is more useful for genes that have nonoverlapping expression.

Several published methods (Hauptmann and Gerster, 1994; Jowett and Lettice, 1994) have used the substrate Fast Red to produce a red colored product. Although this works well for short color reactions (less than an hour), for the longer reaction times required to detect low to moderate abundance transcripts in chick embryos the tissue is stained nonspecifically, possibly because of the chemical instability of this substrate. We have had success with the alkaline phosphatase substrate kit II from Vector Laboratories which yields a brown precipitate (Fig. 1D).

1. Make probes against the two target RNAs, one labeled with fluorescein and the other with DIG, exactly as described in Section IV,B.
2. Carry out whole mount *in situ* hybridization with a mixture of the DIG and fluorescein-labeled probes and detect the fluorescein-labeled probe with the AP-coupled anti-fluorescein antibody and a BCIP/NBT color reaction. The method is exactly as described in Sections IV,C and IV,D. Because detection of the second RNA may be compromised by the first color reaction, it is advisable to detect the less abundant RNA first.
3. Inactivate the AP activity by treating with 0.1 *M* glycine–HCl, pH 2.2, 0.1% Tween 20 for 10 min at room temperature and then wash twice for 5–10 min with PBT.
4. Detect the DIG-labeled probe, starting at step 4 in Section IV,D, using substrate kit II as the substrate for AP. This will generate a brown product.

VI. Double Detection of RNA and Protein

An alternative to detecting two RNAs is to detect an RNA and a protein by combining *in situ* hybridization with immunocytochemistry. This approach can take advantage of well-characterized antibodies that mark defined cell types, such as the neural crest or neurons, to identify the expressing cells or to map spatial domains relative to neuroanatomical landmarks.

The *in situ* hybridization is carried out first, exactly as described earlier, and the color reaction product is fixed (e.g., with 4% paraformaldehyde in PBS for 2 hr). Immunocytochemistry is then carried out using standard conditions for the antibody being used. We have used an HRP-coupled secondary antibody, followed by a color reaction with diaminobenzidine, to generate a brown product (Fig. 1E). Many alternatives exist, including the use of other substrates or fluorescent or AP-coupled antibodies. It should be kept in mind that sheep anti-DIG antibodies are used in the *in situ* hybridization, so anti-sheep antibodies should not be used for the immunocytochemical detection of antigen.

This method will only work if the antigen is recognized after the *in situ* hybridization procedure; this has been successful for a variety of antibodies (HNK1 and anti-brachyury). If the antibody does not work, several changes to the protocol may be beneficial:

1. Omission of the proteinase treatment. This will, however, reduce the *in situ* hybridization signal and can only be used for abundant RNAs.

2. The use of different fixatives. Although crosslinking fixatives, such as paraformaldehyde and glutaraldehyde, are optimal for *in situ* hybridization, other fixatives can be sufficiently effective, e.g., we have had success with 2% trichloroacetic acid.

3. It may be possible to carry out the immunocytochemistry first, but it is very important to take rigorous precautions against ribonucleases during this procedure. The inclusion of 5 mg/ml heparin as a ribonuclease inhibitor may help.

VII. Combined DiI Labeling and *in Situ* Hybridization

The detection of gene expression is often very useful for following cell lineages during tissue morphogenesis and cell migration. However, because gene expression can be dynamically regulated, it may not be a reliable marker and so it is important to directly prove the lineage relationship between expressing cells at different stages of development. Moreover, important information may be obtained by determining the location of cells at stages prior to their upregulating the molecular marker. This can be achieved by marking populations of cells with DiI, photoconverting the fluorescence, and carrying out *in situ* hybridization (Izpisùa-Belmonte *et al.*, 1993; Nieto *et al.*, 1995) (Fig. 1F), as follows.

1. Microinject DiI to label target cells and incubate the embryos until the appropriate stage.

2. Fix embryos in 4% paraformaldehyde at 4°C overnight.

3. Rinse with PBS, 0.1 M Tris–HCl, pH 7.4, and then with 0.5 mg/ml diaminobenzidine in 0.1 M Tris–HCl, pH 7.4, for 30 min each at 4°C.

4. Place each embryo in a depression slide, overlay a coverslip, and illuminate for 10–20 min under an epifluorescence microscope using a rhodamine filter set. Refocus every 5 min. Stop the illumination when a brown precipitate is first observed so as to not obscure the signal for *in situ* hybridization; the photoconverted signal is consequently an underestimate of the number and intensity of DiI-labeled cells.

5. Rinse the embryos in 0.1 M Tris–HCl, pH 7.4, for 30 min and place in methanol, in which they are stable for up to a week.

6. Carry out *in situ* hybridization, starting at step 5 in Section IV,C.

VIII. *In Situ* Hybridization to Tissue Sections

The method for *in situ* hybridization to tissue sections involves steps identical (probe preparation, embryo fixation) or with simple adaptations (pretreatments, hybridization, washing, and the immunocytochemical detection of probe) to those used in whole mount hybridization. It should be kept in mind that the protocol described here has largely been derived from the whole mount protocol described earlier and has not been optimized.

A. General Precautions

As described for whole mounts, precautions should be taken to avoid ribonucleases degrading cellular RNA prior to hybridization. In addition to using autoclaved PBS, avoid using any slide holders that have been exposed to ribonucleases.

B. Preparation of Tissue Sections and Subbed Slides

In the method described next, tissue sections are prepared by embedding fixed embryos in paraffin wax, cutting sections, and drying them onto slides that have been subbed with TESPA. An alternative is to cut cryostat sections. To maximize the signal it may be advantageous to cut thick sections.

1. Dissect the embryos and fix them in 4% paraformaldehyde in PBS overnight at 4°C.
2. Wash the embryos with PBS twice for 10 min.
3. Dehydrate by taking embryos through methanol series in PBT (25% methanol, 50% methanol, and 75% methanol) then twice in 100% methanol, for 10 min each. Later stage embryos should be washed longer to ensure complete dehydration.
4. Equilibrate embryos with toluene, three times for 20 min, then with molten paraffin wax at 60°C, three times for 20 min, occasionally agitating the vial. Take precautions to avoid breathing toluene fumes.
5. Transfer the embryos to glass embryo slides (preheated to 60°C), orientate them with a warmed needle under a dissection microscope, and allow the wax to set. Paraffin wax blocks can be stored indefinitely at 4°C until required for use.
6. On a microtome, cut 6-μm sections as ribbons which are then floated on a bath of distilled water at 50°C until the creases disappear and are collected on TESPA-subbed slides.
7. Dry the sections onto the slides at 37°C overnight. They can be stored desiccated at 4°C.

Subbed slides are prepared as follows:

1. Dip the slides in 10% HCl/70% ethanol, followed by distilled water and 95% ethanol for 1 min each and then air dry.
2. Dip the slides in 2% TESPA (3-aminopropyltriethoxysilane) in acetone for 10 sec.

3. Wash twice with acetone and then with distilled water.
4. Dry at 37°C.

C. Prehybridization Treatments

Prior to hybridization, the sections are dewaxed, permeabilized by proteinase K treatment followed by refixation, and dehydrated. The probe is then spread over the sections under a coverslip. This protocol does not include a prehybridization blocking step, and we have not tested whether this step would reduce background. The same general considerations apply as for whole mount hybridizations, with the additional factor that overdigestion with proteinase can lead to the sections falling off the slides. Except where otherwise stated, the slides are placed in holders suitable for 250-ml slide dishes and 200–250 ml of the solutions is used.

1. Dewax the slides in Histoclear, twice for 10 min, and then place them in 100% methanol for 2 min to remove most of the Histoclear.
2. Transfer the slides through 100% methanol (twice), 75%, 50%, and 25% methanol/PBT, for 1–2 min in each solution, then wash twice in PBS for 5 min.
3. Immerse the slides in fresh 4% paraformaldehyde in PBS for 20 min.
4. Wash the slides with PBS, three times for 5 min.
5. Drain the slides and place horizontally on the bench. Overlay the sections with 10 μg/ml proteinase K (freshly diluted in PBS from a 10-mg/ml stock in distilled H_2O) and leave for 5 min.
6. Shake off excess liquid and wash the slides with PBS for 5 min.
7. Repeat the fixation of step 3; the same solution can be used.
8. Wash the slides twice with PBS for 5 min. Dehydrate by passing through 25%, 50%, 75% methanol/PBT, then twice in 100% methanol, for 1–2 min in each solution. Allow to air dry.
9. Apply the hybridization mix to the slide adjacent to the sections (~5 μl per cm^2 of the coverslip is sufficient) and gently lower a clean coverslip so that the mix is spread over the sections. The hybridization mix and probe are made exactly as described in Section IV,B.
10. Place the slides horizontally in a box containing tissue paper soaked in 50% formamide, 5× SSC, seal the box, and incubate overnight at 55–65°C.

D. Posthybridization Washing and Immunocytochemical Detection

The slides are washed and immunocytochemistry is carried out under identical conditions as described for whole mount hybridization. It may be possible to reduce the times given for these steps without affecting background.

1. Place the slides in a slide rack and immerse in prewarmed 2× SSC, 0.1% CHAPS at 55–65°C until the coverslips fall off. Gentle encouragement with forceps may be necessary.

2. Wash with 2× SSC, 0.1% CHAPS, twice for 30 min at 55–65°C.

3. Wash with 0.2× SSC, 0.1% CHAPS, twice for 30 min at 55–65°C.

4. Wash with KTBT, twice for 10 min at room temperature.

5. Quickly drain each slide and place horizontally in a sandwich box containing moist tissue paper. Take care that the sections do not become dry and quickly overlay them with 20% sheep serum in KTBT. Seal the box and incubate for 2–3 hr.

6. If desired, the antibody can be preabsorbed as described in Section IV,D.

7. Remove the 20% serum from the embryos, replace with the diluted antibody, and incubate in a moist box at 4°C overnight.

8. Wash with KTBT for 5 min, three times, and then for 30 min, three times.

9. Wash with NTMT, three times for 5 min.

10. Incubate in the dark with NTMT containing 4.5 μl NBT, 3.5 μl BCIP per ml. Occasionally monitor, and when sufficient signal has developed, stop the color reaction by washing with PBT.

11. Fix the signal by immersing the slides in 4% paraformaldehyde in PBS for 2 hr, dehydrate quickly through a graded methanol series followed by Histoclear, and mount under a coverslip using Permount mounting agent. Photography is carried out as described in Section IV,E.

IX. Troubleshooting Guide

We do not routinely carry out negative controls, such as a sense strand probe, for *in situ* hybridization as the observation of distinct, nonoverlapping patterns with different antisense probes is equally valid evidence against nonspecific binding. It is possible that cross-hybridization could occur to related genes, especially if the probe includes sequences for conserved motifs, such as homeodomains or kinase domains. In this case, the best control is to use a nonoverlapping and more divergent sequence, such as the 3′-untranslated region. Cross-hybridization may be eliminated by increasing the stringency of hybridization and washing, and/or by including a posthybridization ribonuclease treatment, although the latter will also decrease the specific signal considerably. However, the more common problems with *in situ* hybridization are not due to cross-hybridization to related genes, but rather a nonspecific background or a low signal.

There are many possible causes of a high background, and it is essential to carry out appropriate positive and negative controls to ascertain which step(s) is the cause. For example, omit the probe, use a probe or batch of pretreated embryos known to give good results, or omit the antibody. The most common problems, in our experience, have been due to the probe, to inadequate washing, or to poor batches of the color-developing reagents. The root cause of some background problems might be a low signal, necessitating a long color development such that a moderate background becomes limiting. It is therefore worth also testing some of the possible cures of a poor signal. Some of the possible cures to potential sources of a high background are listed next.

1. Probe: Check that the probe does not include the poly(A) tail or plasmid sequence and is not GC rich. Check that the probe RNA (after limited hydrolysis) is not too small or too large (0.2–1 kb should be fine). If none of these are a likely problem, test a probe from a different region of the cDNA.
2. Pretreatment: Open any enclosed cavities (e.g., the neural tube) prior to hybridization.
3. Hybridization and washing: Use a lower concentration of probe. Hybridize and wash at a higher stringency. Include a ribonuclease step in the posthybridization washing (however, this will decrease the signal). Wash for longer.
4. Antibody: Preabsorb the antibody with embryo powder. Preblock the embryos for longer. Wash for longer.
5. Color development: Inhibit endogenous phosphatases with levamisol. Use a different substrate or batch of substrate.

A low signal can simply be due to a low level of expression, but if low backgrounds are achieved, then the color development can be carried out for up to several days to amplify the signal. In our experience, the best strategy is to initially use as long a probe as possible and reduce the size of the RNA to ~500 bp instead of testing short fragments. Even probes including conserved motifs (such as zinc fingers, homeodomains, or kinase domains) often give specific signals; this can be ascertained with appropriate controls. Even under optimal conditions, the probe does not penetrate far into the embryo, and this can be a limiting factor if the expression is in an internal tissue. The following ways can be used to increase the *in situ* hybridization signal.

1. Probe: Use longer probe sequences. Check that the probe RNA (after limited hydrolysis) is not too small or too large (0.2–1 kb should be fine).
2. Pretreatment: For later stage embryos, increase access to target tissues by dissecting the embryo (e.g., transverse or longitudinal bisection) or by hybridizing sections. Optimize the proteinase K treatment.
3. Hybridization and washing: Hybridize and wash at a lower stringency.
4. Color development: It has been reported that including polyvinyl alcohol in the color reaction mixture increases sensitivity (Barth and Ivarie, 1994). Although this has not been effective in our hands, it may be worthwhile to test this option.

Acknowledgments

We thank Robb Krumlauf and Linda McNaughton for the chick *Hoxb-9* clone used to produce Fig. 1D. M.A.N. is supported by Grant DGICYT-PB92-0045 from the Spanish Ministry of Education and Science. K.P. and D.G.W. are supported by the Medical Research Council.

References

Barth, J., and Ivarie, R. (1994). Polyvinyl alcohol enhances detection of low abundance transcripts in early stage quail embryos in a nonradioactive whole mount *in situ* hybridization technique. *BioTechniques* **17,** 324–327.

Conlon, R. A., and Herrmann, B. G. (1993). Detection of messenger RNA by *in situ* hybridization to postimplantation embryo whole mounts. *In* "Methods in Enzymology" (P. M. Wassarman and M. L. DePamphilis, eds.), Vol. 225, pp. 373–383. Academic Press, San Diego, CA.

Harland, R. M. (1991). In situ hybridization: An improved whole mount method for *Xenopus* embryos. *Methods Cell Biol.* **36,** 685–695.

Hauptmann, G., and Gerster, T. (1994). Two colour whole mount *in situ* hybridization to vertebrate and *Drosophila* embryos. *Trends Genet.* **10,** 266.

Izpisùa-Belmonte, J. C., De Robertis, E. M., Storey, K. G., and Stern, C. D. (1993). The homeobox gene *goosecoid* and the origin of organiser cells in the early chick blastoderm. *Cell (Cambridge, Mass.)* **74,** 645–659.

Jowett, T., and Lettice, L. (1994). Whole mount *in situ* hybridizations on zebrafish embryos using a mixture of digoxigenin- and fluorescein-labelled probes. *Trends Genet.* **10,** 73–74.

Nieto, M. A., Sargent, M. G., Wilkinson, D. G., and Cooke, J. (1994). Control of cell behavior during vertebrate development by *slug,* a zinc finger zone. *Science* **264,** 835–839.

Nieto, M. A., Sechrist, J., Wilkinson, D. G., and Bronner-Fraser, M. (1995). Relationship between spatially restricted *Krox-20* gene expression in branchial neural crest and segmentation in the chick embryo hindbrain. *EMBO J.* **14,** 1697–1710.

Wilkinson, D. G. (1992). Whole mount *in situ* hybridization of vertebrate embryos. *In* "*In situ* hybridization: A Practical Approach" (D. G. Wilkinson, ed.), pp. 75–83. IRL Press, Oxford.

CHAPTER 12

Micromass Cultures of Limb and Other Mesenchyme

Karla Daniels, Rebecca Reiter, and Michael Solursh[1]

Department of Biological Sciences
University of Iowa
Iowa City, Iowa 52242

I. Introduction
II. Micromass Culture Technique
    A. Materials and Solutions
    B. Isolation and Culture
    C. Critical Aspects of the Technique
    D. Microtiter Micromass and Defined Medium
    E. Coculture of Mesenchyme and Ectoderm
    F. Micromass on Nucleopore Filters
    G. Quantification of Chrondrogenesis
III. Use of Micromass Cultures in Teratology
IV. Discussion and Perspectives
    References

I. Introduction

The micromass culture technique was initially developed to study chondrogenesis and consists of high density dot cultures of dissociated limb bud cells (Ahrens *et al.*, 1977). Undifferentiated limb mesenchyme in culture at a density greater than confluency will form cartilage but similar cultures at subconfluent density do not (Umansky, 1966; Caplan, 1970). Initially, large numbers of embryos were needed to isolate the millions of cells necessary for a single experiment. The development of the micromass culture technique allowed a 20- to 25-fold increase in the number of replicate cultures that could be established from the same

[1] Deceased.

number of isolated limb bud cells. The high density cultures form a three-dimensional, multilayered organization of mesenchyme with close cell associations and entrap nascent pericellular and extracellular matrix molecules (ECM) to potentiate differentiation.

The sequence of chondrogenic events within micromass cultures recapitulates the sequence observed *in vivo*. In the limb, the first appearance of pattern is the formation of cellular aggregations or condensations in the core of the limb (Fell, 1925). The aggregates continue to enlarge mainly by assimilating surrounding mesenchyme (Ahrens *et al.*, 1977, 1979) followed by chondrogenic differentiation to form the cartilage template establishing the basic pattern of the limb (reviewed by Maini and Solursh, 1991). Segregated from the chondrogenic core, myoblasts migrating from the somite aggregate to form the dorsal and ventral muscle masses. The same series of events is reprised in micromass culture with the formation of aggregations after 1 day (Fig. 1A) followed by formation of cartilage nodules after 4 days (Fig. 1B). The chondrocytes become more widely separated as cartilage ECM is synthesized. In micromass, as in the limb, the myoblasts are excluded from the forming cartilage nodules and usually lie on the dorsal surface of the micromass (see Fig. 4).

In addition to limb bud cells, the micromass method has been used to study craniofacial mesenchyme (Wedden *et al.*, 1986), dedifferentiated chondrocytes, and periosteal cells. Nonchrondrogenic micromass has also been used for chick embryonic neurons to test possible teratogens (see below). The micromass faithfully reproduces three basic concepts in developmental biology: pattern formation, morphogenesis, and differentiation *in vitro* (see Ettinger and Doljanski, 1992) and will surely be extended to other developing systems.

II. Micromass Culture Technique

A. Materials and Solutions

The staging of the embryos is crucial to the successful outcome of differentiation. Staging is done according to the developmental stages of the chick as described by Hamburger and Hamilton (1951).

1. A 37°C shaker water bath and a CO_2 incubator.

2. Instruments: curved blunt forceps, two fine forceps, microscissors, and a test tube holder (sterilized in 70% alcohol for 20 min).

3. Laboratory equipment: 25-ml Ehrlenmeyer flask, 60- and 100-mm petri dishes, Pasteur and serological pipettes, 15- and 50-ml conical centrifuge tubes, and a hemacytometer.

4. Solutions at room temperature:

    a. Puck's saline G (PSG; Puck *et al.*, 1958)

    b. Ca^{2+}, Mg^{2+}-free Puck's saline G (CMF-PSG)

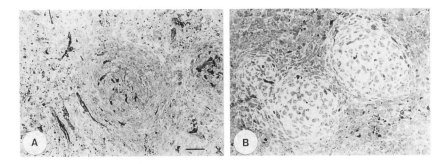

Fig. 1 *En face* thick plastic sections of 1-day (A) and 3-day (B) micromass cultures. Prechondrogenic mesenchyme aggregate and form condensations within 24 hr of culture. Condensation proceeds to overt chondrogenic differentiation which is evident by the formation of cartilage nodules (B). Within the nodules, the aggregated cells are pushed apart by the nascent secretion of ECM and nodules continue to enlarge by the assimilation of surrounding mesenchyme. Bar: 100 μm.

    c. 0.1% trypsin–0.1% collagenase (Worthington) with 10% chick serum in CMF-PSG. The trypsin–collagenase solution can be prepared as a stock and stored in 2-ml aliquots at −20°C.

    d. Complete serum-containing medium [usually Ham's F_{12} (chondrogenic) or Dulbecco's MEM (myogenic) basal medium supplemented with 10% fetal calf serum and antibiotics depending on the experiment; see chemically defined media below].

    5. After digestion, the limb bud cell suspension is filtered to remove undigested clumps. A convenient apparatus for this step can be made in the laboratory. Drill a 17-mm-diameter hole in a silicone stopper (No. 5, Bellco). Cut the bottom from a 17 × 100-mm polypropylene culture tube and push the tube through the stopper. Impale an 18-gauge needle through the stopper. With gloved hands, cut Nitex No. 20 (No. 10 can also be used; Tetko, Inc.) into 1.5 × 6-in. strips. Boil the strips in 0.5% NaHCO₃ to cleanse and rinse well in double distilled water. Fold the Nitex so that it is double layered and secure it to the bottom of the tube with a 2-mm O ring cut from silicon tubing. The Nitex and the needle tip should be at the small end of the stopper. Autoclave the whole apparatus in a beaker in 0.5 in. of double distilled water. After use, disassemble the apparatus, rinse the fabric in distilled water, and repeat as just described.

B. Isolation and Culture

    1. Crack eggs into a 100-mm petri dish.

    2. Remove the embryo from the yolk sac with blunt forceps. When isolating younger embryos (<stage 22), use microscissors to cut the membranes around the embryo, then remove with curved forceps. Place collected embryos in PSG and check developmental stages.

3. After all the embryos have been collected, transfer to fresh PSG to reduce blood cell contamination.

4. Use fine forceps to remove wing buds: use one pair to steady the embryo and the other to pinch off the limb from the body wall. Be careful to take only the limb without any adherent body wall tissue.

5. Transfer wing buds CMF-PSG. If the limb is to be further subdivided, the wing buds are transferred to PSG for dissection (see Fig. 2; Paulsen *et al.*, 1994). Development of the limb proceeds proximal to distal so along this axis each step in chondrogenic differentiation is represented. The distal tip of the stage 25 limb is undifferentiated but chondrogenic with <0.05% myoblast contamination. Micromass cultures from distal tip mesenchyme differentiate into a homogenous sheet of cartilage and are useful for analysis of chondrocyte biochemistry.

Dissociation is basically a two-step process: incubation of the limb buds with enzyme and pipetting up and down with a long-tip Pasteur pipette. The goal is to obtain a single cell suspension with the least amount of damage to the cells.

6. Transfer the limbs to a 25-ml Erlenmeyer flask.

7. Remove excess CMF-PSG.

8. Add 2 ml of the thawed trypsin–collagenase.

9. Dissociate by shaking in rotary water bath with slow rotation for 10 min at 37°C.

10. Use Pasteur pipette to draw wings up and down to disperse aggregates.

11. Add 2–5 ml of complete medium.

12. Transfer cell solution to 15-ml tube and centrifuge the tube at 100–200 g for 4 min to pellet the cells.

13. Carefully remove as much supernatant as possible without disturbing the cell pellet. Add 2–5 ml of complete medium and resuspend the pellet.

14. Place the Nitex apparatus into a 50-ml conical tube using a test tube holder. Attach a 10-cc syringe to the Luer tip of the needle. Pour the cell suspension into the polypropylene tube to passively filter through the Nitex. Any residual solution can be drawn through the filter by pulling air into the syringe.

15. Using a hemacytometer, count an aliquot of the cell suspension. Adjust the cell concentration to 2×10^7 cells/ml.

16. Pipette 0.1 ml of complete media around the edge of each tissue culture dish. Humidifying the culture dish reduces the chance of dehydration of the micromass during cell attachment.

17. Dispense 10-μl dots (2×10^5 cells) onto the center of the dish, being careful not to get any air bubbles in the dot. Vortex the remaining cell suspension occasionally.

18. Put dish in the incubator for 1 hr.

19. Flood the dish with 2 ml of warmed complete medium. Change the media every day.

C. Critical Aspects of the Technique

Several points are critical to the success of setting up a micromass. (1) Isolate limb buds from the appropriate stage. Mesenchyme from stage 19 and younger embryos will aggregate but will not form cartilage nodules; however, stage 20 mesenchyme will form nodules. Maximal chondrogenesis is achieved by mesenchyme isolated from stage 23–24 mesenchyme (Solursh and Reiter, 1980) whereas older embryos (stage 26) show a marked reduction in the size and number of nodules. (2) As in any enzymatic digestion, extended exposure to proteases results in decreased cell attachment and/or cell death. As new stock solutions are made or enzyme lots are used, the time of digestion must be empirically determined and adjusted accordingly. (3) The addition of culture media to the perimeter of the dish abolishes concerns about dehydration of the 10-μl dot during the attachment of the fragile embryonic cells. (4) Add culture media slowly to the edge of the dish to generate the least amount of shear force across the micromass, particularly in cocultures of micromass and ectoderm.

D. Microtiter Micromass and Defined Medium

This technique extends the usefulness of the micromass culture model by adapting it to a 96-well microtiter plate. This facilitates the handling of large numbers of cultures and biochemical analyses by standard ELISA methods (Paulsen and Solursh, 1988). Limb bud mesenchyme is isolated as described earlier except the final cell concentration is diluted to 2.33×10^6 cells/ml. Put 150 μl of the cell solution (3.5×10^5 cells) into each well of the flat-bottomed, tissue culture-treated microtiter plate. This concentration is sufficient to achieve a high density over the entire well (Fig. 2).

High density cultures undergo chondrogenesis in the absence of serum (fig. 2; Paulsen and Solursh, 1988). Using the microtiter micromass with chemically defined media dramatically reduces the quantities of expensive reagents needed for growth factor studies and isolates the actions of certain agents from interaction with serum proteins. Paulsen's defined medium consists of 60% Ham's F_{12} and 40% Dulbecco's MEM (high glucose) supplemented with 5 μg/ml insulin, 100 nM hydrocortizone, 5 μg/ml chick transferrin (conalbumin), and antibiotics.

E. Coculture of Mesenchyme and Ectoderm

The interaction of epithelia and mesenchyme is fundamental to the development of tissues and organs. High density cultures are combined with ectoderm to study tissue interactions controlling chondrogenesis and the development of pattern.

1. Micromass cultures of limb bud mesenchyme are established as described earlier in 35-mm dishes.

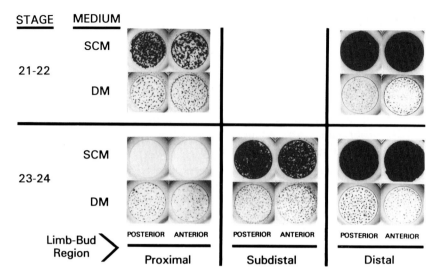

Fig. 2 Microtiter micromass culture of chick limb bud mesenchyme from the stages and regions indicated. Cultures were grown in serum-containing medium (SCM) or defined medium (DM) for 4 days prior to Alcian blue histochemistry. From Paulsen *et al.* (1994), by copyright permission of Wiley-Liss, Inc.

2. The following day, ectoderms are removed from appropriately staged limb buds (stage dependent on experiment) by digestion in 0.43% trypsin–0.25% pancreatin for 15–30 min at 4°C (Solursh *et al.*, 1981).

3. The loosened ectoderms are transferred to horse serum diluted 1:1 in CMF-PSG and are removed using fine tungsten wire needles.

4. Transfer ectoderms to micromass culture dish.

5. The media level is lowered so only a thin layer covers the cultures. Spread the ectoderm over the surface of the micromass with tungsten needles.

6. Place the dish in the incubator for 2 hr to allow the ectoderm to settle down and attach.

7. Taking care not to dislodge the ectoderm, add 0.5 ml of complete medium so that surface tension holds the ectoderms in place. After an additional 4 hr, add another 0.5 ml of medium.

In Fig. 3A, the inhibition of chondrogenesis by the ectoderm is clearly seen by the absence of Alcian blue staining. If the apical ectodermal ridge is present, increased cell proliferation in the mesenchyme will occur, resulting in an outgrowth (Fig. 3b; Solursh *et al.*, 1981). To monitor the precision of ectoderm isolation, cocultures of chick micromass and quail ectoderm are advantageous since quail cells can be identified by the nucleolar marker (see Chapter 2).

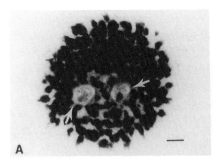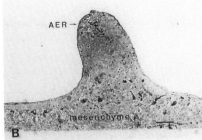

Fig. 3 (A) A 4-day micromass stained with Alcian blue at pH 1.0 demonstrates the rapid accumulation of sulfated proteoglycans in the extracellular matrix. The inhibition of chondrogenesis by the limb ectoderm is apparent by the absence of Alcian blue staining below pieces of ectoderm (arrows). (B) Day 4 micromass cocultured with ectoderm including the apical ectodermal ridge (AER). Mesenchyme under the AER rapidly proliferate, causing an outgrowth away from the substrate. From Solursh *et al.* (1981). Bar: A, 500 μm; B, 100 μm.

F. Micromass on Nucleopore Filters

In the 1950s, transfilter cultures were used to demonstrate the transfer of developmental signals across membrane filters. This technique was improved by using straight-pore Nucleopore filters of varying pore sizes to distinguish between signals mediated by a diffusable signal (pore size 0.2 μm) or by direct cell–cell contact (pore size 0.8 μM) (Wartiovaara *et al.*, 1972). This technique has been used to demonstrate both the induction of chondrogenesis in the mesencephalic neural crest by retinal pigmented epithelium (Smith and Thorogood, 1983) and the short range interactions that occur during the generation of the pattern of cartilage nodules and myoblasts in micromass (Fig. 4; Schramm *et al.*, 1994).

1. Straight-pore polycarbonate filters (6–10 μm thick, 13 mm in diameter containing either 0.1- or 0.8-μm pores; Costar or Poretics Corp.) are autoclaved in double distilled water and allowed to air dry.

2. The filter is sandwiched between two sterile 13-mm Millipore Teflon O rings.

3. A 10-μl micromass culture is placed on the upper surface of the filter and allowed to attached for 1 hr in the incubator.

4. The top O ring is then removed, the filter is inverted, and the O ring is returned. A second culture is plated opposite the first using the original cell suspension that had been stored at 4°C. This second culture can be either high density or subconfluent depending on the experiment.

5. The second culture is allowed to attach for 2 hr. The filter is removed from the O rings and is placed on a support (sterile silicon tubing ring) placed in the bottom of a 24-well tissue culture dish. Each well is fed 1.5 ml of medium and is replaced daily (see Fig. 4).

1. Assemble sterile filter and O rings.

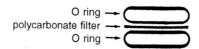

O ring →
polycarbonate filter →
O ring →

2. Place 10 μl micromass on upper filter surface.
   Allow one hr for attachment.

3. Remove upper O ring. Invert filter.
   Replace O ring.

3. Place second culture on upper filter surface.
   Allow 1-2 hr for attachment.

4. Transfer to 24-well dish.

Filter →
Silicon ring →

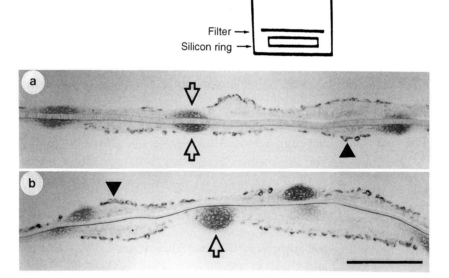

Fig. 4 Transfilter micromass cultures. Large-pore transfilter cultures (a) show that Alcian blue-stained cartilage nodules (open arrows) are aligned across the filter. The alignment of nodules is apparently random across small-pore filters (b). Myogenic cells (arrowheads) on the surface of the micromass are identified by immunoperoxidase staining of the monoclonal antibody MF-20. From Schramm *et al.* (1994). Bar: 100 μm.

G. Quantification of Chondrogenesis

During differentiation, chondrocytes rapidly accelerate the production of highly sulfated proteoglycans (PG). Sulfated PG can be assayed by histochemistry, spectrophotometry, and metabolic [^{35}S]sulfate incorporation. Each method has advantages and limitations, and the method chosen is dependent on the experimental question and design.

Standard assays for chondrogenesis, except radiolabeling, are based on the precipitation of cartilage proteoglycans by the cationic dye, Alcian blue, which at pH 1 will specifically bind sulfated proteoglycans (Lev and Spicer, 1964). To study the pattern, size, and number of cartilage nodules within a micromass culture, Alcian blue histochemistry is used. Details of this procedure are found in Schramm *et al.* (1994). Any fixation that immobilizes PG can be used. This flexibility may be important for subsequent immunohistochemistry. The monoclonal antibodies MF-20 and QH1 (Developmental Studies Hybridoma Bank, NICHD Contract 1-HD-6-2915), localized by immunoperoxidase (Vectastain kit, Vecta Labs), have been used to identify the distribution of myoblasts and quail endothelial cells in micromass cultures. This assay provides both qualitative and quantitative (with morphometry and image analysis) analyses of both homotypic and heterotypic cell interactions.

The greatest advantage of spectrophotometric measurement of Alcian blue precipitation of proteoglycans is the rapid analysis of multiple cultures. This assay is the standard in teratology laboratories where multiple culture conditions may be tested in a single experiment. When combined with the microtiter micromass technique, the assay can be done entirely in a 96-well plate. After fixation and precipitation, the Alcian blue dye is extracted from the cultures using a chaotrophic solution of 4 M guanadine–HCl and the optical density is read at 595 nm. The extractability of the Alcian blue differs among manufacturers. Alcian blue distributed by K & K laboratories (a division of ICN) gives reproducible results with the least background. Immunohistochemistry using alkaline phosphatase as a colorimetric substrate can also be extracted, with the optical density read at 405 nm. Details of these procedures can be found in Paulsen and Solursh (1988).

Incorporation of [^{35}S]sulfate into nascent proteoglycans allows individual proteoglycans to be identified utilizing gel filtration, differential precipitation, and protein electrophoresis. Also, radiolabeling allows analysis of synthesis over time in culture and the separate isolation of PG from the media, the ECM, and the cell residue. Details of this procedure can be found in Paulsen *et al.* (1988).

III. Use of Micromass Culture in Teratology

The purpose of teratogenicity testing is to detect substances that are toxic to the embryo at doses that are not toxic to the adult. An *in vitro* model should elicit processes normal to embryogenesis such as cell proliferation, pattern formation, morphogenetic movement, inductive tissue interactions, and differentiation. The culture concentration of suspected teratogens should be comparable to concentrations found in maternal blood. The micromass culture system fulfills all these requirements and therefore is a popular screening assay for teratogens. Rapid screening of multiwell plates (Hassell and Horigan, 1982) can be achieved by monitoring quantifiable end points that simultaneously measure both growth and differentiation. The micromass system has been modified to include the quantitation of DNA synthesis by radioactive thymidine incorporation to discriminate between true inhibition of cartilage differentiation from inhibition of cell proliferation and nonspecific cytotoxicity. Micromass cultures established from embryonic chick brain and limbs have been used to test insecticides (Farage-Elawar and Rowles, 1992), herbicides (Tsuchiya *et al.,* 1991), and mycotoxins (Wiger and Stormer, 1990).

IV. Discussion and Perspectives

The success of the micromass culture system is found in its faithful recapitulation of *in vivo* differentiation. The system is versatile, allowing multiple manipulations. The effect of high cell density, where cell–cell interactions are favored, can be compared with cultures of single cells where cell–matrix interactions are favored (reviewed by Daniels and Solursh, 1991). The regulatory mechanisms of chondrogenesis (cell–cell and cell–matrix signaling) ultimately lead to the control of response elements in ECM genes. Building on the details of micromass chondrogenesis already published, further studies will identify the signaling pathways to cartilage-specific genes controlled by growth factors, "morphogens," and their receptors during limb development. This model may therefore provide insights in how molecular interactions lead to macroscopic pattern formation in the limb.

References

Ahrens, P. B., Solursh, M., and Reiter, R. S. (1977). Stage related capacity for limb chrondrogenesis in cell culture. *Dev. Biol.* **60,** 69–82.

Ahrens, P. B., Solursh, M., Reiter, R. S., and Singley, C. T. (1979). Position-related capacity for differentiation of limb mesenchyme in cell culture. *Dev. Biol.* **69,** 436–450.

Caplan, A. I. (1970). Effects of the nicotinamide-sensitive teratogen 3-acetylpyridine on chick limb bud cells in culture. *Exp. Cell Res.* **62,** 341–355.

Daniels, K., and Solursh, M. (1991). Modulation of chondrogenesis by the cytoskeleton and extracellular matrix. *J. Cell Sci.* **100,** 249–254.

Ettinger, L., and Doljanski, F. (1992). On the generation of form by the continuous interactions between cells and their extracellular matrix. *Biol. Rev. Cambridge Philos. Soc.* **67,** 459–489.

Farage-Elawar, M., and Rowles, T. K. (1992). Toxicology of carbaryl and aldicarb on brain and limb cultures of chick embryos. *J. Appl. Toxicol.* **12,** 239–244.

Fell, H. B. (1925). The histogenesis of cartilage and bone in the long bones of the embryonic fowl. *J. Morphol. Physiol.* **40,** 417–459.

Hamburger, V., and Hamilton, H. L. (1951). A series of normal stages in the development of the chick embryo. *J. Morphol.* **88,** 49–92.

Hassell, J. R., and Horigan, E. A. (1982). Chondrogenesis: A model system for measuring the teratogenic potential of compounds. *Teratogen., Carcinog., Mutagen.* **2,** 325–331.

Lev, R., and Spicer, S. S. (1964). Specific staining of sulfate groups with Alcian blue at low pH. *J. Histochem. Cytochem.* **12,** 309.

Maini, P. K., and Solursh, M. (1991). Cellular mechanisms of pattern formation in the developing limb. *Int. Rev. Cytol.* **129,** 91–133.

Paulsen, D. F., and Solursh, M. (1988). Microtiter micromass cultures of limb-bud mesenchymal cells. *In Vitro Cell Dev. Biol.* **24,** 138–147.

Paulsen, D. F., Langille, R. M., Dress, V., and Solursh, M. (1988). Selective stimulation of in vitro limb bud chondrogenesis by retinoic acid. *Differentiation (Berlin)* **39,** 123–130.

Paulsen, D. F., Chen, W.-D., Pang, L., Johnson, B., and Okello, D. (1994). Stage-and region-dependent chondrogenesis and growth of chick wing-bud mesenchyme in serum-containing and defined tissue culture media. *Dev. Dyn.* **200,** 39–52.

Puck, T. T., Cieciura, S. J., and Robinson, A. (1958). Genetics of somatic mammalian cells. III. Long-term cultivation of euploid cells from human and animal subjects. *J. Exp. Med.* **108,** 945–956.

Schramm, C., Reiter, R., and Solursh, M. (1994). Role for short range interactions in the formation of cartilage and muscle masses in transfilter micromass cultures. *Dev. Biol.* **163,** 467–479.

Smith, L., and Thorogood, P. (1983). Transfilter studies on the mechanism of epithelio-mesenchymal interaction leading to chondrogenic differentiation of neural crest cells. *J. Embryol. Exp. Morphol.* **75,** 165–188.

Solursh, M., and Reiter, R. S. (1980). Evidence for histogenic interactions during *in vitro* limb chondrogenesis. *Dev. Biol.* **78,** 141–150.

Solursh, M., Singley, C. T., and Reiter, R. S. (1981). The influence of epithelia on cartilage and loose connective tissue formation by limb mesenchyme cultures. *Dev. Biol.* **86,** 471–482.

Tsuchiya, T., Burgin, H., Tsuchiya, M., Winternitz, P., and Kistler, A. (1991). Embryolethality of new herbicides is not detected by the micromass teratogen tests. *Arch. Toxicol.* **65,** 145–149.

Umansky, R. (1966). The effect of cell population density on the developmental fate of reaggregating mouse limb mesenchyme. *Dev. Biol.* **13,** 31–56.

Wartiovaara, J., Lehtonen, R., Nordling, S., and Saxén, L. (1972). Do membrane filters prevent cell contacts? *Nature (London)* **238,** 407–408.

Wedden, S. E., Lewin-Smith, M. R., and Tickle, C. (1986). The patterns of chondrogenesis of cells from facial primordia of chick embryos in micromass culture. *Dev. Biol.* **117,** 71–82.

Wiger, R., and Stormer, F. C. (1990). Effects of ochratoxins A and B on prechondrogenic mesenchymal cells from chick embryo limb buds. *Toxicol. Lett.* **54,** 129–134.

CHAPTER 13

Autonomic and Sensory Neuron Cultures

Rae Nishi

Department of Cell and Developmental Biology
Oregon Health Sciences University
Portland, Oregon 97201

I. Introduction
II. Materials
    A. Solutions and Media
    B. Materials for Dissection
    C. Materials for Dissociation and Culture
III. Methods
    A. Dissection of Ganglia
    B. Dissociation of Ganglia
    C. Culturing Neurons
IV. Critical Aspects of the Procedures
    A. Dissection
    B. Dissociation
    C. Culturing
V. Results and Discussion
VI. Summary and Conclusions
    References

I. Introduction

Beginning with the studies of the outgrowth of axons by Harrison (1910), the maintenance of nervous tissue *in vitro* has facilitated studies of neuronal differentiation. Two major advantages of this method are the ability to study the behavior of neurons in isolation from the body of the organism, and the ability to directly and continuously observe developmental processes. Although primary neuronal cell culture was once considered difficult and mysterious, it is now widely accepted as another technique by which the nervous system can be studied. In addition the expansion of commercial services for culture, including the marketing of a wide variety of culture media, vessels, sera, and neurotrophic factors, has made the technique readily available to anyone who is willing and able.

Among the most readily isolated yet relatively homogenous populations of neurons are those from autonomic (parasympathetic and sympathetic) and sensory (dorsal root) ganglia. Each ganglionic source has special advantages and disadvantages, which this chapter will attempt to summarize. Parasympathetic ganglia are the most homogenous of the three types of peripheral ganglia because they typically innervate a single target organ. Parasympathetic neurons are virtually all cholinergic and they all receive cholinergic presynaptic input, usually from a single nucleus in the central nervous system. Unfortunately, the number of neurons within a parasympathetic ganglion are small, and the number of any particular ganglion per organism is one or two. The two largest parasympathetic ganglia in the chick are the ciliary ganglion (6000–8000 neurons) and the ganglion of Remak (number unknown, but $\geqslant 10,000$). This chapter focuses on methods for the culture of ciliary ganglia (Nishi and Berg, 1979, 1981; Eckenstein *et al.*, 1990). Many more neurons can be obtained from lumbar sympathetic and dorsal root ganglia because 10–16 ganglia can be obtained from each embryo and each ganglion contains several thousand neurons. The difference between these two sources is largely functional—sympathetic neurons receive cholinergic input from the spinal column and innervate organs, blood vessels, and enteric neurons, whereas dorsal root ganglion neurons receive no synapses but process information from the periphery into the central nervous system. Both sympathetic and dorsal root ganglion neurons require trophic support from the neurotrophin family of molecules; sympathetic neurons are all supported by nerve growth factor (NGF), whereas dorsal root ganglia have subpopulations of neurons that require NGF, brain-derived neurotrophic factor, or neurotrophin 3. In contrast, ciliary ganglion neurons do not respond to neurotrophins, but do require the ciliary neurotrophic factor (CNTF).

Thus although all types of ganglionic neurons are useful for studying general neuronal properties such as growth cone motility, axonal outgrowth, neuronal metabolism, and membrane channels, each ganglion is also especially suited to specific types of studies. For example, ciliary ganglion neurons have often been used for studies of *in vitro* neuromuscular junction formation because their cholinergic properties ensure a high rate of synapse formation on striated muscle myotubes. On the other hand, sympathetic and dorsal root ganglion neurons are more useful for biochemical studies requiring large numbers of neurons because of their ease of dissection and their high number per embryo. Obviously, the determination of which type to use will be dictated by the type of studies that are to be pursued. The following details the methods of dissection and culture of these three types of peripheral neurons and discusses critical aspects of culture in order to try to circumvent some of the most commonly made mistakes made by novices.

═══ II. Materials

A. Solutions and Media

HEPES-buffered Earles balanced salt solution (HEBSS):

Dissolve EBSS powder without $NaHCO_3$ from a culture medium supplier
   (e.g., GIBCO/BRL) in 90% of final volume

Add HEPES (Sigma) to a final concentration of 15 mM

Compensate for remaining lack of $NaHCO_3$ by adding NaCl to 11 mM

pH to 7.2; sterilize by filtering through a 0.2-μm filter

Note: by substituting HEPES for $NaHCO_3$ the solution will maintain its pH
   at atmospheric $[CO_2]$; the normal $[Ca^{2+}]$ in EBSS prevents fragile embryonic
   tissue from coming apart

Modified Puck's solution with glucose (MPG):

5× MP stock		1× MPG
NaCl	36 g/liter	20 ml 5× MP
KCl	2 g/liter	1 ml 10% glucose
Na_2HPO_4	6.75 g/liter	79 ml distilled H_2O
NaH_2PO_4	1.02 g/liter	
1 ml 0.5% phenol red		
pH to 7.2; sterilize by filtering through a 0.2-μm filter		

Complete medium:

88 ml Eagles' minimal essential medium (MEM; GIBCO/BRL)

1 ml 100× sterile glutamine (GIBCO/BRL)

1 ml sterile 100× penicillin/streptomycin (GIBCO/BRL)

10 ml heat-inactivated sterile horse serum (GIBCO/BRL)

Note: Thaw, mix the 100× glutamine and 100× pen/strep solutions together,
   and store them in 2- or 4-ml aliquots at −20°C; the horse serum is also
   stored in 10- to 20-ml aliquots at −20°C

0.15 M borate buffer, pH 8.4

Sterile distilled water

Sterile laminin stock (usually 1 mg/ml from Collaborative Ressearch Products,
   Upstate Biotechnology Inc., or GIBCO/BRL)

B. Materials for Dissection

One straight, blunt-ended 4- to 6-in. long forceps

One curved, blunt-ended 4- to 6-in. long forceps

Two Dumont No. 5 forceps

Two No. 2 iridectomy knives

One straight, 4-in. long scissors (for sympathetic dissection only)

One straight, 3- to 4-in. long iridectomy scissors (for dorsal root ganglion dissection only)

Two 100× 20-mm sterile glass petri dishes

One 60× 15-mm sterile glass petri dish

Sterile, cotton-plugged 9-in. Pasteur pipettes

Sterile 15-ml polystyrene conical centrifuge tube with cap

Chicken eggs, preferably 8 days of incubation at 100°F (E8) for ciliary ganglia, E10 for sensory ganglia, and E13 for sympathetic ganglia

Low power dissecting microscope (3–70× magnification) that can illuminate preparations from above or below

C. Materials for Dissociation and Culture

15-ml polystyrene conical centrifuge tube containing dissected and cleaned ganglia (as described earlier)

Sterile 2.5% trypsin (GIBCO/BRL)

Complete medium with 10% heat-inactivated horse serum (as described earlier)

Sterile 9-in. Pasteur pipettes with cotton plugs

Amber latex Pasteur pipette bulb

Water bath set at 37°C

Tabletop clinical centrifuge

24-well tissue culture plate (if using other vessels, correct amounts for the surface area)

III. Methods

A. Dissection of Ganglia

1. Suggested Age of Embryos to Use for Dissections

a. Ciliary Ganglia

The best cultures of ciliary ganglion neurons are obtained from embryonic day (E) 7.5 to 8 chicks (Hamburger–Hamilton stage 34). At this stage the chicks do not yet have pin feathers and two-thirds to all of the scleral papillae have formed around the eye. Stage 34 is prior to the time of cell death, so 6500–8000 neurons can be recovered per ganglion. In comparison, the volume of the ganglion at stage 40 (E14) is four to six times larger, even though the number of neurons is half that of stage 34, indicating that the number of nonneuronal cells has significantly increased. The trypsin protocol described does not work well with ganglia ≥E14.

b. Lumbar Sympathetic Ganglia

The lumbar sympathetic ganglia are most readily found, dissected, and cultured at E12–E14. Although the sympathetic chain can be identified at earlier stages, the populaton is mixed in that it contains both differentiating neuroblasts and postmitotic neurons. After embryonic day 14 the ganglia become increasingly difficult to dissociate with trypsin and contain increasingly more nonneuronal cells.

c. Dorsal Root Ganglia

Dorsal root ganglia can be isolated and cultured between E8 and E12. The E8 ganglia are often used in the explant culture as a bioassay for NGF, but they adhere less well to the substratum than neurons from older ganglia. E10–E12 ganglia produce more robust, larger neurons and survival appears to be better with fewer nonneuronal cells than at E8.

2. General Protocol Common to All Dissections

a. Sterilize the instruments in 70% ethanol for >20 min.
b. Squirt each egg twice with 70% ethanol (allow ethanol to dry between applications).
c. Crack the egg and pull the shell off with the straight, blunt forceps; remove the embryo with the curved forceps by hooking them around the neck.
d. Place embryo into a 100-mm petri dish that is about two-thirds full of cold EBSS; remove all embryos at once.
e. Using the curved forceps, cut the heads off E7.5–E10 embryos by pinching the neck between the forceps tips; cut heads off E12–E13 embryos with small scissors.

3. Dissection of Ciliary Ganglia

a. Collect all the heads from E7.5–E8 embryos into a fresh 100-mm petri dish containing HEBSS. Place the dish with heads on the stage of a dissecting microscope with the light coming from above; position the 60-mm petri dish containing 10 ml of cold MPG near the microscope with the lid off.
b. Working at the lowest magnification possible (3–4×), use the Dumont No. 5 forceps to turn a head so that the beak points up. Holding the head down with one pair of forceps pinned in the neck, use the other pair to pinch through the skin and extraocular tissue around the orbit of the eye. Work about three-fourths

of the way around, pinching and cutting through the skin and muscle, but not piercing the eye.

c. Place one pair of forceps in the orbit of the eye against the beak and place the other pair of forceps against the eye and gently rotate the eye away from the orbit. Look for the optic nerve. A ganglion suspended by its pre- and postganglionic nerve can be seen just below the optic nerve. That is the ciliary ganglion. Keep rotating the eye until the optic nerve breaks (Fig. 1A).

d. Turn the loose eyeball over so that the optic nerve and the choroid fissure can be seen. The ciliary ganglion should be between the optic nerve and the fissure. It is small, white, and round. A nerve will often be attached.

e. Remove the ganglion by grabbing the postganglionic nerve (the one that attaches the ganglion to the eye); transfer the ganglion to the 60-mm petri dish.

f. After all the ganglia have been collected, position the 60-mm dish with the ganglia under the scope, increase the magnification (to about 10×), and push all the floating ganglia down below the surface tension of the solution with the forceps. The ganglia will then sink to the bottom. Bring all the submerged ganglia together in the center of the dish by gently swirling the dish.

g. Using the iridectomy knives in a "scissoring" action, trim the extra mesodermal tissue off the ganglia and cut the nerves as close as possible to the ganglion. This will minimize nonneuronal contamination of the cell culture. Once the ganglia have been cleaned, push them to a different part of the dish and count them.

4. Dissection of Lumbar Sympathetic Ganglia

a. Turn the body of the embryo so that the back side is up and cut along the outside of the spinal column to remove the strip of body wall that contains the

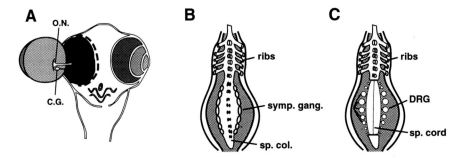

Fig. 1 Location of ganglia after dissection of embryos. (A) The ciliary ganglion (C.G.) can be seen just under the optic nerve (O.N.) when the eye is rotated out of its socket. (B) The lumbar sympathetic ganglia (symp. gang.) can be seen as condensations along the side of the spinal column (sp. col.) after all adhering organs and blood vessels have been removed from the body wall. The sympathetic ganglia are not to scale. They are actually smaller and have connectives between the ganglia. (C) The dorsal root ganglia (DRG) can be seen embedded in mesenchymal tissue on either side of the spinal cord (sp. cord) after the ventral half of the spinal column is removed. The peripheral nerves exiting the ganglia join together to form the lumbar plexus.

lumbar spinal column; transfer a strip of the spinal column/cord to a petri dish filled with HEBSS and clean organ parts and blood vessels away from the internal face.

b. Transfer the cleaned strip to a 60-mm dish containing 10 ml sterile MPG. Turn the strip so that the internal face is up; the outline of the spinal column and, along its side, the sympathetic chain (Fig. 1B) should be visible. Run an iridectomy knife blade along the outside of the sympathetic chain to cut the postganglionic nerves. Similarly, cut the preganglionic nerves by slicing between the chain and the spinal column.

c. Grab the sympathetic chain at one end with a pair of Dumont No. 5 forceps and pull up using the iridectomy knife to free the ganglia from adherent tissue. Set the chain down in the bottom of the same dish; discard the spinal column once all the sympathetic ganglia have been removed.

d. Using the iridectomy knives, cut the ganglia free from the chain, cutting the connectives as close to the ganglion as possible. With transillumination the ganglia can be readily distinguished from connectives by the texture (ganglia contain small clear and bright spheres, whereas connectives look like bundles of cables).

5. Dissection of Lumbar Dorsal Root Ganglia

a. Collect all beheaded chick embryo bodies in one dish filled with HEBSS. Turn them so their backs are up and, using fine dissecting scissors, cut out the strip of body wall containing the lumbar spinal column away from the limbs. Place the strips in another dish with HEBSS.

b. Clean the strips free of organs and blood vessels. Holding the body wall so that the internal (ventral) side is up, insert one pair of Dumont No. 5 forceps into one side of the spinal column and use the other pair of forceps to pinch and cut along the side of the column. Repeat along the opposite side until the ventral spinal column cartilage can be "peeled" away from the dorsal half, exposing the spinal cord.

c. Once the spinal cord is exposed, the dorsal root ganglia are very easily seen between each segment of the spinal column (Fig. 1C). Each ganglion can be "plucked" out by pinching the peripheral nerve, pinching the central nerve, grabbing the ganglion by either nerve stump, and transferring the ganglion to another dish containing MPG. Alternatively, by removing the spinal cord, most of the ganglia will come attached by the dorsal roots. Cut the ganglia away from the cord.

B. Dissociation of Ganglia

1. Add 2.4 ml MPG to the centrifuge tube containing the ganglia. Add 0.1 ml 2.5% trypsin to the MPG (final trypsin concentration is 0.1%) and gently agitate the tube to mix the trypsin into the solution. Incubate ganglia in a water bath at 37°C for 20 min.

2. Spin ganglia down to the bottom of the tube by centrifuging for 2 min at 200–250 g. Carefully remove the supernatant with a Pasteur pipette. Add 3 ml complete medium with serum and triturate using a cotton-plugged 9-in. Pasteur pipette with a tip that has been fire-polished so that it is approximately half its original diameter.

3. Spin cells down in clinical centrifuge at 200–250 g for 5 min. Remove the supernatant with a Pasteur pipette (do not use an aspirator because the cells may be accidentally sucked out).

4. Resuspend cells at desired concentration.

C. Culturing Neurons

1. Preparation of the Substratum (Should Be Done 1–2 Days Prior to Dissection and Dissociation)

a. Make the polylysine solution up fresh each time the plates are prepared. Dissolve the poly-D-lysine in borate buffer, pH 8.4, at a concentration of 0.5 mg/ml. Sterilize the solution by passing it through a 0.2-μm filter mounted on a syringe. Add 0.5 ml of polylysine solution per well. Incubate at room temperature for 4–18 hr.

b. Wash each well three times with 1 ml of sterile distilled water (thorough washing is important because borate is toxic to cells).

c. Dilute the laminin to 20 μg/ml in the sterile balanced salt solution and add 0.25 ml to each well of the 24-well plate. Incubate at 4°C overnight. Allow the plate to come to room temperature before aspirating the laminin solution off and replacing with medium. Ideally, the plates should be used the day after adding the laminin solution, but they can be left up to a week at 4°C wrapped in plastic wrap (Saran wrap, cling wrap) to minimize evaporation.

2. Medium

The basic medium that is used for both ciliary and lumbar sympathetic ganglia is Eagles' minimal essential medium supplemented with 50 U/ml penicillin, 50 μg/ml streptomycin, 2 mM glutamine, and 10% (v/v) heat-inactivated horse serum. The penicillin, streptomycin, and glutamine can be purchased as sterile 100× stock solutions from commerical vendors (e.g., GIBCO/BRL, Microbiological Associates, Sigma). Because sera available for cell culture tend to be very variable and differ greatly in their quality, different lots of horse serum from several different vendors should be pretested for their ability to support long-term (10–14 days) neuronal cell survival in the presence of an appropriate neurotrophic factor (see below), and then purchasing a large quantity and storing it at −20°C. Serum that is already heat inactivated can be purchased from some vendors. If the serum is not heat inactivated, then incubate at 100-ml bottle at 56°C in a water bath for 30 min and spin at 40,000 g in a refrigerated centrifuge for 45 min to remove precipitated material.

Ciliary, sympathetic, and dorsal root ganglion neurons cannot survive in cell culture without the addition of neurotrophic factors. Although crude sources of trophic factors (e.g., 5% chick embryo extract) can be used, it is preferable to use a purified or recombinant trophic factor, especially to limit the proliferation of nonneuronal cells. Fortunately, a number of molecules that support sympathetic, dorsal root, or ciliary ganglion survival have now been identified (Table I; Fig. 2). With the exception of growth-promoting activity, all of the trophic factors listed in this chapter are now commercially available or available for research purposes through material transfer agreement from private companies. The neurotrophic factors should be used at a concentration that is greater than or equal to the saturating concentration. The cells should be fed every 3 days.

3. Reducing the Number of Nonneuronal Cells

Nonneuronal cell contamination can be a problem if the ganglia contain a large number of satellite cells and fibroblasts (e.g., dorsal root ganglia or ciliary ganglia >E8) or if the medium contains molecules that are mitogenic to the nonneuronal cells. The number of nonneuronal cells that are plated can be

Table I

Molecules That Support the Survival of Autonomic and Sensory Neurons in Cell Culture

Molecule	Specificity[a]	Linear concentration range	Saturating concentration
Stage 7 nerve growth factor (NGF)[b]	symp; some DRG	0.1–0.5 μg/ml	$\geq$1 μg/ml
Stage 2.5 NGF[c]	symp; some DRG	0.01–0.5 ng/ml	$\geq$1 ng/ml
Ciliary neurotrophic factor[d]	CG; symp; DRG	0.1–1.0 ng/ml	$\geq$1 ng/ml
Growth-promoting activity[e]	CG; symp; DRG	1.0–10 pg/ml	$\geq$0.1 ng/ml
Acidic fibroblast growth factor (aFGF)[e]	CG; symp; DRG	0.01–0.1 ng/ml	$\geq$1 ng/ml
Basic fibroblast growth factor (bFGF)[e]	CG; symp; DRG	0.01–0.1 ng/ml	$\geq$1 ng/ml
Brain-derived neurotrophic factor[f]	Some DRG	0.01–0.5 ng/ml	$\geq$1 ng/ml
Neurotrophin 3[g]	Some DRG	0.01–0.5 ng/ml	$\geq$1 ng/ml

[a] symp, sympathetic ganglion; DRG, dorsal root ganglion; CG, ciliary ganglion.
[b] Chun and Patterson (1977); available from Collaborative Biomedical Products; GIBCO/BRL; Upstate Biotechnology, Inc.; Sigma Chemical Co.
[c] Greene (1977a,b); available from Collaborative Biomedical Products; GIBCO/BRL; Upstate Biotechnology, Inc.; Sigma Chemical Co.
[d] McDonald et al. (1991); Manthorpe et al. (1986); Alomone Labs.
[e] Eckenstein et al. (1990); FGFs are available from Collaborative Biomedical Products; GIBCO/BRL; Upstate Biotechnology, Inc.; Sigma Chemical Co.; Calbiochem.
[f] Leibrock et al. (1989); Alomone Labs.
[g] Hohn et al. (1990); Alomone Labs.

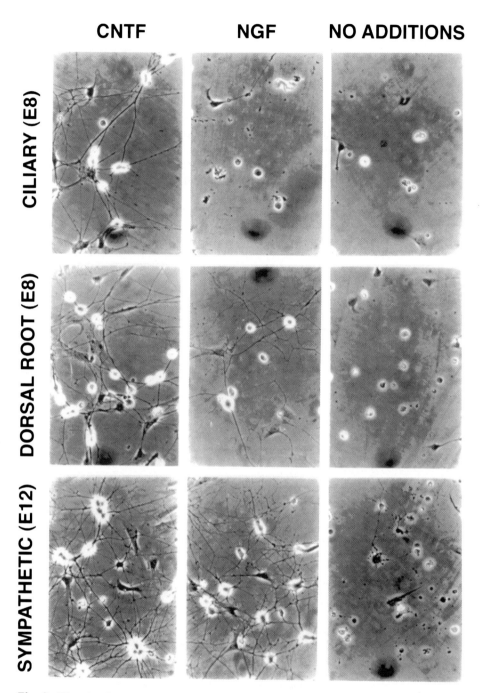

Fig. 2 Dissociated sympathetic, ciliary, and dorsal root ganglin neurons in culture. The responses of sympathetic, ciliary, and dorsal root ganglion neurons to nerve growth factor (NGF) and ciliary neurotrophic factor (CNTF) are shown after 48 hr in cell culture. Note that there is no neuronal survival in the absence of a trophic factor (no addition). This figure has been modified from Eckenstein *et al.* (1990).

significantly reduced by carefully cleaning the ganglia free of attached nerve and adherent mesenchymal tissue. The mitogenicity of the medium can be controlled by using horse serum instead of fetal calf serum and by using defined trophic factors instead of embryo extract to support neuronal survival. Interestingly, the use of aFGF or bFGF in supporting ciliary or sympathetic neuron survival does not seem to induce proliferation of the ganglionic nonneuronal cells (R. Nishi, unpublished results). Preplating the cell suspension for 1 hr at 37°C also helps eliminate fibroblast contamination but may also decrease the yield of neurons. Antimitotic drugs such as cytosine arabinoside will kill rapidly dividing cells such as fibroblasts, but will not kill more slowly dividing cells such as satellite cells from the ganglion. In addition, chick neurons may also be nonspecifically killed by antimitotic agents. If an antimitotic agent must be used, then use lower than suggested concentrations of cytosine arabinoside ($<10^{-5} M$) or use antimitotic agents that are less toxic (fluorodeoxyuridine + uridine at $10^{-5} M$).

IV. Critical Aspects of the Procedures

A. Dissection

As soon as the organism is killed, anoxia produces a number of degenerative processes which can be minimized if the solutions in which the tissues are bathed are kept cold and if the ganglia of interest are isolated as rapidly as possible. Because embryonic tissues are extremely fragile and soft with little color contrast for identifying structures, it is often helpful to immerse them completely in isotonic saline to buoy the structures and preserve morphology. The saline used for dissection should contain divalent cations to promote tissue integrity and the buffer should not be bicarbonate because the pH will become alkaline if left at atmospheric CO_2 concentrations for extended periods of time. The sticking of tissues to dissecting instruments can be minimized if the instruments are cleaned after each use by carefully rubbing them over the surface of soap embedded with an abrasive (Lava soap).

B. Dissociation

The best yields of viable neurons are obtained when one is extremely careful about each step of the dissociation. Likewise, in order to obtain maximal reproducibility it is wise to adhere rigorously to the times suggested for enzyme incubation, trituration, and centrifugation. Crude trypsin contains proteolytic activities that work well to dissociate tissue, but if digestion conditions are not carefully controlled, trypsin can reduce neuronal viability. For example, the optimum pH for trypsin is 8.0; however, tissue dissocation is better controlled at physiological pH where the enzyme activity is reduced. As a consequence, bicarbonate-buffered solutions should not be used for trypsin incubations because the solution will rapidly lose CO_2 at 37°C and become more alkaline. Trypsin lots can be very variable, even when purchased from the same source, e.g., 2.5% sterile trypsin solution purchased from GIBCO/BRL varying anywhere from 0.06 to 0.125% works best in digesting ganglia without reducing viability. The strength of mechanical dissociation used can also cause cell damage. The variables in mechanical dissociation are the bore of the pipette used, the device used to move fluid into the pipette, and the number of times the ganglia must be passed through the pipette. For the protocol just given, the opening of a 9-in. Pasteur pipette is fire polished and reduced in diameter by about one-half, an amber latex bulb is used for moving fluid, and the ganglia should be pipetted up and down 40–90 times. If the ganglia dissociate in less than 30 trips up and down, then the trypsinization or the strength of trituration (i.e., the bore of the pipette or the speed of the trituration) is too much, and many cells will be damaged. If it takes more than 100 times, then the trypsin is too weak or the bore of the pipette is not closed down enough.

C. Culturing

The two most important variables in culturing neurons are the substratum on which the neurons are grown and the medium in which they are cultured. Although a variety of substrata have been used for plating neurons, the most consistently supportive of neuronal attachment and neurite outgrowth for autonomic and sensory neurons is laminin. Laminin is commercially available from a number of sources such as GIBCO/BRL, Collaborative Research, and UBI. When purchasing laminin pay close attention to the bioassay data; the best lots of laminin for neurite outgrowth are the ones that test best in a cell attachment assay. Although most manufacturers supply laminin in a phosphate-buffered saline, it actually has a longer storage life if it is put in 20% glycerol and stored at −80°C. Once thawed, leave the laminin solution at 4°C. Because laminin is a very large molecule (M_r 10^6 Da), repeated freeze–thawing causes a loss of cell attachment and neurite outgrowth activity. The protocol described earlier attaches laminin to a tissue culture plastic that has been precoated with poly-D-lysine. In the experience of this author, more laminin adheres to poly-D-lysine, probably because many laminin preparations are contaminated with heparin sulfate proteoglycans. Poly-D-lysine is used instead of poly-L-lysine because of its greater resistance to proteolysis.

Most peripheral neurons require neurotrophic factors to survive in cell culture. In many cases, several structurally distinct molecules have been reported to support the survival of specific neuronal populations, and the list is still growing. Obviously, the choice of neurotrophic support will profoundly influence the properties of the neurons that survive in culture. For example, although sympathetic neuron survival can be supported by CNTF, CNTF has also been reported to induce cholinergic properties in noradrenergic neurons. Most mammalian neurotrophic factors will support the survival of chick neurons. On the other hand, not all antibodies against mammalian molecules will cross-react to the chick. For example, although mouse NGF supports chick sympathetic neuron survival, blocking antibodies to mouse NGF will not block endogenous chick NGF. Finally, an essential fact to keep in mind is that many trophic factors are very labile and hence cannot be kept for very long once they have been diluted into complete medium. Trophic factors should be aliquoted into one-time use volumes and stored at −80°C (long-term storage) or at −20°C (e.g., short-term storage between feedings). The factors should be thawed and added to the culture medium just prior to feeding.

One last important consideration is the type of tissue culture vessel in which the neurons will be plated. This will largely be dictated by the purpose for which the cultures are being established. If the aim is to observe the behavior of neurons with time-lapse photography or electrophysiology, then the smallest single culture plate available is a 35-mm dish. Neurons can be confined to a smaller area of the 35-mm dish by using a modified tabletop lathe to drill a 5- to 10-mm hole in the center of the dish, under which a glass or plastic coverslip is mounted with paraffin or Sylgard (Dow Corning). Such a vessel is also useful for limiting volumes used when performing immunocytochemistry or *in situ* hybridization (a typical volume is 50–75 μl). If the aim is to compare the survival of the neurons in response to a variety of putative trophic molecules, then a 24- or 48-well tissue culture plate facilitates culturing the neurons under a variety of conditions. As the number of wells in a plate increases, the ability to view the neurons with good phase contrast optics decreases. Multichamber culture slides are also available (Nunc) but the neurons tend to grow only in the corners of the chambers (they probably get washed out of the center of the chambers when the cultures are fed). This is most often a problem with ciliary ganglion neurons and less of a problem with sympathetic and E10 dorsal root ganglion neurons.

V. Results and Discussion

One day after plating all of the viable neurons should be attached directly to the substratum and not merely on top of nonneuronal cells. Cellular debris should be minimal. The cell bodies should look smooth and phase bright, and many neurites should already have initiated and extended several cell body diameters. Poor attachment and stunted neurite outgrowth indicate that the substratum or the medium supplementation (presence of appropriate trophic factors) is not optimal; rough, phase dark cell bodies with a large amount of cellular debris indicate that the dissociation was too rough. Cultures that survive the first 48 hr after plating can usually be maintained for many days, provided that trophic factors are replenished by feeding and that no toxic substances are inadvertently introduced.

Because the amount of material is limited, primary cultures of autonomic and sensory ganglia are most useful for studies requiring observations of the behavior of single cells. Techniques used for such studies are immunocytochemistry, *in situ* hybridization, electrophysiological recording, electron microscopy, time-lapse photography, cell counting, single cell PCR, and single cell injection. Extraction techniques that measure the average behavior of all the cells within the culture must be very sensitive or one must be willing to dissect many ganglia in order to obtain enough material for analysis. For example, techniques such as RNase protection and PCR are preferable to Northern blotting for analysis of mRNA levels in cultures of primary peripheral neurons.

Although cell culture greatly facilitates the visualization and manipulation of neurons, it is important to keep in mind that it is a highly artificial environment for neuronal development. Seemingly small changes like switching to a new lot of serum or a different formulation of basal medium can significantly change the response of neurons. As a result, culture conditions should be set up with all possible controls at each plating in order to interpret each experiment. In addition, a larger number of trials may be required before data obtained by cell culture are "believable." One typically must see the same result three to five times before it can be believable. If unknown circumstances cause an experiment to produce highly variable results, then it is worth investigating what the essential variable is by systematically varying every parameter of the experiment until conditions are optimized to produce consistent results. If possible, all results obtained in cell culture should eventually be tested *in vivo* to determine the physiological sigificance of the findings.

VI. Summary and Conclusions

This chapter has provided a rather detailed protocol for the dissection, dissociation, and culture of autonomic and sensory neurons from the chicken embryo. These protocols are by no means absolute. Many other laboratories that routinely culture these neurons may use techniques that differ significantly from the ones detailed in this chapter. All of the protocols described in this chapter can also be applied to quail embryos, which develop more rapidly but are of comparable size to chicken embryos until about E9. The list of suppliers for the various reagents described in these protocols is also limited. Many other vendors of cell culture products are probably equally reliable.

References

Chun L. L. Y., and Patterson, P. H. (1977). Role of nerve growth factor in the development of rat sympathetic neurons in vitro. I. Survival, growth and differentiation of catecholaminergic production. *J. Cell Biol.* **75,** 649–704.

Eckenstein, F. P., Esch, F., Holbert, T., Blacher, R. W., and Nishi, R. (1990). Purification and characterization of a trophic factor for embryonic peripheral neurons: Comparison with fibroblast growth factors. *Neuron* **4,** 623–631.

Greene, L. A. (1977a). Quantitative *in vitro* studies on the nerve growth factor (NGF) requirement of neurons I. Sympathetic neurons. *Dev. Biol.* **58,** 96–105.

Greene, L. A. (1977b). Quantitative *in vitro* studies on the nerve growth factor (NGF) requirement of neurons II. Sensory neurons. *Dev. Biol.* **58,** 106–113.

Harrison, R. G. (1910). The outgrowth of the nerve fiber as a mode of protoplasmic movement. *J. Exp. Zool.* **9,** 787–846.

Hohn, A., Leibrock, J., Bailey, K., and Barde, Y.-A. (1990). Identification and characterization of a novel member of the nerve growth factor/brain-derived neurotrophic factor family. *Nature (London)* **344,** 339–341.

Leibrock, J., Lottspeich, F., Hohn, A., Hofer, M., Hengerer, B., Masiakowski, P., Thoenen, H., and Barde, Y.-A. (1989). Molecular cloning and expression of brain-derived neurotrophic factor. *Nature (London)* **341,** 149–152.

Manthorpe, M., Skaper, S. D., Williams, L. R., and Varon, S. (1986). Purification of adult rat sciatic nerve ciliary neuronotrophic factor. *Brain Res.* **367,** 282–286.

McDonald, J. R., Ko, C., Mismer, D., Smith, D. J., and Collins, F. (1991). Expression and characterization of recombinant human ciliary neurotrophic factor from *Escherichia coli. Biochim. Biophys. Acta* **1090,** 70–80.

Nishi, R., and Berg, D. K. (1979). Survival and development of ciliary ganglion neurones grown alone in cell culture. *Nature (London)* **277,** 232–234.

Nishi, R., and Berg, D. K. (1981). Two components from eye tissue that differentially stimulate the growth and development of ciliary ganglion neurons in cell culture. *J. Neurosci.* **1,** 505–513.

CHAPTER 14

Retinal Cultures

Deborah Finlay, George Wilkinson, Robert Kypta, Ivan de Curtis,[1] and Louis Reichardt

Howard Hughes Medical Institute and
Department of Physiology
University of California
San Francisco, California 94143

I. Introduction
II. Obtaining Primary Cells
    A. Retinal Dissection
    B. Trypsinization
    C. Retinal Ganglion Cell Isolation
    D. Dissection of the Retina
    E. Preparation of Retinal Cell Suspension
    F. Percoll Gradient
    G. Retinal Explants: Flat Mounts and Retinal Strips
III. Cell Culture
    A. Retinal Cell Culture
    B. Transient Transfection of Chicken Retinal Neurons
    C. Staining for β-Galactosidase Expression
IV. Neuronal Cell Assays
    A. Preparation of Substrates
    B. Cell/Substratum Adhesion Assay
    C. Crystal Violet Stain
    D. Neurite Outgrowth Assay
V. Concluding Remarks
    References

I. Introduction

The avian retina has proven to be a very useful tissue for analysis by cell biologists and biochemists. Its principle advantages are that the eye is very large

[1] Present address: Dept. Biology and Technology, San Raffaele Hospital, via Olgettina 60, 20132 Milano, Italy.

METHODS IN CELL BIOLOGY, VOL. 51
Copyright © 1996 by Academic Press, Inc. All rights of reproduction in any form reserved.

265

in early chick embryos; that it is easy to dissect and is well separated from other neuronal populations; and that it is composed of only a few classes of neurons. In addition, retinal neurons are hardy and therefore easy to culture.

Dissociated retinal neurons are currently used *in vitro* to study the adhesive properties of neurons and changes in adhesiveness during development (DeCurtis *et al.*, 1991; De Curtis and Reichardt, 1993; Hall *et al.*, 1987; Neugebauer *et al.*, 1991); fate determination, survival, and differentiation of neuronal precursors (Watanabe and Raff, 1992; Reh, 1992); and navigation by advancing growth cones (Snow and Letourneau, 1992).

Explanting pieces of retina gives two advantages over culturing dissociated retinal neurons. The first is that all the axons which emerge from retinal strip explants originate from a single class of retinal cell, the retinal ganglion cell (Halfter *et al.*, 1983). Second, it is possible in explant pieces of retina to keep track of the relative retinal location of all the neurons in the explant. This is important because the pattern of axonal outgrowth from retinal explants will vary depending on the location in the retina from which the neurons were obtained (Halfter *et al.*, 1983). For example, investigators have found differences in outgrowth behavior between the axons of retinal ganglion cells in explants obtained from nasal retina compared to the axons of temporal retinal ganglion cells (Raper and Grunewald, 1990; Walter *et al.*, 1987).

Many techniques for studying the chick retina exist in the primary literature. Criteria for staging the embryonic chick are described in Hamburger and Hamilton (1992). Also, Mey and Thanos (1992) review the development of this brain region in detail. More about neuronal cell culture may be found in Banker and Goslin (1992).

Space restrictions limit this chapter to a discussion of methods used in our laboratory. These methods have been separated into sections dealing with obtaining primary cells, cell culture, and cell assays. There is some unavoidable overlap among these sections. Where overlap occurs it is best to follow the particular instructions included with a given method.

II. Obtaining Primary Cells

This section describes the basic dissection used to obtain retinal cells for the majority of assays, as well as a slightly modified protocol for explant cultures. In addition, a protocol for the enrichment of retinal ganglion cells has been included.

The dissection itself is fairly similar in all the following protocols. Figure 1 describes the basic steps in obtaining the retina. Extra care is required in the actual removal of the retina from the vitreous humor when flat mounting the retina for explant (see specific details in that protocol). The procedure that can be the most trying in this dissection is the complete removal of the retinal pigment epithelium (RPE). The retina and the RPE are maintained in close proximity

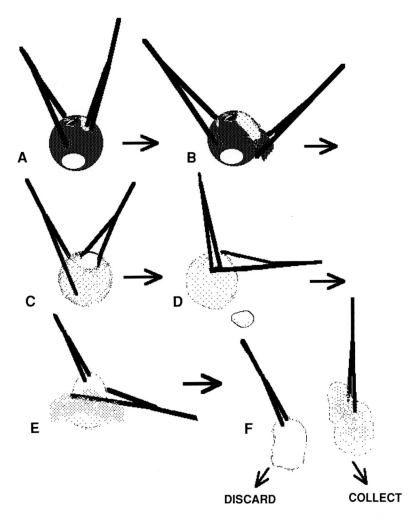

Fig. 1 Dissection of an embryonic day 7 retina. (A and B) Peel away RPE from the back of the eye. (C) Remove the lens. (D) Grasp the vitreous humor with one pair of forceps and hold the retina with the other. (E) Pull the virteous humor out from the retina. (F) Discard the virteous humor and collect the retina into holding media.

by cation-dependent interactions. Therefore, incubating the chick eyes in divalent free holding medium at 37°C prior to RPE removal is important for success.

Although the basic dissection varies little, some noteworthy differences do exist in the preparation of the cell suspension (found both here and in the section on cell culture). The standard trypsinization protocol, combined with preplating the retinal cells (as described in the cell culture section), is sufficient for most adhesion or neurite outgrowth assays. For transfection, however, the enzymatic digestion is eliminated, replaced by trituration alone, with the intent of leaving small clumps of cells. This modification aids cell survival. In contrast, the ganglion cell enrichment protocol requires rigorous enzyme digestion to obtain a single cell suspension adequate for the separation of cells by density. Reviewing all of the methods in this chapter should facilitate the proper dissection for a given application.

A. Retinal Dissection

This procedure is modified from Hall *et al.* (1987) (for flat mounting, see the modified protocol).

Materials

70% ethanol

Two pairs of No. 5 forceps

Two 60- or 100-mm dissecting dishes for dissecting eyes from head

One additional 35-mm dissecting dish per four to six eyes

One 15-ml conical tube

Dissecting scope (with overhead light source)

Holding medium:

100 U/ml penicillin and streptomycin (pen/strep)

0.5% glucose in Ca^{2+} and Mg^{2+}-free phosphate-buffered saline (PBS-CMF)

Sterile filter and store at $-20°C$ in 10-ml aliquots.

1. Rinse eggs with 70% ethanol. Place embryos into petri dish with forceps and decapitate. Remove eyes, transfer eyes into holding medium, and carefully trim off as much as possible of the connective tissue. Sort four to six eyes per 35-mm dish and incubate for 20 min at 37°C. Warming of the eyes facilitates the removal of the RPE from the retina. Be careful not to incubate too long at this temperature as it will reverse this effect. Temperature is most important for older embryos, embryonic day 9 and older. Placing batches of eyes in the incubator at 20-min intervals is recommended for large dissections.

2. Remove the warm eyes from the incubator. Rotate the eye lens down and hold it with one pair of forceps. Insert the tip of the remaining forceps between the pigment epithelium (dark layer) and the retina. Separate away some pigment epithelia from gashes received in the dissection process. If this is not possible, carefully pierce the pigmented layer and peel away from the retina. (Alternatively, one can start with the eye upright, remove the lens, and peel the RPE down from around the lens.) Since the RPE is most likely to stick to the rim of the lens and the optic nerve head, take extra care in pinching it off the retina at these spots.

3. Removal of the retina.

a. For eyes from E6 and older: Remove the lens. Grasp the vitreous humor (gelatinous ball) through the lens hole and scrape the retina off by holding it in place with one pair of forceps at the lens opening and pulling the vitreous humor through them (Fig. 1). Keep the dissection area clear by discarding the RPE and vitreous humor from the dissection dish.

b. For embryos less than E6 or situations where the vitreous humor is extruded from the eye during the dissection: Cut through the cell layers and place the resulting strip retinal side up on the dish. The retina cells can then be peeled away from the RPE. Occasionally, the vitreous humor will pop out of the eye during the dissection. When the dissection proceeds without the vitreous humor, the orientation of the cell layers can become confused. Overhead lighting combined with a dark opaque background under the dish give the retina a translucent appearance which very clearly distinguishes it from the sclera.

4. Place the retinae in a 15-ml conical tube with PBS holding media. Retinae can be accumulated in this tube on ice until the trypsinization step and cell culture.

B. Trypsinization

Materials

        Trypsinization buffer

           0.5% trypsin (bovine pancreatic grade III, Sigma No. T8253)

           0.5% glucose

           in PBS-CMF

        Defined medium

           50 ml F12 (GIBCO) with:

           20 mM glutamine

           100 U/ml pen/strep

           1× modified Bottenstein's additives (see below)

           0.1 mg/ml conalbumin (Sigma type II No. C-0880)

        Modified Bottenstein's additives (100×):

           0.5 mg/ml insulin (Sigma Cat. No. I 1882)

           10 mg/ml human transferrin (Sigma Cat. No. 51147)

           300 nM selenous acid (J.T. Baker Cat. No. 4-0310)

           in PBS-CMF

        Filter to sterilize, aliquot, and store at −20°C.

1. Trypsinize tissue by adding 1 ml trypsin solution to retina in 5 ml holding medium (0.1% trypsin final). Incubate in a 37°C water bath for ~3–5 min with occasional mixing. When the retinae start to fall apart, add 2 ml fetal calf serum

to stop digestion. *Note:* This method is fine for under 20 or so retinae. For larger numbers, add 0.5 mg/ml DNase. Also, the incubation should be monitored closely, it may take up to 10 min for sufficient DNase digestion.

2. To wash, spin cells in a clinical centrifuge at 1000 *g* for 5 min. Aspirate the supernatant and add 3 ml medium. Triturate with a sterile Pasteur pipette until cloudy (maximum of 10 times). Add media to bring cells to desired concentration.

C. Retinal Ganglion Cell Isolation

The following protocol is modified from one developed by Dr. Jim Johnson (Wake Forest University School of Medicine, see Johnson, 1989), which in turn is modified from Sheffield *et al.* (1980).

This protocol has been optimized for the isolation of retinal ganglion cells (RGCs) from embryonic day 6–7 (E6–7) and embryonic day 12 (E12) chick retinae (DeCurtis *et al.*, 1991). The separation of RGCs from other cells depends on differences between the density of these cells compared to the other retinal cells. Therefore, in order to obtain a good separation, it is particularly important to try to obtain the best possible suspension of single cells after dissociation of the retinae. For a good isolation of RGCs, particular care is needed during the preparation of the cell suspension and the preparation of the Percoll gradient.

Digestion with trypsin is an important step, and optimal trypsinization conditions have to be determined by testing. Usually 8–15 min of trypsinization are required for good dissociation. If trypsinization is insufficient, cell aggregates will be present, resulting in a poor separation. On the other hand, excessive trypsinization will result in a loss of too many cells and poor recovery. Retinae from different ages are also differently sensitive to trypsin. In particular, E12 retinae are more sensitive to overtrypsinization than E6–7 retinae.

D. Dissection of the Retina

Materials

See Section II,A.

1. For each preparation, use up to 40 E6–7 retinae or 14 E12 retinae. After removal of the eyes from the embryos, incubate the eyes for several minutes in PBS-CMF to facilitate the separation of the neural retina from the pigmented epithelium.

2. Dissection proceeds as described in Section II,A.

E. Preparation of Retinal Cell Suspension

Materials

0.2% hyaluronidase (Sigma, type IV) or 0.1% hyaluronidase (Worthington)
0.1% trypsin (Worthington

0.01% DNAase I (Sigma, type IV)

F12 culture medium

0.2% soybean trypsin inhibitor

Fetal calf serum (FCS)

1. Incubate the E6-7 and E12 retinae, which are collected in the 15-ml conical tube, for 5 min at 37°C in 5 ml of 0.2% hyaluronidase (Sigma, type IV) in PBS. This step is required to reduce cell aggregation induced by hyaluronic acid present in residual vitreous humor.

2. Centrifuge for 3 min at 500 g to recover retinae. Wash once with PBS-CMF and centrifuge again for 3 min at 500 g.

3. After hyaluronidase treatment, resuspend the tissue pellet in 10–15 ml of 0.1% trypsin (Worthington) and 0.01% pancreatic DNAase I (Sigma, type IV). Trypsinize for 7–10 min in a 37°C water bath, mixing every 2 min to resuspend the tissue pellet.

4. It is possible that large tissue clumps may form during the trypsinization due to the release of DNA from broken cells. These must be eliminated before pelleting the trypsinized cells. This is done by adding a second aliquot of DNAase (stock 100× = 10 mg/ml DNAase I) at the end of the trypsin incubation. Mix the cell suspension a few times by inverting the tube to help disrupt the aggregates.

5. Add 0.2 volumes of fetal calf serum to inhibit the trypsin. This should be done as soon as possible after the end of trypsinization.

6. Centrifuge cells for 3 min at 500 g. Resuspended gently in 15 ml of F12 culture medium and centrifuge once more.

7. Resuspend the final pellet in 2 ml of F12 culture medium containing 0.2% soybean trypsin inhibitor and 0.05% DNAase I, and triturate 10 times up and down through a fire-polished Pasteur pipette with the tip held near the bottom of the 15-ml conical tube.

8. After trituration, the cell suspension should appear homogeneous and free of visible clumps. Dilute the cell suspension with F12 medium to about 12 ml.

F. Percoll Gradient

Materials

Percoll stock: 9 parts of Percoll (Pharmacia, Cat. No. 17-0891-01) and 1 part of 10× PBS-CMF

F12 medium with 1× modified Bottenstein's additives

Modified Bottenstein's additives (100×):

0.5 mg/ml insulin (Sigma Cat. No. I 1882)

10 mg/ml human transferrin (Sigma Cat. No. 51147)

300 nM selenous acid (J.T. Baker Cat. No. 4-0310)

in PBS-CMF

Filter to sterilize, aliquot, and store at −20°C.

1. The Percoll gradient is prepared as follows, starting from the bottom of a 50-ml tube:

Layer 5: 4 ml F12 plus 5.65 ml Percoll stock

Density = 1.0900 g/ml

Layer 4: 4 ml cell suspension + 2 ml F12 + 3.8 ml Percoll stock

Density = 1.0600 g/ml

Layer 3: 4 ml cell suspension + 4 ml F12 + 1.75 Percoll stock

Density = 1.0380 g/ml

Layer 2: 4 ml cell suspension + 4 ml F12 + 0.842 ml Percoll stock

Density = 1.0171 g/ml

Layer 1: 9 ml F12

Density = 1.0086 g/ml

Add each new layer by *very careful and slow* pipetting along the edge of the tube. Avoid mixing the layers while preparing the gradient.

2. Load the gradient into a clinical centrifuge with a swinging bucket rotor and centrifuge for 30 min at 500 g and 4°C. To avoid perturbation of the preformed gradient, a slow start and a slow stop of the run are recommended. Two bands will be visible in the final gradient. Fraction I, enriched in retinal ganglion cells [as assayed by enrichment of the G4 antigen (DeCurtis *et al.*, 1991)], usually occurs close to the boundary between layers 2 and 3 (1.017 < d < 1.038). Fraction I typically contains about 5% as much protein as Fraction II. Fraction II is more visible than Fraction I and is located within layers 4 and 3 of the gradient. When separation is not optimal, Fraction I from E6-7 cells forms a band right above Fraction II within layer 3 of the gradient.

3. Collect the two bands separately using a fire-polished Pasteur pipette. Usually each band is collected in a volume of about 5 ml.

4. Wash the cells once by bringing the volume of each fraction to 50 ml with F12 medium and centrifuging for 10 min at 500–1000 g.

5. Resuspend the pellets in F12 medium with modified Bottenstein's additives. The cells are now ready for culture or biochemical analysis.

G. Retinal Explants: Flat Mounts and Retinal Strips

It is very difficult to prepare undamaged explants, and this affects the consistency of axonal outgrowth. This method [modified from Halfter *et al.* (1993) and Halfter and Deiss (1984)] is most useful, therefore, in studies in which it is important to keep track of the original location of the retinal neurons.

Materials

Two or three pairs of No. 5 forceps; one pair should have blunt tips

Two dissecting dishes: one with a hard plastic bottom and the other coated with Sylgard (Dupont)

Two Pasteur pipettes, shaped in a Bunsen burner to have ball endings (optional)

Dissecting scissors, 1/4 in.

Sterile razor blade or a scalpel

Blotting paper

Nitrocellulose; for fluorescent studies use black nitrocellulose, e.g., Millipore AABP 04700 6- or 24-well tissue culture plates, precoated with substrate (see Section IV)

Holding media: Hank's buffered salts solution

Defined culture media: 50 ml F12 (GIBCO), 20 mM glutamine, 100 U/ml pen/ strep, 1× modified Bottenstein's additives, and 0.4% methylcellulose (Sigma Cat. No. M7027)

Modified Bottenstein's additives (100×):

0.5 mg/ml insulin (Sigma Cat. No. I 1882)

10 mg/ml human transferrin (Sigma Cat. No. 51147)

300 nM selenous acid (J.T. Baker Cat. No. 4-0310)

in PBS-CMF

Filter to sterilize, aliquot, and store at −20°C.

0.8% methylcellulose (2×): Methylcellulose is difficult to get into solution. We prepare a 2× stock (0.8% methylcellulose) by prewarming 100 ml F12 to 37°C and then adding to 0.8 g sterile, dry methylcellulose. The methylcellulose should dissolve after several hours of stirring with gentle heat or stirring overnight with no heat. To prepare the final medium, add the 2× methylcellulose to an equal volume of F12 containing 2× of the other additives (pen/ strep, modified Bottenstein's additives, and glutamine).

1. Dissect whole eyes from E5-6 embryos and place in holding medium. Incubate at 37°C for 20 min. This will make the rest of the dissection much easier. Perform all subsequent steps in this medium.

2. Remove the connective tissues (whitish) and RPE (black) from the eyes. Remove the lens. This procedure results in a translucent epithelium (the retina) attached to a gelatinous ball (vitreous humor).

3. Remove the vitreous by inserting the blunt forceps into the vitreous through the opening left by the lens. Straddle the tines of a second forceps across the blunt forceps and gently peel back the retina. The retina will begin to curl within several minutes, so mount it promptly (steps 4–6). It is important to keep the

orientation of the retina straight. The photoreceptor side is the *outside* of the retina. The retina usually curls up toward the ganglion cell layer (inside).

Alternative to steps 1–3: Decapitate E5-6 embryos and place the heads into holding medium. Bracing the head with one pair of forceps, insert the blunt forceps through the lens into the vitreous and remove them together. Gently remove the eye from the head, and dissect the retina from the connective tissues and RPE.

4. Transfer the retina to a second, fresh dish with a hard plastic bottom (the "mounting dish"). This dish must be kept clean of debris, which would otherwise stick to the nitrocellulose. Use dissecting scissors to cut the retina as desired. For a whole mount retina, make four cuts from the peripheral retina inward, taking care to avoid the region of the optic nerve which appears as a thickened strip. For retinal strips, cut out a large, unwrinkled patch of retina (Fig. 2). Remove any unsuitable retina from the mounting dish.

5. Place a precut piece of nitrocellulose into the mounting dish in the proper orientation: photoreceptor side down. Float the retina onto the nitrocellulose. It is important to mount the retina smoothly, without wrinkles. Gently roll it flat with the tines of the forceps or with the blunted Pasteur pipettes. *Note:* the retina is very fragile, any areas touched with the forceps will be damaged! Fasten the retina to the nitrocellulose at the edges by pressing down with the forceps tips. Keep contact to a minimum!

6. Remove the retina fastened to the nitrocellulose from the mounting dish and place it on blotting paper to dry. This is the most critical part of the procedure. The retina must be dry enough to adhere firmly to the nitrocellulose, but not so dry as to cause cell death. The time should be worked out by trial and error. It is always less than 30 sec. For whole mount retinas, this is the end of the procedure. Place the mounted retina into medium and culture.

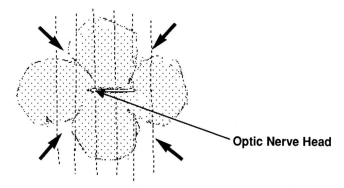

Fig. 2 Flat-mounted whole retina. The arrows indicate the four cuts made in the retina which allow it to be mounted flat. The dashed lines indicate the orientation of the cut for retinal slices with respect to the optic nerve head.

7. To make retinal strips, transfer the mounted retina back into the mounting dish. Hold down the retina with forceps and cut 1-mm strips with a fresh, sterile razor or scalpel (Fig. 2). If the retina pulls away from the nitrocellulose, either the retina was mounted improperly (steps 4, 5, or 6) or the blade is not sharp enough.

8. Transfer the strips to wells precoated with substrate (see Section IV) and containing culture medium. Under a microscope, position the strips, retina side down, on the bottom of the wells. Gently press down on the strips to ensure attachment. This is a critical step as well. Pushing down too hard will smash part of the strip, but nothing will grow if the strip is not attached properly! This is easiest to judge in a retina that has been properly mounted and cut. Alternatively, use small steel weights to hold the ends of the strips down (see Baier and Bonhoeffer, 1992).

III. Cell Culture

After dissection, the choice of tissue culture method depends, once again, on the intended application. This section describes a preplating step which enriches for neuronal cells, a general culture method using defined media, and a method of transient transfection.

For experiments requiring maintenance of the cell–cell relationships within the tissue, explant methods, such as those described in the last section, are the appropriate choice. However, for many purposes, dissociated cell culture provides an environment that may be controlled and modified in a much more flexible manner. Preplating the dissociated retina on uncoated tissue culture plastic is a simple method of enriching for the mixed neuronal cell population.

Retinal neurons generally survive and differentiate better in culture in the presence of 1 to 10% serum. However, defined medium is of great advantage for most short-term assays. The controlled environment allows studies of substrate, cell, and neurotrophin actions without contaminating proteins in the assay. The defined medium described in this chapter was modified from Bottenstein *et al.* (1980; see also Bottenstein, 1992).

Transient transfection of DNA into the embryonic retina can be used to study cellular processes in an environment which more closely resembles the situation *in vivo*. For example, Vardimon and colleagues have studied the developmental control of glucocorticoid receptor transcriptional activity by the transient transfection of glucocorticoid-inducible reporter constructs (Ben Dror *et al.*, 1993). In this system, correct transcriptional regulation requires contact between glia and neurons. Our group is using transient transfection of cDNAs encoding dominant negative forms of proteins to test their potential involvement in neurite outgrowth. Using the same expression vector as this group, but different conditions for transfection, we have optimized a method for high levels of expression in retinal neurons from embryonic day 7 retinae. The method uses lipofectamine and is adapted from the manufacturer's protocol (GIBCO). Transfection works well for E6-9 retinae, but cells at older ages do not survive well. Transient transfection and expression of a protein require a long incubation time and high survival rates to be successful. To increase survival during the relatively harsh transfection conditions, the cells are triturated without enzymatic treatment. The absence of antibiotics and serum is essential for efficient transfection.

A. Retinal Cell Culture

This procedure is modified from Hall *et al.* (1987).

Materials

Defined medium: 50 ml F12 (GIBCO), 20 mM glutamine, 100 U/ml pen/strep, 1× modified Bottenstein's additives, and 0.1 mg/ml conalbumin (Sigma type II No. C-0880)

Modified Bottenstein's additives (100×):

0.5 mg/ml insulin (Sigma Cat. No. I 1882)

10 mg/ml human transferrin (Sigma Cat. No. 51147)

300 nM selenous acid (J.T. Baker Cat. No. 4-0310)

in PBS-CMF

Filter to sterilize, aliquot, and store at −20°C.

1. After trituration and spinning, resuspend the cells in defined media.

2. To remove nonneuronal cells, plate cells on an uncoated tissue culture dish (Falcon No. 3003) at about 1×10^6/ml. Incubate for 45 min at 37°C and 5% CO_2.

3. Tap the plate *gently* and remove the neuron containing the supernatant off the plate with a sterile pipette. The majority of nonneuronal cells will remain attached to the dish.

4. Count and resuspend cells in defined media to the desired concentration for the intended assay.

B. Transient Transfection of Chicken Retinal Neurons

Materials

6-well plate (Falcon, 3846)

Holding medium: calcium- and magnesium-free PBS, 0.5% glucose, and 100 U/ml pen/strep

OPTIMEM I reduced serum medium (GIBCO/BRL Cat. No. 39185)

Poly-L-lysine (2 ml of 0.01 mg/ml in PBS containing 1 mM Ca^{2+} and 1 mM Mg^{2+})

Plasmid DNA (2 μg): β-Galactosidase (β-Gal) expression vector (p6R, a gift from K. Yamamoto, UCSF).

Experimental vector containing gene of choice driven by the Rous sarcoma
virus LTR with SV40 polyadenylation sequences

LipofectAMINE reagent (GIBCO/BRL Cat. No. 18324-012)

5% fetal calf serum

100 U/ml pen/strep

1. Dissect E7 retinas (about one retina per transfection) as described earlier
except *do not use trypsin or any other cell dissociation solutions*. Dissociate in
holding medium by trituration with a Pasteur pipette until the cells are in *clumps*
of about 20–100 cells. *This is important.* Single cells do not readily survive the
transfection conditions.

2. Wash the cells once in OPTIMEM I *without* antibiotics and resuspend in
the same medium to estimate the number of cells. Plate approximately 2 million
cells per well of a six-well plate. The plates should be coated with poly-L-lysine
for 5 min, followed by two washes with PBS with 1 mM Ca^{2+} and 1 mM Mg^{2+}.
Once again, use OPTIMEM I without added serum and without antibiotics.
Allow the cells to attach and recover for 2–3 hr.

3. Using polystyrene culture tubes (12 × 75 mm, Fisher), dilute 2 μg plasmid
DNA to 0.1 ml medium; in separate tubes, dilute varying amounts of Lipofect-
AMINE in 0.1 ml medium. [Using catacholamine acetyl transferase (CAT) and/
or luciferase assays, several common promoters have been tried, with only the
Rous sarcoma virus LTR giving good results for retinal neurons.] Try a range
of 2–30 μl of LipofectAMINE in 0.1 ml medium. The optimal amount is about
15 μl for the RSV–β-Gal construct.

4. Combine the two solutions and incubate for 30 min at room temperature.
During the incubation, rinse cells with fresh medium and remove. Add 0.8 ml
of medium to the DNA–lipofectamine mixture and add the total mixture (1 ml)
gently to the rinsed cells. Incubate for 2–10 hr. Shorter times will increase the
survival of the cells. From 5 to 16 hr works well for the surviving cells, provided
they do not become contaminated. If the cells do become contaminated, change
the medium only once more.

5. Remove the transfection mixture and add 2 ml fresh medium supplemented
with 5% fetal calf serum and antibiotics (the addition of serum to increase cell
viability is optional). Incubate the cells for a further 12–16 hr, remove medium
again, and add fresh medium. Assay the cells for expression 8–20 hr later.
Alternatively, allow the cells to recover for 12–16 hr and replate as single cells.
Expect the majority of the cells not to survive replating.

C. Staining for β-Galactosidase Expression

This procedure is modified from Harlow and Lane (1988).

Materials

Paraformaldehyde stock: 6% paraformaldehyde in PBS

Bromochloroindolyl-β-D-galactopyranoside (BCIG) staining solution:

Dissolve 4.9 mg BCIG in 0.1 ml dimethylformamide.

Add to 10 ml PBS containing 1 mM magnesium chloride and 3 mM potassium ferricyanide.

Filter to sterilize.

1. Wash cells 1× with PBS with 1 mM Ca^{2+} and 1 mM Mg^{2+}. Fix by adding paraformaldehyde stock diluted 1:1 with PBS for a 3% final concentration. Incubate for 10 min at room temperature.

2. Rinse cells with PBS and add staining solution for 10–60 min. Stop the reaction by washing with water.

IV. Neuronal Cell Assays

The following two assays measure the neuronal behaviors of cell adhesion and neurite outgrowth. As described in Hall *et al.* (1987), these two assays are almost identical in preparation. The common steps involve preparation of the substrate, dissection and preplating of the cells, and preparation of the inhibiting or activating antibodies and chemicals. The first part of this section lists a number of substrates and the conditions for plating them. The substrates can be as complicated as a cell layer or as simple as a peptide for both of these assays. Therefore, a literature search may be necessary to find the correct conditions for a particular substrate. Also, replacement of tissue culture plates by acid-cleaned coverslips or slides will facilitate immunofluorescence analysis and videomicroscopy.

The two assays differ in the number of cells plated per well. Between 25,000 and 50,000 cells should cover a well. This is an appropriate number to use for studying cell adhesion. In measuring neurite outgrowth, however, a lower number of cells per well, between 1000 and 5000, are necessary in order to be able to adequately count the neurites. For adhesion assays, defined media provides a clean experiment by eliminating exogenous proteins that may bind to the substrate changing the experimentally defined conditions. Neurite outgrowth experiments can also be done in defined media, however, adding serum to longer assays aids in cell survival. Frequently only 1% serum is sufficient to sustain overnight cultures. We have found that this low amount of serum rarely interferes with our assays.

A. Preparation of Substrates

Materials

> Linbro/Titertek nontissue culture plastic 96-well plates
> Blocking solution: 10% BSA (Fraction V RIA grade, Sigma No. A7888) in PBS with or without divalents

Positive control: 1 mg/ml poly-D-lysine in 0.1 M borate buffer, pH 8.5 (boric acid/NaOH), or 1 mg/ml polyornithine in distilled H_2O

Protein or cellular substrate as described below.

a. Cellular Substrates

1. Plate substrate cells in a 96-well plate a day or more before the assay is to take place and allow the cells to become confluent. Plate enough wells for triplicates of all experimental conditions. Include a triplicate of wells coated with 1% BSA only for the negative binding control.

b. Protein Substrates

1. Coat the plate with test proteins the night before the assay. Include 1% BSA as a negative control and poly-D-lysine or polyornithine as a positive control. Do everything in triplicate. Use 0.075 ml per well (smaller volumes will result in uneven protein distribution). Dilute the protein in the appropriate buffer as follows:

Laminin	PBS-CMF
Collagen IV	PBS-CMF
Fibronectin	PBS-CMF
Vitronectin	PBS-CMF
Thrombospondin	PBS + 1 mM Ca^{2+} and 1 mM Mg^{2+}
Fibrinogen	PBS + 1 mM Ca^{2+} and 1 mM Mg^{2+}
Collagen I	0.1 N acetic acid

The concentration of the substrate protein is an important variable of these assays and should be determined for a given experiment through a concentration curve. Concentrations ranging from 5 mM/ml to 20 μg/ml are appropriate for most assays. (Occasionally concentrations as high as 50–100 μg/ml have been used for neurite outgrowth). Incubate for 3 hr at 37°C or wrap the coated plates in plastic wrap and incubate overnight at 4°C.

2. Rinse the wells once with PBS and add 0.1 ml blocking solution per well, except for the positive control wells. Block protein-coated wells using the BSA solution with or without divalents depending on the substrate listed earlier. Use BSA in PBS + CA^{2+} and Mg^{2+} for collagen I. Incubate at 37°C for at least 3 hr.

B. Cell/Substratum Adhesion Assay

Materials

Protein substrate-coated 96-well plate(s) in blocking buffer or cell substrate-coated 96-well plate(s), confluent

Multipipettor

Clinical centrifuge with plate spinner adapters

Inverted tissue culture microscope

Fixative:

2% glutaraldehyde, 5% sucrose, in PBS

Filter to sterilize

or

6% paraformaldehyde in PBS

Filter to sterilize, use at 3% final concentration.

Note: Sterile conditions are necessary only for lengthy incubations.

1. Prepare antibodies, peptides, etc. for perturbing adhesion. There should be enough for 0.05 ml per well at twice the final concentration desired in the assay. For cell layer substrates go on to step 2.

For protein substrates only: Wash the plate.

Remove the BSA by inverting and shaking the plate. Fill the wells with the appropriate PBS, then remove the solution. Repeat for a total of five washes. After the last wash, aspirate off any remaining PBS.

2. Add 0.05 ml medium, with or without antibodies, into each well. Put the plate in the tissue culture incubator to warm and equilibrate before adding the cells.

3. Resuspend the cells in defined media at $0.5-1.0 \times 10^6$ per ml. Using the multiwell pipettor, add 0.05 ml of cell suspension to each well, i.e., between 25,000 and 50,000 cells per well. Mix the cells frequently to prevent settling.

4. Centrifuge the cells onto the plate at about 1000 g for 1 min.

5. For a standard inhibition of the adhesion assay, incubate between 60 and 90 min at 37°C. If assaying for *activation* of adhesion, incubate at 37°C for between 10 and 60 min.

6. After incubation, remove nonadherent cells with 37°C media. Using an eight-well multipipettor, pipette 0.05 ml down the left and the right sides of the wells. Gently aspirate off the medium using a glass Pasteur pipette with a micropipette tip attached. Using a tissue culture microscope, check that all the cells are removed from the BSA-treated wells and that cells still remain on the positive control. If cells are still present on the BSA control wells, wash again. Add 0.1 ml of fresh medium to each well.

7. Add 0.1 ml fixative to each well. Incubate for 15 min at room temperature or 4°C overnight. Stain with crystal violet as described next.

C. Crystal Violet Stain

This procedure is modified from Bodary *et al.* (1989).

Materials

ELISA plate reader (capable of reading A_{540})

Crystal violet solution: 200 ml methanol and 5 g crystal violet (Sigma Cat. No.

c0775); filter through Whatman No. 1 paper, dissolve, and bring to 1 liter with distilled H_2O

Lysis solution: 1% SDS in distilled H_2O

1. Remove fix and add 0.05 ml of the crystal violet solution for 15 min at room temperature.
2. Wash with distilled H_2O.
3. Add 0.05 ml lysis solution and incubate on a rotating platform for about 15–60 min until all the cells are lysed.
4. Read the A_{540} in an ELISA plate reader.
5. Obtain averages of all triplicates and then calculate the percentage of cells attached for all experimental wells using the following formula:

$$\frac{A_{540} \text{ (experimental well average)} - A_{540} \text{ (BSA-coated well average)}}{A_{540} \text{ (poly-D-lysine or polyornithine-coated well average)} - A_{540} \text{ (BSA-coated well average)}}$$

See Hall et al. (1987) for an example of data accumulated by this method.

D. Neurite Outgrowth Assay

Materials

Protein substrate-coated 96 well plate(s) in blocking buffer or cell substrate-coated 96 well plate(s), confluent

Multipipettor

Clinical centrifuge with plate spinner adapters

Inverted tissue culture microscope

Fixative:

2% glutaraldehyde, 5% sucrose, in PBS Plus 1 mM Ca^{2+} and 1 mM Mg^{2+}

or

6% paraformaldehyde in PBS, filter to sterilize, and use at 3% final concentration

1. Follow steps 1 and 2 from the cell adhesion protocol. Since these assays require many hours, it is best to adhere to sterile conditions. Therefore, all solutions should be sterile filtered, including antibodies. Microfiltration devises are available from Costar, Millipore, Nalgene, and others for this purpose.

2. Resuspend the cells to a final concentration of 20,000–100,000 cells/ml. Add 50 μl per well, i.e., 1000–5000 cells added per well. The choice of media can vary here to include from 0 to 10% serum. As mentioned earlier, the addition of serum may increase cell viability in longer assays. However, proteins in the serum may interfere with outgrowth assays.

3. Centrifuge the cells onto the plate at about 1000 *g* for 2 min.

4. Incubate in 5% CO_2 at 37°C for 6–24 hr.

5. At the end of the assay, add an equal volume of fixative to each well. Incubate from 15 min at room temperature to overnight at 4°C.

6. Neurite outgrowth may be quantified in a number of ways:

a. For conditions that result in the definite presence or absence of neurites compared to controls, take representative photographs of experimental and control results. Photographs are sufficient for definitive results.

b. Most commonly the result will require quantifying the percentage of neurons with neurites. For the purpose of counting, a neurite is defined as a projection that is at least the length of two cell body diameters.

c. It is also useful to measure neurite lengths which provide an estimate of the rate of neurite growth. Usually from 60 to 100 neurites per triplicate are quantified to record statistically significant data. In our laboratory, neurite length is measured using an inverted Olympus IMT2 microscope with Nomarski optics. Microscope images are collected with a cooled CCD camera (Photometrics, series 200) equipped with a 1024 × 1024 pixel CCD imaging device (Texas Instruments, TC215) and are stored on a hard disk in a VAX 3200 computer. The process length is determined using the Prism program (Chen *et al.,* 1989). See Varnum-Finney and Reichardt (1994) for an example of data accumulated with this method. A simple but much more time-consuming alternative is to use camera lucida. It is also possible to photograph the cells and measure the neurite lengths from the developed pictures.

V. Concluding Remarks

This chapter has presented several methods used in our laboratory for the purpose of culturing and assaying chick retinal neurons. The ease of dissection, abundance, and hardiness of these neuronal cells makes them good choices for studying many problems in cellular, developmental, and neurobiology.

Acknowledgments

We thank Kristine Venström and Cristina Weaver for comments on the manuscript. Work in the author's laboratory has been supported by US PHS Grants NS 19090 and PO1-16033; LFR is an investigator of the Howard Hughes Medical Institute.

References

Baier, H., and Bonhoeffer, F. (1992). Axon guidance by gradients of a target-derived component. *Science* **255,** 472–475.
Banker, G., and Goslin, K., eds. (1992). "Culturing Nerve Cells." MIT Press, Cambridge, MA.

Ben Dror, I., Havazelet, N., and Vardimon, L. (1993). Developmental control of glucocorticoid receptor transcriptional activity in embryonic retina. *Proc. Natl. Acad. Sci. U.S.A.* **90**(3), 1117–1121.

Bodary, S. C., Napier, M. A., and McLean, J. W. (1989). Expression of recombinant platelet glycoprotein IIbIIa results in a functional fibrinogen-binding complex. *J. Biol. Chem.* **264**(32), 18859–18862.

Bottenstein, J. E. (1992). Environmental influences on cells in culture. *In* "Practical Cell Culture Techniques: Neuromethods" (G. B. Alan, A. Boulton, and A. W. W. Baker, eds.), Vol. 23, pp. 63–85. Humana Press, Totowa

Bottenstein, J. E., Skaper, S. D., Varon, S. S., Sato, G. H. (1980). Selective survival of neurons from chick embryo sensory ganglionic dissociates utilizing serum-free supplemented medium. *Exp. Cell Res.* **125**(1), 183–190.

Chen, H., Sedat, J. W., and Agard, D. A. (1989). Manipulation, display, and analysis of three dimensional biological images. *In* "The Handbook of Biological Confocal Microscopy" (J. Pawley, ed.), pp. 127–135. IMR Press, Madison, WI.

DeCurtis, I., and Reichardt, L. F. (1993). Function and spatial distribution in developing chick retina of the laminin receptor alpha 6 beta 1 and its isoforms. *Development* **118**(2), 377–388.

DeCurtis, I., Quaranta, V., Tamura, R. N., and Reichardt, L. F. (1991). Laminin receptors in the retina: Sequence analysis of the chick integrin alpha 6 subunit. Evidence for transcriptional and posttranslational regulation. *J. Cell Biol.* **113**(2), 405–416.

Halfter, W., and Deiss, S. (1984). Axon growth in embryonic chick and quail retinal whole mounts in vitro. *Dev. Biol.* **102**(2), 344–355.

Halfter, W., Newgreen, D. F., Sauter, J., and Schwarz, U. (1983). Oriented axon outgrowth from avian embryonic retinae in culture. *Dev. Biol.* **95**(1), 56–64.

Hall, D. E., Neugebauer, K. M., and Reichardt, L. F. (1987). Embryonic neural retinal cell response to extracellular matrix proteins: Developmental changes and effects of the cell substratum attachment antibody (CSAT). *J. Cell Biol.* **104**(3), 623–634.

Hamburger, V., and Hamilton, H. L. (1992). A series of normal stages in the development of the chick embryo. *Dev. Dyn.* **195**, 231–272.

Harlow, E., and Lane, D. (1988). "Antibodies: A Laboratory Manual." Cold Spring Harbor Lab., Cold Spring Harbor, NY.

Johnson, J. E. (1989). Retinal cultures used to assay CNS neurotrophic factors. *In* "Nerve Growth Factors" (R. A. Rush, ed.), p. 111. Wiley, New York.

Mey, J., and Thanos, S. (1992). Development of the visual system of the chick—A review. *J. fur Hirnforschung* **33**(6), 673–702.

Neugebauer, K. M., Emmett, C. J., Venström, K. A., and Reichardt, L. F. (1991). Vitronectin and thrombospondin promote retinal neurite outgrowth: Developmental regulation and role of integrins. *Neuron* **6**(3), 345–358.

Reh, T. A. (1992). Cellular interactions determine neuronal phenotypes in rodent retinal cultures. *J. Neurobiol.* **23**(8), 1067–1083.

Sheffield, J. B., Pressman, D., and Lynch, M. (1980). Cells isolated from the embryonic neural retina differ in behavior in vitro and membrane structure. *Science* **209**, 1043–1045.

Snow, D. M., and Letourneau, P. C. (1992). Neurite outgrowth on a step gradient of chondroitin sulfate proteoglycan (CS-PG). *J. Neurobiol.* **23**(3), 322–336.

Varnum-Finney, B., and Reichardt, L. F. (1994). Vinculin-deficient PC12 cell lines extend unstable lamellipodia and filopodia and have a reduced rate of neurite outgrowth. *J. Cell Biol.* **127**(4), 1071–1084.

Walter, J., Kern-Veits, B., Huf, J., Stolze, B., and Bonhoeffer, F. (1987). Recognition of position specific properties of tectal cell membranes by retinal axons in vitro. *Development* **101**, 685–696.

Watanabe, T., and Raff, M. C. (1992). Diffusible rod-promoting signals in the developing rat retina. *Development (Cambridge, UK)* **114**(4), 899–906.

CHAPTER 15

Migration and Adhesion Assays

Thomas Lallier

Department of Cell Biology
University of Virginia
Charlottesville, Virginia 22908

I. Introduction
II. Materials
    A. Chemicals
    B. Solutions
III. Assay Methods
    A. Cell Adhesion Assay
    B. Cell Migration Assay
    C. Substrata Preference Assay
IV. Conclusions
    References

I. Introduction

Cells derived from avian embryos serve as useful models for studying the interactions between cells and the extracellular matrix (ECM). In Chapters 3 and 12–14, several procedures have been described for the isolation of specific cell types from avian embryos. These methods can be adapted, with relative ease, to allow the isolation of cells from other tissues. This chapter focuses on how cell–ECM interactions can be measured and manipulated *in vitro*. Three procedures are described in detail: (1) a centrifugal cell adhesion assay, (2) a cell migration assay, and (3) an ECM molecule preference assay.

II. Materials

The following companies are sources for several commonly used ECM components. This list is meant to be useful to investigators looking to purchase ECM molecules: Sigma Chemical (St. Louis, MO), Collaborative Biomedical Products (Bedford, MA), and GIBCO/BRL (Gaithersburg, MD).

For function blocking experiments involving avian integrins, the anti-β1 integrin function blocking monoclonal antibody JG22E is available through the Developmental Studies Hybridoma Bank in Iowa.

A. Chemicals

Bovine serum albumin (BSA; Cat. No. A2153), ovalbumin (Cat. No. A5398), sodium phosphate (monobasic, Cat. No. S0751), sodium phosphate (dibasic, Cat. No. S0876), sodium chloride (Cat. No. S9888), sodium bicarbonate (Cat. No. S6014, phenol red (Cat. No. P0290, calcium chloride (Cat. No. C4901), ethylenediaminetetraacetic acid (EDTA; Cat. No. EDS), and magnesium chloride (Cat. No. M8266) were obtained from Sigma.

B. Solutions

1. Substrata Coating Solution (SCS)

10 mM sodium bicarbonate, pH 7.4, 100 mM sodium chloride containing extracellular matrix molecule (i.e., laminin or fibronectin) at a final concentration of 10–100 μg/ml.

Collagen type I should be diluted in ice-cold buffer to prevent premature gelling. Store at 4°C.

2. Tissue Culture Media (MEM)

MEM with 10% fetal calf serum or the preferred medium of choice.

3. Substrata Blocking Solution (SBS)

MEM, pH 7.4, with 1 mg/ml heat-inactivated BSA or ovalbumin

BSA or ovalbumin can be heat inactivated in a 10-mg/ml stock solution by heating to 60°C for 1 hr. In this solution, MEM can be replaced with phosphate-buffered saline (PBS) or the serum-free tissue culture medium of choice. Store at 4°C.

4. Phosphate-Buffered Saline (PBS)

To make 1 liter, dissolve 8.2 g NaCl, 1.15 g Na_2HPO_4, and 0.2 g NaH_2PO_4 in distilled H_2O, adjust pH to 7.4. Store at room temperature.

5. 500 mM EDTA Stock

> To make 100 ml, dissolve 14.6 g of EDTA in distilled H_2O neutralized to pH 7.0–8.0 with 10 M NaOH. Store at room temperature.

III. Assay Methods

A. Cell Adhesion Assay

> The following assay is a centrifugal cell adhesion assay modified from McClay *et al.* (1981). This assay allows for the quantitation of cell adhesion using relatively small numbers of cells. The removal force is perpendicular to the site of attachment and can be controlled directly by varying the centrifugal speed employed. The results are highly reproducible and are not subject to the variabilities inherent in both "swirling" and "washing" adhesion assays.

1. Specific Materials

> Polyvinyl chloride (PVC) and polystyrene 96-well plates were obtained from Falcon (Cat. No. 3912; Cat. No. 3915). Double-sided carpet tape was obtained from 3M (Cat. No. 140). Minimal essential media (MEM) was obtained from GIBCO (Cat. No. 410-100EB). L-[^{3}H]- and L-[^{14}C]leucine (sterile in 2% ethanol) were obtained from ICN (Cat. No. 20032E; Cat. No. 10088E).

a. Common Equipment

Tabletop centrifuge with swinging buckets for 96-well plates

Metal vise with a 8 × 4-cm minimum area

Liquid scintillation counter

Scintillation vials

Cork bore (7 mm diameter)

Dry ice/methanol bath

Forceps

18-gauge needle

Scissors

b. Custom equipment

Modified dog nail clippers (Figs. 1A and 1B)

Stainless-steel "chuck" for microassay plates (Figs. 1C and 1D).

2. Procedure

a. Radiolabeling of Cells

The population of cells to be tested are grown to a nonconfluent state in a 35-mm tissue culture dish. If these cells are abundant, 10^4–10^5 cells per assay

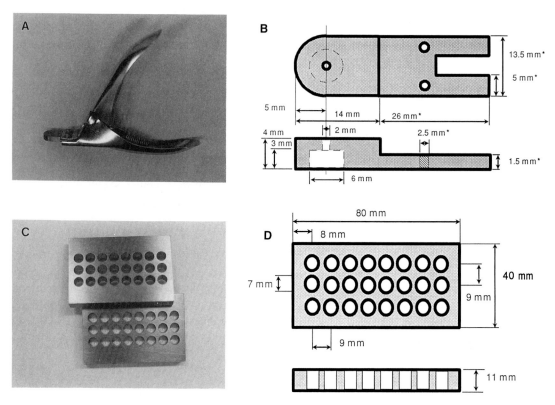

Fig. 1 Special equipment for adhesion assay. (A) Modified dog nail clippers used to remove the ends of assay wells. (B) Modified head for dog nail clippers. Large commercially available dog nail clippers can be purchased at most pet shops. The stationary top ring, designed to hold the dog nail during cutting, should be removed and replaced with a solid brass (or stainless steel) fitting, milled to the specifications in the diagram. The measurements with asterisks (*) will vary depending on the exact configuration of the clippers purchased. The 2.5-mm-diameter hole is threaded for a screw and should match the specifications of the "host" clippers. The 6-mm hole (only partially through the head) allows for ease in reproducibly cutting the same volume of fluid and cells. The small 2-mm hole allows for easy ejecting of the bottom of the clipped well with a blunted 18-gauge needle (top view above, side view below). (C and D) Steel "chuck" for clamping assay plated together. This can be made of either stainless steel or brass. The measurements for the holes and their placement are critical. Note that the holes go entirely through the block (D: top view above, side view below).

plate will give best results. For rare cells, as few as 10^3 cells per assay plate can be measured reliably. Cells are grown on fibronectin substrata (coated 25 μg/ml in a 35-mm tissue culture dish) in order to facilitate later cell removal. These cells are labeled by adding 10–100 μCi of L-[^{3}H]leucine to 1 ml of tissue culture media and incubating overnight. (A stock solution of L-[^{3}H]leucine at 1 mCi/ml in sterile distilled H_2O is convenient for later dilutions). Serum in the media does not appreciably affect the incorporation of the isotope.

b. Preparation of Adhesion Assay Plates

1. Cut the edges off the PVC 96-well plates and cut into quarters so that there are four assay plates of 8×3 wells. A typical experiment uses 24 plates (12 substrata plates and 12 covers).

2. Cover half of the assay plates with double-sided carpet tape (with the backing retained). Trim off the excess tape. Rub the assay plate, tape side down, on a flat surface to achieve even adherence of the tape to the plate. These are the bottom assay plates (Fig. 2A).

3. Label the bottom of the central six wells with a black lab marker (other colors are soluble in methanol). Remove backing from the tape. Heat a 7-mm cork bore with a Bunsen burner and gently touch the heated metal to the tape covering the center six wells. This will burn holes through the tape. Be careful not to let the metal touch the sides of the PVC wells or it will burn a hole through them as well. This will cause the wells to leak fluid, making them unusable.

4. Place three assay plates into polystyrene 96-well plates so that the sticky edges of adjacent plates do not touch. Coat wells with an ECM molecule of interest by placing 50 μl of SCS per well. Label plates by writing directly onto the tape with a black lab marker. Place the assay plates in humid chambers to prevent the coating solution from evaporating. Coating the wells overnight at 4°C works best, but incubating for as little as 2 hr at room temperature will result in comparable results for solutions at concentrations of ECM molecules greater than 10 μg/ml (Fig. 2C).

5. Rinse wells twice with PBS to remove nonadherent protein.

6. Incubate wells with 200 μl SBS for 2 hr at 37°C. The protein in the SBS will bind to any uncoated regions of plastic within the well, thus blocking nonspecific cell attachment to the plate.

c. Preparation of Radiolabeled Cells

Rinse labeled cells (from step A) five times with SBS. Remove cells from substrate. This can be done by incubating the cells in 5–10 mM EDTA in SBS for 5–20 min (depending on the cell type). The cells should become rounded and can be removed easily by gentle trituration. This method has the advantage of not destroying the surface receptors of the cells. Alternatively, cells can be removed from the substrate by incubation with 0.25% trypsin for 5–20 min. Cells should be transferred to a sterile polypropylene test tube. Gentle trituration of the cells with a Pasteur pipette will yield a suspension of single cells.

d. Centrifugal Cell Adhesion Assay

Have standing by:

Test Solution. This solution will vary with each experiment, but is generally SBS containing antibodies, enzymes, or competitive inhibitors for adhesion.

Scintillation vials. Twelve vials per plate of six wells will be needed: six for adherent cells (substrata side) and six for nonadherent cells.

Methanol/Dry Ice Bath.   Bath should contain at least a liter of methanol and several pounds of dry ice. Add dry ice to methanol until the dry ice fails to produce bubbles. This will quickly freeze water. This bath can be reused several (20 or more) times, so do not discard after the experiment.

1. Rinse wells of substrata-coated plates twice with SBS and fill with 200 μl/ well of test solution. Place three assay plates into a polystyrene 96-well plate so that their taped edges do not touch (Fig. 2D).

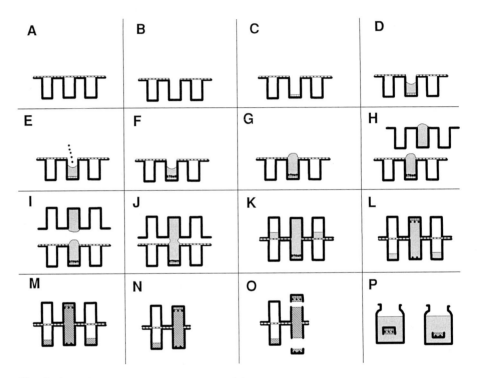

Fig. 2 Procedural steps for adhesion assay. (A) Side view of a bottom assay plate (cut away). Tape is placed over all the wells and the edges are trimmed. (B) A hole is burnt through the tape covering the center six wells using a heated cork borer. (C) A substrata molecule is adsorbed to the bottom of the center six wells. (D) The central wells are partially filled with SBS. (E) Labeled cells are added to the central wells. (F) The cells are brought into contact with the substrata by centrifugal force. (G) The central wells are further filled with test solution until the menisci bulge. (H) The central six wells of a second plate (the cover) are filled with SBS until the menisci also bulge (but only slightly). (I) The cover plate is inverted over the substrata plate so that the central six wells of both plates now align. (J) The cover plate is lowered into proximity with the substrata plate, such that the menisci meet. (K) The cover plate is brought into contact with the substrata plate, to be sealed by the metal vise. Note that the excess solution tends to fill the empty wells in the cover plate. (L) The chamber is inverted and subjected to a centrifugal force. Note that some of the cells are now attached to the substrata whereas others are adjacent to the cover. (M) The chamber is "quick" frozen in a methanol/dry ice bath. (N) One row of wells is cut off the assay plate. (O) The ends of the assay wells, both substrata and cover, are clipped off using modified dog nail clippers. (P) The well ends are placed into scintillation vials for counting.

2. Lay out top assay plates and fill the central six wells with test solution. The top assay plates should be filled so that each well has a small positive meniscus (i.e., the solution should bulge up slightly in the well).

3. Load cells into plates by placing an aliquot of the cells (50 μl) into each of the central six wells on the bottom assay plate (Fig. 2E).

4. Bring cells into contact with the substrate. This is commonly done by placing the open bottom assay plates, in their polystyrene 96-well plates, into a bench top centrifuge and subjecting them to a centrifugal force of 150 g for 5 min (Fig. 2F).

5. Seal assay plates as follows:

    a. Place the bottom assay plate (containing the labeled cells) into one of a pair of stainless-steel chucks.

    b. Add test solution to the central six wells so that there is a bulging positive meniscus (Figs. 2G and H).

    c. Invert the top assay plate and lower it so that the central six wells of the two plates align (Fig. 2I).

    d. Bring the two plates together so that the menisci touch (Fig. 2J). Continue lowering the cover plate so that six fluid-filled chambers are formed. Excess test solution should flow into the empty wells on the top assay plate (Fig. 2K).

    e. Place the second steel chuck over the top assay plate, and place the entire assay unit into the sheet metal vise, pressing together firmly.

    f. Remove joined assay plates (assay unit) and incubate at desired temperature for desired time. This will vary with the experiment. It has been found that significant adherence occurs within 5 min, but that experiments standardized to 15 min simplify the manipulations. For incubations at 37°C or room temperature, allow for receptor clustering and cytoskeletal interaction. Incubations at 4°C allow for measurements of receptor–ligand interaction.

6. Remove nonadherent cells. Invert assay unit so that the labeled wells are now visible. Place the assay unit in centrifuge and spin for 5 min (Fig. 2L). The removal force used will vary from cell to cell. For avian neural crest cells, cells are removed by subjecting them to a force of 50 g. This parameter can also be varied within an experiment in order to compare the strength of attachment between substrata or cells types. Too forceful a centrifugation of cells may lead to cell lysis.

7. After spinning cells off of the substrata, note which wells have air bubbles. Air bubbles destroy the reliability of those wells. Large air bubbles tend to lyse cells during the spin-off process, releasing their labeled contents to the media. Small air bubbles tend to buoy up cells, giving them an apparent high adhesion to the substrate.

8. Quick freeze cells by placing them rapidly into a methanol/dry ice bath. Use black lab markers as this ink is more stable in methanol than blue or red.

9. Clip plate tops and bottoms as follows:

   a. Remove one row of eight wells from the side of the now frozen assay plate (Fig. 2N).
   b. Using the modified dog nail clippers, clip off the bottoms of the six central wells from the bottom and top assay plates (Fig. 2O). Be careful to match bottoms and tops for later analysis. A blunted 18-gauge needle is useful for pushing well bottoms out of the nail clippers. Forceps are also useful for retrieving misplaced well bottoms.
   c. Place the clipped well bottoms into separated labeled scintillation vials. Fill vials with scintillation fluid and measure radioactivity using a scintillation counter (Fig. 2P).

10. Data analysis.

Each well is a separate assay chamber, such that if the tops and bottoms are matched, accurate calculations of the percentage of cells bound can be performed:

$$\%\text{cells bound} = \frac{\text{counts per minute (cpm) bottom} \times 100\%}{\text{cpm bottom} + \text{cpm top}}.$$

3. Comments

This cell attachment assay can be used to measure the attachment of any cell, even very rare ones, to either other cells or extracellular matrix molecules. Some cells, especially large embryonic cells, lyse under moderate centrifugal forces (25 g). The first experiment performed on any cell should be to test the cells resilience during centrifugation. Cells should be allowed to adhere under increasing g forces, starting with settling under a force of 1 g on a bench top, followed by a long (1 hr) 1 g removal force. Once the force used to bring cells into contact with their substrata is established, the removal force should be optimized. Attachment and removal forces that allow between 70 and 90% of the cells to remain attached in the absence of adhesion inhibitory agents are generally used.

B. Cell Migration Assay

The following assay has been used extensively to compare the ability of various ECM components to promote the migration of neural crest cells *in vitro* (Fig. 3) (Perris *et al.,* 1989). It should be noted that this assay relies on three related events: the ability of a piece of explanted tissue to attach en mass to a specific ECM component, the ability of individual cells within the explanted tissue to overcome cell–cell interactions and attach exclusively to the ECM molecule, the ability of the ECM molecule to promote cell motility in a directed fashion. Researchers often evaluate the results from these types of experiments in relation to only the third event. However, the third event is dependent on the first two

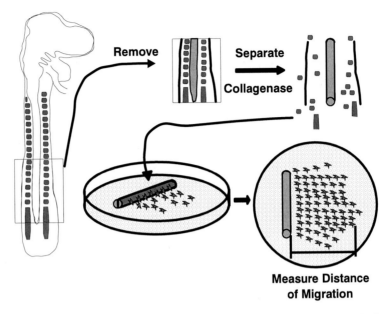

Fig. 3 Migration assay procedure. A cell migration assay based on measurements of avian neural crest cell migration. Neural tubes (containing premigratory neural crest cells) are isolated using collagenase. These explants are allowed to adhere to the substrata molecule adsorbed to the bottom of a 35-mm polystyrene tissue culture dish. After 12 to 18 hr, the migration distance of the cells at the leading edge of single cells is measured.

events. Therefore care should be used when evaluating the results of experiments based on comparing the migratory promotion of two ECM molecules.

The simplest and technically least demanding way to measure cell movement is to photograph the cells shortly after adding them to the substrata and again after a predetermined interval of time. More accurate measurements can be made using time-lapse video equipment and/or computer-aided image analysis software packages. For most studies, this added level of accuracy and expense is not necessary. For this reason, this chapter describes only the method for measuring cell movement via the simpler photographic approach.

1. Specific Materials

35-mm polystyrene tissue culture dishes
Inverted microscope

2. Procedure

1. Prepare substrata by SCS (described earlier) containing the molecules of interest and allow them to adsorb onto plastic overnight at 4°C. Polystyrene 35-

mm dishes normally require 500 μl of solution and should be placed within a sealed humid chamber.

2. Block the remaining protein-binding sites on the polystyrene dish by adding SBS (described earlier) for 2 hr at 37°C. Rinse the dishes three times with PBS prior to the addition of tissue explants.

3. Prepare avian tissue explants as described in Chapters 3 and 12–14.

   a. Add individual cells to dishes in 500 μl or greater volumes of tissue culture media and allow to adhere undisturbed for several hours. The dish should be rinsed several times with tissue culture media or PBS and filled with 500 μl or greater volumes of tissue culture media.

   b. Place tissue explants in the dish with minimal amounts of media. This can be accomplished by adding the tissue to the dish in a few drops of media and removing any excess by applying suction to the tilted dish. Using an inverted microscope, inspection should reveal cells attaching to the substrata along the edges of the explant after 1 to 2 hr. At this point, gently add 500 μl or greater of tissue culture media.

4. Fields of view can now be marked using red or blue lab markers on the bottom of the tissue culture dish. The explants or cells should be photographed at this time; these photographs are used as the initial time point for cell movement. The advantage of polaroid pictures for these experiments is the greater ease with which subsequent photos can be framed and aligned. The generally lower picture resolution in polaroid pictures is of little importance in day to day retrieval. The use of inverted microscopes greatly enhances the ease of photography and reduces the risk of contamination of the culture dishes.

5. Photographs of the explants should be taken at convenient intervals: from every 1 to 2 hr if measuring the rate of cell movement or after 18 hr to allow time for significant cell movement. Using 2% paraformaldehyde in PBS for 10 min, cultured cells can be fixed after the last time point to allow for later data collection.

6. Cell movement can be measured in several ways. In each, the photograph of the time point to be evaluated is compared to that of the initial photograph. This can be done simply by tracing the initial photograph onto clear plastic sheets and using these overlays to evaluate the test photograph. Several points should be noted here:

   a. Use care if photocopying the initial photograph onto a transparent plastic sheet since not all photocopiers produce true 100% size reproductions.

   b. The use of three stationary marks within the field of view will greatly increase the ease in aligning later photographs.

   c. Avoid changes in magnification, especially if manually developing photographs from standard film.

7. The amount of cell movement on a specific substrata can be measured in several ways:

a. The shortest distance between the cells at the leading edge of moving cells is measured back to the closest initial position. Here multiple cells (up to hundreds) within a few explants can be evaluated and averaged to achieve an accurate measurement.

b. The area enclosing all of the cells from a given explant, less the area originally occupied by the explant, can be found. Using this method, many explants (20 or more) are required in order to achieve an accurate estimate of cell movement. It is also important to normalize these data for explants of different sizes.

c. Individual cells can be tracked and their paths accurately determined and measured by either time-lapse or short interval photography. While this method is undoubtedly the most accurate measure of cell movement, it has certain limitations. Time-lapse video microscopy can only examine one field of view at a time. Therefore, only a relatively small number of cells can be evaluated over a given (up to 24-hr) period. This method limits the amount of data that can be obtained in a week to seven explants, while method (a) can evaluate hundreds of explants in a given day.

C. Substrata Preference Assay

The last assay described in this chapter has been used to successfully compare the ability of two substrates to promote both cell attachment and migration. Several versions of this method are described, one involving specifically manufactured equipment which produces substrata with alternating lanes containing two different substrata molecules (Walter *et al.*, 1987), and less expensive alternative versions.

1. Materials

35-mm polystyrene tissue culture dishes
Silicon mold (Fig. 4, the generous gift of Dr. Fredrick Bonnhoeffer)
Rhodamine–BSA (Sigma, Cat. No. A-2289)
Fluorescein–BSA (Sigma, Cat. No. A9771)
Inverted fluorescence microscope

2. Nitrocellulose Solution

2 cm^2 is dissolved in 100 ml methanol.

Procedure 1

This procedure is illustrated in Fig. 5.

1. Coat 35-mm polystyrene dishes with nitrocellulose by adding 100 μl of the nitrocellulose solution to each dish and allowing it to air dry. These dishes can be stored for several months in a dry container.

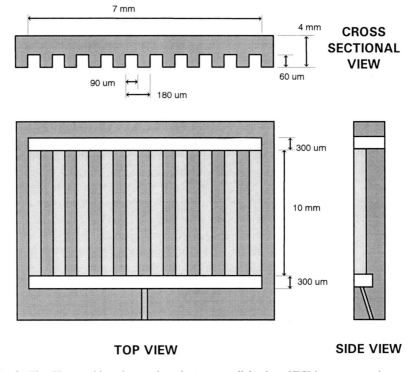

Fig. 4 The silicon mold used to produce the even parallel stripe of ECM components (not to scale).

2. Sterilize the silicon mold by immersion in 70% ethanol and allow it to air dry. Place the silicon mold in contact with the bottom of a 35-mm polystyrene tissue culture dish previously treated with nitrocellulose. The region of the dish containing the substrata field should be marked on the underside of the dish using a blue lab marker (this allows for later removal of the mark using ethanol).

3. Fill the mold by placing a 100-μl drop of the SCS (described earlier) containing the first substrata molecule at one end of the mold and drawing the solution under the mold by applying suction. After 10 min, draw more of the solution under the mold; this process is repeated three times to maximize the amount of substrata molecule bound to the dish. The first SCS should be mixed with a marker in order to distinguish between the two substrata later in the experiment. Adding rhodamine–BSA to a final concentration of 1 μg/ml works well as a marker.

4. Rinse the lanes of the first substrata by drawing 100 μl of PBS through the mold. Block the remaining protein-binding sites on these lanes by drawing 100 μl of SBS (described earlier) through the mold as described in step 3.

5. Remove any remaining fluid under the mold by vacuum and carefully remove the mold from the 35-mm dish.

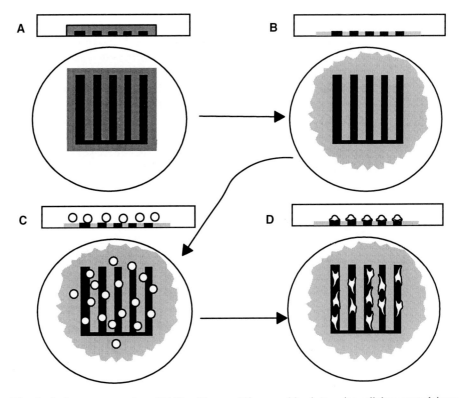

Fig. 5 Stripe assay procedure. (A) The silicon mold is pressed firmly to a nitrocellulose-coated tissue culture dish. The mold is filled with the first substrata molecule and is mixed with rhodamine–BSA as a marker for this substrata. After adsorption, the solution is removed and replaced with a substrata blocking solution. (B) The mold is removed, and the substrata field is overlayed with the second substrata molecule. The newly coated region of the plate is blocked by adding SBS. (C) Individual cells are allowed to attach randomly to the substrata field. (D) After several hours of incubation, the cells move from a random placement to one of being aligned along one substrata molecule.

6. Add the second substrata to the substrata field by placing a 100-μl drop of the second SCS on the demarcated area for 1 hr. All remaining protein-binding sites are then blocked by adding 100 μl of SBS to the substrata field. It is important to restrict the region of the dish exposed to fluid to a minimum. This ensures that a maximal number of cells will adhere to the substrata field and not to extraneous regions of the dish.

7. Remove all fluid from the dish and add the cells to be tested in a 100-μl drop to the substrata field. If a single cell suspension is used, approximately 10,000 cells should be added to the field and allowed to adhere for 1 hr. If tissue explants are used, place them within the substrata field as described in Section III,B. Fill the dish with 1 ml of tissue culture media and place in a 37°C incubator.

8. Fix cells at any later time using 2% paraformaldehyde in PBS for 10 min and analyze using an inverted fluorescence microscope.

4. Alternative Procedures

Several other techniques have been used to confront cells with multiple substrata in a way that presents borders where cells encounter both molecules and must make a choice. One such technique requires the application of one substrata molecule using a camel's hairbrush. Here regions of one molecule are "painted" directly onto the tissue culture dish (Perris *et al.*, 1989). The use of rhodamine–BSA mixed into the first SCS aids in defining the location of this substrata. The second substrata is adsorbed as described in step 6. One drawback to this approach is the lack of a blocking step between substrata coatings so that the second substrata is present wherever the first is adsorbed.

A second approach (Fig. 6) requires no special equipment at all and has the advantage of comparing substrata in combination. One drawback of this and the previous method is that it does not confront every cell with a choice of substrata on which to adhere.

1. Mark the underside of a 35-mm polystyrene dish to delineate four quarters, with 90° intersections at the center of the dish. Using a blue lab marker for this allows the marks to be removed later using ethanol.

2. Place the dish upright in a humid chamber on a level surface with an object (glass pipette or three stacked microscope slides) under one edge of the dish so

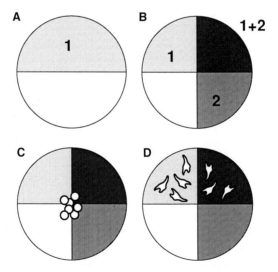

Fig. 6 Alternate substrata preference assay. (A) One substrata molecule is allowed to adsorb to one-half of a tissue culture dish. This is accomplished by tilting the dish. (B) A second substrata molecule is allowed to adsorb to one-half of a tissue culture dish. By rotating the dish 90° and again tilting it, four substrata fields are produced. (C) Cells are allowed to attach to the intersection point of the four substrata fields. (D) After several hours of incubation, the cells have localized to the region of the dish containing substrata molecule 1, ignoring the presence of substrata molecule 2.

that the dish is now tilted with one line parallel to the object used to establish the tilt.

3. Fill the dish with the first SCS solution containing 1 μg/ml rhodamine–BSA, such that only one-half of the dish is covered with fluid. Incubate for 1 hr in a sealed humid chamber (to prevent evaporation).

4. Remove the solution and rotate the dish 90°. The second SCS solution containing 1 μg/ml fluorescein–BSA is added as in step 3.

5. Remove the solution. Place the dish on a level surface and incubate in SBS for 1 hr. At this point the dish contains four quadrants containing substrata 1, substrata 2, substrata 1 mixed with substrata 2, and one without any substrata.

6. Add cells to the dish so that they come in contact with all four quadrants. If testing tissue explants, place the explants as close to the intersection of the four quadrants as possible. Incubate cells at 37°C.

7. Fix cells at any later time using 2% paraformaldehyde in PBS for 10 min and analyze using an inverted fluorescence microscope.

IV. Conclusions

The techniques described in this chapter provide researchers with several means of measuring cell–ECM interactions on embryonic avian cells. These techniques should provide a good basis for formulating experiments to investigate the role of cell–ECM interactions in development. It is important to reemphasize the limitations of these assays. Cell migration and substrata preference are both dependent on cell adhesion and can never be assayed in isolation. It is also important to remember that the context within which an ECM molecule is presented to a cell may have dramatic effects on cell interactions with that cell. Most ECM components interact with each other, as well as growth factors, and are unlikely to be found in isolation within the embryo. Although a large amount of data concerning cell–ECM interactions *in vitro* have been compiled, their role *in vivo* is still largely unknown and much work in this area is required.

Acknowledgment

I thank Joe Ramos for his comments on this manuscript.

References

McClay, D. R., Wessel, G. M., and Marchase, R. B. (1981). Intercellular recognition: Quantitation of initial binding events. *Proc. Natl. Acad. Sci. U.S.A.* **78,** 4975–4979.

Perris, R., Paulsson, M., and Bronner-Fraser, M. (1989). Molecular mechanisms of neural crest cell migration on fibronectin and laminin. *Dev. Biol.* **136,** 222–238.

Walter, J., Kern-Veits, B., Huf, J., Stolze, B., and Bonhoeffer, F. (1987). Recognition of position-specific properties of tectal cell membranes by retinal axons *in vitro*. *Development (Cambridge, UK)* **101,** 685–696.

CHAPTER 16

Cell Division and Differentiation in Avian Embryos: Techniques for Study of Early Neurogenesis and Myogenesis

John Sechrist and Christophe Marcelle

Developmental Biology Center
University of California
Irvine, California 92717

  I. Cell Cycle and Cell Specialization
 II. Cell Division and Neural Differentiation
III. Cell Division and Somite Differentiation
 IV. Primary Methods Selected to Detect Dividing Cells
       A. [³H]Thymidine Autoradiography
       B. Bromodeoxyuridine Immunohistochemistry
  V. Selected Histological Procedures
       A. Preparation of Chick Embryos for Experimental Manipulation
       B. Embryo Collection
       C. General Fixatives and Histological Solutions
       D. Embedding Procedures
       E. Staining Procedures
       F. Antibody Labeling on Sectioned Material
       G. Preparation of Emulsion-Coated Autoradiographs
      References

I. Cell Cycle and Cell Specialization

Cell division and differentiation have long been recognized as two fundamental processes in the development of multicellular organisms. Early cytologists provided morphological descriptions of mitotic activity and changes in cytoplasmic

Copyright © 1996 by Academic Press, Inc. All rights of reproduction in any form reserved.

organelles based on light microscopic observations of developing embryos. To-day, it is remarkable that the elegant pictures they contributed can now largely be explained in molecular terms (Alberts *et al.*, 1994). The cell cycle consists of a mitotic phase (M phase) in which the chromosomes condense and separate as the nucleus divides and an interphase during which there is growth in size, replication of DNA (S or synthetic phase), and other elaborate preparations for the next division. Before and after the S phase are the gap phases (G_1 and G_2, respectively) or a specialized pause of varied length, known as G_0. In young embryos, all cells divide rapidly to provide an adequate cell population for the different organ systems that will form. The regulatory mechanisms which control the number of cell divisions in any given tissue are not only crucial for producing a normal multicellular organism but also may contribute significantly to species differences.

During and after the gastrulation stage of development, a few nerve cell precursors begin to exit the cell cycle (to enter a long G_0 phase) followed later by exiting skeletal muscle precursors. One characteristic that many neuroblasts and skeletal myoblasts have in common is that their terminally differentiated state is postmitotic. This contrasts with other embryonic tissues that make cell-specific proteins while continuing to proliferate. Although it was originally assumed that division and differentiation were incompatible (Cajal, 1960; Okazaki and Holtzer, 1966; Balls and Billet, 1973), it later became clear that in many cell types, such as sympathetic neuroblasts, erythroblasts, cardiac myoblasts, and chondroblasts, tissue-specific proteins are synthesized while cells continue to divide (see Rothman *et al.*, 1978; Rohrer and Thoenen, 1987). Although some have suggested that DNA synthesis and mitosis are essential precursors to cell differentiation (Holtzer *et al.*, 1975), more recent evidence argues against an obligatory coupling of a terminal mitotic division and differentiation (see Alberts *et al.*, 1994).

The ability to introduce exogenous molecules or to detect selected endogenous ones with a variety of radioactive or fluorescent markers provides a unique opportunity to further explore old questions about the relationship of cell differentiation and cell division. The primary intent of this chapter is to describe and illustrate how [³H]thymidine autoradiography and bromodeoxyuridine (BrdU) immunohistochemistry have been used alone or in combination with antibody staining and *in situ* hybridization to analyze cell division and differentiation in birds. Early avian neurogenesis and skeletal muscle differentiation have been chosen as models to exemplify this methodology. We also provide a variety of techniques from classical and contemporary histology that are necessary to use in conjunction with cell division and cell differentiation markers, but have broader applications as well. Particular emphasis will be devoted to that part of the methodology which is unique to avian species as opposed to fish, amphibians, or mammals.

II. Cell Division and Neural Differentiation

The nature of the early neural epithelium. To study the sequence of events that occur during the cell cycle in the early chick, numerous investigators have applied a variety of informative techniques, such as reduced silver staining, radioactive labeling, antibody staining, or analysis of specific gene expression patterns (Holmes, 1943; Cajal, 1960; Sechrist, 1969; Sidman, 1970; Sechrist and Bronner-Fraser, 1991; Henrique *et al.,* 1995). The pseudostratified columnar epithelium of the neural plate, neural folds, and early neural tube appears to primarily be an undifferentiated stem cell population which undergoes rapid cell division. As neuroblasts exit the cell cycle and extend their axons, they accumulate near the outer margin of the neural wall, resulting in the formation of three layers (Fig. 1A, see color insert), most frequently named (from inner to outer) the ventricular, intermediate, and marginal zones (Boulder Committee, 1970).

Homogeneity versus nonhomogeneity of the ventricular zone. The view that the ventricular zone is composed of a proliferating, homogeneous, and undifferentiated population is widely accepted. Early studies with [^{3}H]thymidine (Fujita, 1962, 1963) seemed to confirm this description as most ventricular cells at young developmental stages incorporate DNA precursors given sufficient time (Figs. 1D and G). However, Cajal had described, as early as the 1890s (1960, for English translation), the presence of apolar neuroblasts (i.e., round cells adjacent to the lumen with thread-like neurofibrils, as in Figs. 1B and 1F and Fig. 3), and bipolar neuroblasts (i.e., columnar or spindle-shaped cells with neurofibrils in their apical and basal processes, as in Figs. 3B, 3G, and 3I) in the ventricular zone. Cajal had wrongly stated that the apolar neuroblasts are not germinal or mitotic cells since, as described earlier, they can be labeled with [^{3}H]thymidine. Therefore, the validity of descriptions of early neuroblast differentiation based on neurofibrillar staining or thymidine labeling alone is open to question. An alternative explanation, however, could be that some neuroblasts form neurofilaments during their terminal cell cycle prior to leaving the ventricular zone.

By combining Feulgen (DNA stain), silver staining, and autoradiography, we have observed that neurofibrils could be detected in some dividing or recently divided neural precursors (Figs. 1E–1H) (Sechrist 1968, 1969). Subsequent studies of the developing retina, spinal cord, and brain stem with reduced silver staining (Figs. 1B and 1F), neurofilament antibodies (Figs. 3A–3I), and electron microscopy (Fig. 4) confirmed that the ventricular zone is, at certain times and locations, a mixed, nonhomogeneous cell population since differentiation is detectable prior to movement of neuroblasts into the intermediate zone (Tapscott *et al.,* 1981; Sechrist and Bronner-Fraser, 1991).

Neuroblasts are not always postmitotic. Disagreement regarding the nature of vertebrate neural epithelial cells is not a recent occurrence. Even before the turn of the last century, a question arose regarding the relationship of mitotic (or germinal) cells and the remaining neural epithelial cells. Confirmation that these were actually one cell type in different phases of the cell cycle required an additional 60 years of research and was best shown by [³H]thymidine autoradiography (see Sidman, 1970). Undifferentiated cells with their nuclei in the external half of the neural epithelium synthesize DNA and, within several hours, move toward the ventricular surface to divide. Even though neurofilament production in dividing cells appears to be a selective early marker for several neuroblast populations (retinal ganglion cells, brain stem, and spinal cord motor neurons), an important observation by Bennett and colleagues indicated that caution should be exercised. The dorsal forebrain, optic vesicles, and heart show transient neurofilament staining at early stages (Bennett and DiLullo, 1985). In our hands, reduced silver methods will variably stain both the transient and the subsequent neuronal-specific neurofilament proteins consistently shown by an antibody to an unphosphorylated, intermediate weight neurofilament (NF-M) (Lee et al., 1987).

The first central nervous system neuroblasts differentiate postmitotically. It is now apparent that the first neuroblasts (hindbrain reticular) in the chick become identifiable in a postmitotic bipolar–unipolar sequence [i.e., without any detectable differentiation in the apolar configuration during mitosis (Sechrist and Bronner-Fraser, 1991; see also Cowdry, 1914; Henrique et al., 1995)]. Many reticular neuron precursors exit the cell cycle before closure of the neural tube (Figs. 2A–2E, 3I, 5B–5E) and only then become identifiable as bipolar columnar cells with neurofilament antibodies or other neuron-specific markers (such as transcripts for the vertebrate *Delta* homolog; Henrique et al., 1995). The nature of the very earliest intracellular response of this population or their parent cells to primary neural induction is yet to be determined at a molecular level. The much more familiar apolar–bipolar–unipolar sequence (Figs. 3A–3I) of Cajal (1960) begins a day or more later when motor neuron and then retinal ganglion cell precursors undergo a terminal cell cycle along with the precocious production of neurofilament molecules. The identification of additional molecules such as embryonic cholinesterases (Layer and Sporns, 1987) that might be involved in regulating the transition from a proliferating to a differentiated state is an important pursuit for the near future.

Fig. 2 [³H]Thymidine autoradiographs of the chick brain stem during earliest neurogenesis. (A) A section through the preotic level of a 15 ss embryo (HH 12-) treated 18 hr earlier at the 4–6 ss (HH 8). At this rhombomere 4 level, nearly all cells are labeled, including otic (OT) ectoderm, migrated neural crest (NC), and neural tube (NT) cells with the exception of several (arrow) near the lateral basal lamina. These postmitotic cells and others shown on this plate are young reticular neurons which exit the cell cycle during neural plate and fold stages. (B) A section through the future caudal hindbrain level of a 2,3 ss (HH 7+) embryo treated 7 hr earlier at the definitive streak or early head process stage (HH 4,5). At this young stage, all notochord (N), endoderm, and somite mesoderm (Som) cells are labeled, but a very few dispersed neural fold (NF) cells (arrow) are not. If allowed to develop for sufficient time (see below), the postmitotic cells will differentiate and extend axons. (C and D) Sections through the third and sixth somite levels of an 18 ss (HH 13-)

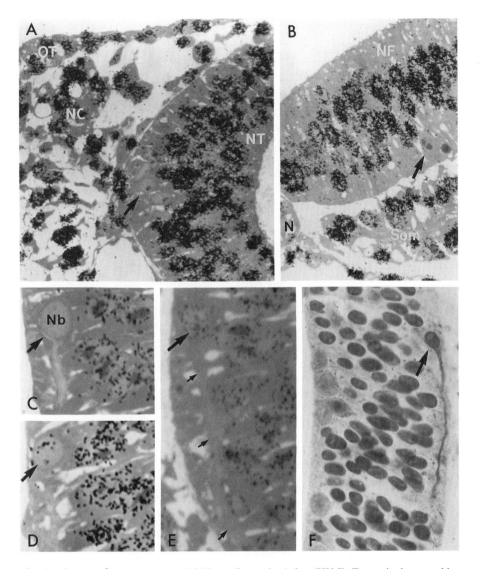

Fig. 2 (*continued*) embryo treated 25 hr earlier at the 1–3 ss (HH 7). Two unipolar neuroblasts (Nb, arrows) with axons illustrate a rostrocaudal gradient in the time cells of a probably equivalent functional type exit the cell cycle. The more caudal cell (D) with some label had not completed DNA replication at the time of treatment unlike the cell that had already done so (C). (E) A section through the fourth somite level of a 20 ss (HH 13) embryo treated 32 hr earlier at the late primitive streak stage (HH 3+, 4). The commissural neuroblast (large arrow) with a long axon (small arrows) is well labeled as were all detectable neuroblasts rostral to this level; an equivalent embryo again confirmed no neuron precursors had completed DNA replication prior to late HH stage 3. (F) Light micrograph of a silver-stained section [Holmes (1943) method] through the lateral wall of the neural tube at the first somite level of a 20 somite embryo (HH 13) with a similar unipolar neuroblast (arrow) to that shown in E. *Note:* The sections in A–E were plastic embedded, toluidine blue-stained whereas F was double embedded in celloidin and paraffin.

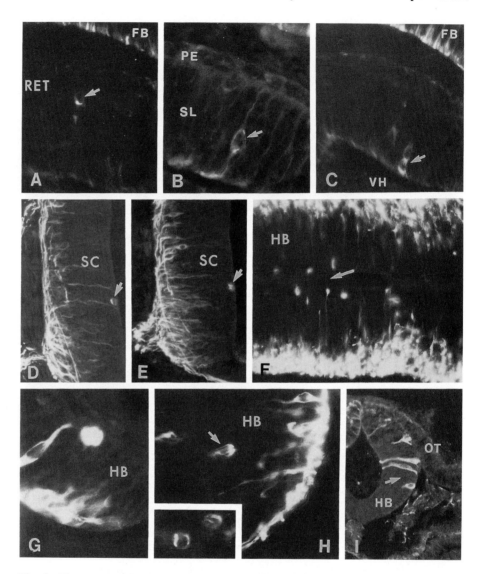

Fig. 3 Fluorescence micrographs of neurofilament (NF-M) immunoreactivity in embryonic retina (RET), spinal cord (SC), and hindbrain (HB) neuroblasts. (A–C) Sections of the retina of a 28 ss (HH 16) embryo showing several of the first NF-M+ ganglion cell neuroblasts (arrows) within the developing sensory layer (SL). There appears to be an apolar premitotic neuroblast (A) adjacent to pigment epithelium (PE) and a postmitotic bipolar (B) and a prospective unipolar (C) pair of neuroblasts near the vitreous humor (VH). The forebrain (FB) still exhibits transient staining of neural epithelial cells at this stage whereas the retina does not. (D and E) Transverse sections of the spinal cord at the forelimb level of a 4-day (HH 22) embryo show an apolar premitotic and apolar postmitotic neuroblast pair (arrows) adjacent to the lumen as well as more advanced NF-M+ neuroblasts close to the marginal layer. Based on the position of the dorsal and ventral roots, the NF-M+ cells in the mitotic zone are nearly always in the basal (ventral) half of the spinal cord.

III. Cell Division and Somite Differentiation

Somite differentiation. Limb and trunk skeletal muscles arise from precursor cells present in the somites. The somites differentiate such that at the level of the fourth or fifth newly formed somite, its ventromedial portion undergoes an epithelio-mesenchymal transition that gives rise to the sclerotome, which contains the precursors of the cartilage and bone of the axial skeleton. The remaining dorsal epithelium of the somite, the dermomyotome, contains precursors for axial and limb skeletal muscles, the dermis, and a portion of the skeletal muscle vascular endothelium (reviewed in Christ and Ordahl, 1995). Concomitant with sclerotome formation, cells at the craniomedial edge of the lip of the dermomyotome ingress ventrally, then elongate caudally to form the myotome (Kaehn *et al.*, 1988), a structure composed of mononucleated myocytes that express myogenic determination factors of the MyoD family and muscular proteins (reviewed in Wachtler and Christ, 1992; Pownall and Emerson, 1992). Later in development the myotome will give rise to axial skeletal muscles. Limb muscles originate from precursors present in the lateral edge of the dermomyotome and which migrate into the early limb mesenchyme (reviewed in Wachtler and Christ, 1992).

The myotome of early avian embryo is composed only of postmitotic cells. Previous studies using tritiated thymidine have shown that the myotome is composed of postmitotic myotomal cells (Langman and Nelson, 1968). We reinvestigated cell division in the differentiating somite by using BrdU labeling in combination with *in situ* hybridization and immunohistochemistry techniques. Stage 18 embryos were labeled with BrdU for 2 hr. Cryostat sections were reacted sequentially with monoclonal antibody MF20, which recognizes the embryonic form of the myosin heavy chain (expressed by myotomal cells), and with the BrdU antibody. In the trunk region of a stage 18 embryo, the MF 20-positive myotome is devoid of replicating cells (Figs. 6A–6C, see color insert). This confirms the work of Langman and Nelson (1968) and demonstrates that the myotome of early avian embryos is composed only of postmitotic cells.

Myogenic precursor migration from the dermomyotome to the myotome takes 4 hr. Because mitosis is observed in the dermomyotome and not in the myotome,

Fig. 3 (*continued*)   (F) Longitudinal section of the ventral hindbrain of a 3-day (HH 19) embryo with NF-M+ mitotic cells on either side of the lumen (arrow). (G and H) Transverse sections of preotic and postotic brain stem levels of a 28 somite (HH 16) embryo showing NF-M+ apolar, bipolar, and unipolar neuroblasts. (G) The bright cells are differentiating facial motor neurons near the ventral midline. (H) The inset shows two premitotic cells to compare with an overlapping daughter cell pair (arrow) several sections away. (I) Transverse section of the hindbrain (HB) at the otic (OT) level of a young 9 ss (HH 10-) embryo. The bipolar and prospective unipolar neuroblasts (arrow) in the lateral wall of the hindbrain are likely to be early postmitotic reticular neurons; apolar neuroblasts near the lumen are not detectable until later stages, as shown earlier. *Note:* These sections were cut from frozen embryos that were gelatin–sucrose embedded.

the former is assumed to be the sole source of axial myotomal cells. Therefore, muscle progenitors actively dividing in the dermomyotome exit the cell cycle before migrating into the myotomal compartment of the somite. How long does it take for a muscle progenitor to migrate from the dermomyotome to the myotome? To address this question, Langman and Nelson (1968) exposed chick embryos to [³H]thymidine for increasing lengths of time. Although they did not observe labeled myotomal cells after short exposures to thymidine, they observed that thymidine treatment for more than 4 hr led to the presence of labeled cells in the myotome. These results indicate that myogenic progenitors labeled in the dermomyotomal compartment of the somite need approximately 4 hr to migrate into the myotome. We confirmed this observation by labeling a 23 somite chick embryo (stage 14 HH) with [³H]thymidine for 5 hr. Semithin sections through the cervical region of this embryo show that two labeled cells can be seen in the dorsomedial part of myotome (Fig. 7A, see color insert).

Mitotically competent muscle progenitors appear in the myotome at E2.5. The demonstration that mitosis is observed only in the dermomyotome and not in the myotome raises a paradox since the dermomyotome is a transient structure which disappears around day 5 of development whereas muscles continue to grow thoughout development and after hatching. Therefore, mitotically competent muscle progenitors must be present in the myotome by the time the dermomyotome disappears. Mitotically competent muscle progenitors, or myoblasts, express the fibroblast growth factor receptor FREK (Marcelle *et al.*, 1994), which can therefore be used as a marker for this cell population in chick and quail embryos (Marcelle *et al.*, 1995). We have demonstrated that a small population of FREK-positive cells appears in the myotomal compartment of the somite at 2.5 days of development, approximately 15 hr after the appearance of the first postmitotic myotomal cells (Marcelle *et al.*, 1995). Although we have evidence that few FREK-positive myoblasts present in the myotome at these early stages of somite differentiation are mitotically active (unpublished results), at E6 the FREK-positive myoblast population is actively dividing (Fig. 7B) (Marcelle *et al.*, 1995). Therefore, the myotomal compartment of the somite is formed by a first wave of postmitotic, MyoD-positive myocytes; 15 hr later a second wave of mitotically competent, FREK-positive muscle progenitors migrates into the myotome. These results do not preclude that FREK-positive myoblasts present in the somite from E2.5 later express MyoD during their differentiation.

Overt differentiation, myogenic determination factor expression, and cell division. During the course of muscle differentiation, the expression of myogenic determination factors (MDF) of the MyoD family is thought to signal the onset of overt muscle differentiation and therefore the commitment of pluripotent progenitors to a myogenic fate. Support for this idea comes from the observation that forced expression of any MDF causes many types of nonmuscle cells to respecify their phenotype to myogenesis (reviewed in Wright, 1992). This unique property has led investigators to suggest that MDFs are "master regulatory genes" whose embryonic expression signals the commitment of pluripotent mesoderm cells to a myogenic lineage (Weintraub *et al.,* 1991; reviewed in Christ and Ordahl, 1995). Terminal muscle differentiation is characterized by the fusion of myocytes into postmitotic, multinucleated myotubes that express muscle-specific proteins. Although it has been demonstrated in a tissue culture system, that MyoD-expressing cells are replicative (Tapscott *et al.,* 1988; Yablonka-Reuveni and Rivera, 1994), it is not clear whether MyoD expression precedes or follows the end of mitotic capacities of muscle progenitors *in vivo.* To address this question, we incubated stage 23 chick embryos with BrdU for 2 hr. We then reacted transverse sections sequentially with a chick MyoD probe and an anti-BrdU antibody (Figs. 7C and 7D). Although a large majority of MyoD-expressing cells are BrdU negative, we observed colocalization of MyoD and BrdU in a few myotomal cells. This indicates that MyoD expression and cell division are not mutually exclusive *in vivo* as well as *in vitro* and confirms that muscle differentiation precedes the end of muscle progenitor cell proliferation.

IV. Primary Methods Selected to Detect Dividing Cells

A. [^{3}H]Thymidine Autoradiography

The application of [^{3}H]thymidine autoradiography to study (primarily mouse) neurogenesis was thoroughly reviewed by Sidman (1970). The methodological principles he discussed are nevertheless relevant to this chapter which is focused primarily on avian species. Even though a variety of newer and faster techniques [mainly BrdU and proliferating cell nuclear antigen (PCNA) labeling] have since been introduced [^{3}H]thymidine labeling of proliferating cells continues to be utilized effectively and appears to be the standard for comparison of cell cycle kinetic analysis (Boswald *et al.,* 1990).

1. Staging Young Chick Embryos

Determining the stage of development at the time of treatment based on incubation time alone is unreliable; seasonal variation and the maturity of the laying hens are just two factors that seem to affect developmental rates. In addition, there is normal variation within the same batch of eggs. To stage embryos over the 1–2 somite stage, it is best to window the eggs and introduce a subblastodermal injection of ink [Pelikan Fount India ink diluted 1:8 in phosphate-buffered saline (PBS)]. This clearly reveals the somite number and other morphological features with the aid of a dissecting microscope. Embryos are usually staged according to the number of somite pairs and/or according to the criteria of Hamburger and Hamilton (HH) (1951). Even though Pelikan Fount India ink is said to be less toxic than others (Stern, 1993), the ink is increasingly difficult to obtain due in part to its carcinogenic properties.

Prior to the 1–2 somite stage, any disturbance of these young avian embryos (HH4–6), whether by injecting isotonic saline, ink for staging, or even making a window, can lead to abnormalities. Therefore, at early stages, we prefer to infer the developmental age retrospectively by collecting and staging untreated embryos at the same time as thymidine-treated embryos and calculating backward from the stage at sacrifice after limited experimental intervals (ranging from hours to 1–2 days). Alternatively, *ex ovo* whole embryo culture can be used in order to accurately stage HH4–6 embryos (Fisher and Fedoroff, 1978; Selleck, this volume). However, this approach is only applicable for survival times of 1–2 days.

2. Procedure for Application of [³H]Thymidine

Tritiated thymidine is available through a variety of suppliers (e.g., Schwarz Bioresearch, New England Nuclear, and Amersham Corporation). The metabolite is labeled in the methyl group and is usually provided in an aqueous solution with a radioactive concentration of 1 mCi/ml. A range of specific activites from 0.36 to 60 Ci/mmol can be purchased depending on the supplier. In our experience, labeling embryos via the yolk sac with [³H]thymidine at 3, 6.7, 25, or 57.2 Ci/mmol specific activity gives satisfactory results; 6.7 Ci/mmol is adequate for routine use.

The procedure for administering [³H]thymidine is determined in part by the age of the embryo and by the objectives of the experiment. A significant difference between avian and rodent species is that one injection in the latter results in a pulse label of less than an hour duration (due to a rapid metabolic breakdown of the labeled thymidine). In contrast, in the chick, the availability of the precursor is usually longer, depending on the dose, embryonic age, and site of application. This difference has important implications for birthdating and cell cycle kinetic analysis. In chick, the relatively long availability of [³H]thymidine often results in a "cumulative labeling" (i.e., a complete labeling of all replicating cells of the embryo) instead of "pulse labeling" (i.e., labeling of a portion of the replicating cells).

To achieve cumulative labeling in the chick, investigators have injected the labeled DNA precursor into the yolk sac via a hole in the shell (Sauer and Walker, 1959; Fugita, 1962,1963). Fujita injected 25 μCi in 0.1 ml of physiologic saline and observed that at E1, the neural epithelium became totally labeled after 5 hr, whereas by E6, 10 hr are needed for the same result. Injection of 30 μCi into the albumen rather than the yolk of 2- to 6-day embryos also results in complete labeling of sympathetic ganglion precursors and other dividing cells (Rothman *et al.*, 1978).

To achieve a pulse labeling of a 1- to 2-day chick embryo, 0.3 μCi of [³H]thymidine diluted in 0.1 ml of saline can be dropped directly onto the vitelline membrane through an opening in the shell (Martin and Langman, 1965; Langman *et al.*, 1966). At low doses, the isotope appears to remain available for only 2–3 hr. Therefore, to cumulatively label these embryos, it is necessary to apply a second treatment (with the same dose) after an additional 2–4 hr. Using this technique in conjunction with a mitotic inhibitor, it was possible to determine that the length of a cell cycle is approximately 8 hr at 2–3 days of development (Langman *et al.,* 1966). At 1–2 days of development, low amounts of [^{3}H]thymidine are recommended as long-term survival rates decrease significantly if doses approach 6 μCi or more (McConnell and Sechrist, 1980).

After somite formation (beginning at stage 12 HH), we have successfully labeled developing embryos by depositing the solutions through a hole in the vitelline and, at later stages, the amniotic membranes. By the sixth to ninth day, some investigators have found that injection directly into the vitelline vein or the chorioallantoic vein may be necessary to reach an evenly distributed and consistent labeling throughout the embryo (Rothman *et al.,* 1978; Dupin, 1984).

In conclusion, to label an embryo at an early stage of development (stage 3–9 HH), the most reliable method is application of the DNA precursor by dripping it onto the vitelline membrane over the embryo in doses between 1 and 5 μCi (diluted in 20–50 μl PBS) with a specific activity of 6.7 μCi/mmol (or equivalent). To cumulatively label with confidence, the most reliable method is to apply a second dose within 2–4 hr. Beyond stage 12 HH (around 48 hr of incubation), doses should be increased to 10–25 μCi.

At these early stages of development, an alternative approach is the direct injection of thymidine into the yolk sac. A single injection of 50 μCi (with or without saline) leads to a complete labeling of HH 4–5 embryos with very infrequent abnormalities; embryos are collected 24–36 hr later (Sechrist and Bronner-Fraser, 1991). The injections are done with eggs blunt side up. The 25-gauge needles attached to a Hamilton microsyringe are inserted into the upper half of the egg or through the lateral part of the air space, taking care to avoid the developing blastoderm. Using this approach, we have observed that around 20% of the embryos are unlabeled after a single injection (whether low or high specific activity-labeled thymidine is used).

3. Autoradiographic Procedure

Our autoradiographic methodology follows the procedure of Kopriwa and LeBlond (1962) with assistance from subsequent reviews and books (Sidman, 1970; Rogers, 1979; Humason, 1979; Hayat, 1989) as well as original articles. Embryos are fixed overnight in an aldehyde mixture of 2% glutaraldehyde–2% paraformaldehyde or in 4% paraformaldehyde. Those fixed with the aldehyde mixture are postfixed in 1–2% osmium tetroxide to preserve the morphology of membranes in semithin plastic sections and to provide the option for doing electron microscopy (Fig. 4). The tissue can be embedded in paraffin, double-embedded in paraffin and celloidin, epoxy resin (Epon 812 or Eponate), or a 15% gelatin–sucrose mixture for frozen sections. Sections may vary in thickness from 1 to 10 μm (also ultrathin for EM) depending on the embedding medium with 1–2 (plastic) or 3–4 (double-embedded) μm being close to optimum.

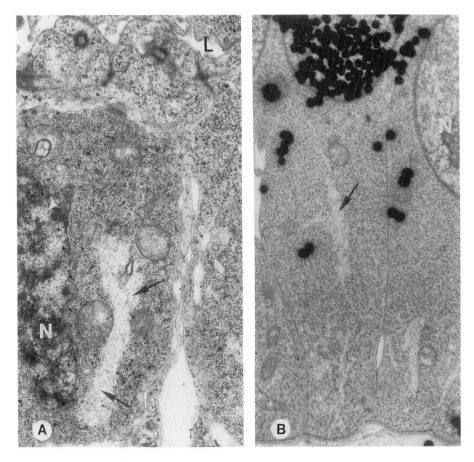

Fig. 4 Electron micrographs of the apical and basal parts of the neural epithelium in the cervical spinal cord. (A) An apolar daughter cell (one of a pair) near the lumen (L) of a 72-hr embryo (HH 18) fixed in 4% glutaraldehyde. To the right of the condensed nucleus (N) is a clear cytoplasmic region (arrows) containing neurofilament aggregates; their size and coiled configuration correspond to the images of postmitotic apolar neuroblasts obtained with reduced silver staining or NF-M antibodies. (B) The basal processes of two neural epithelial cells attached to the forming basal lamina of a 52-hr embryo (HH 13) fixed in 2% glutaraldehyde–2% paraformaldehyde. After 2 hr of treatment with [^{3}H]thymidine, one replicating nucleus is heavily labeled (black crystals) while the other (N) on the right is not. Small microfilament aggregates (arrow) are present in the basal cytoplasm of this premitotic labeled cell which may accumulate further as the cell soon moves toward the lumen to divide.

Some stains can be applied prior to the emulsion application (Holmes-reduced silver method or Feulgen) whereas others (toluidine blue or hematoxylin and eosin) are usually applied afterward since they chemically react with the undeveloped emulsion (which results in a background "fog"). Since toluidine blue staining of sections after emulsion application does not give satisfactory results, we have found that after prestaining, an intervening layer such as a carbon film prevents chemical reaction and gives excellent results (Sechrist and Upson, 1974).

Slides are dipped in Kodak NTB-2 emulsion. The slides are dried and stored in a light-tight box for 1–3 weeks prior to developing with Kodak D-19. The slides can be mounted in Permount after dehydration or in an aqueous medium (Gel-mount, Biomeda) depending on the staining procedure. Plastic sections with toluidine blue stain can be viewed and then stored for years without a coverslip or oil immersion photographs can be taken with direct application of oil onto the dried emulsion followed by careful removal of any excess immersion oil.

4. Interpretation of Grain Counts

When 100% of replicating cells are labeled after cumulative application of thymidine, those cells which completely lack silver grains (Figs. 1H and 2A–2C) can be assumed to have left the cell cycle, having undergone their terminal S phase prior to treatment. Cells with reduced grain count may have nearly completed the terminal S phase at the time of treatment and then divided (Fig. 2D) or may have divided one final time after S with each daughter inheriting half of the label (Figs. 1C and 1G). If the length of treatment is less than a full cycle, some unlabeled ventricular cells may have not reentered S or may already be postmitotic (Figs. 1A and 4B). After cumulative labeling, long-term birthdating can be performed in the chick by looking for unlabeled nuclei (Langman and Haden, 1970). However, it is far easier to do this with pulse label and then look for heavily labeled nuclei, indicating that the cells were the daughters of a cell in the terminal S phase which became labeled just before dividing (McConnell and Sechrist, 1980).

The disadvantages of the [³H]thymidine labeling procedure include the necessity to use radioactivity and the lengthy nature of the procedure. This has resulted over the years in the use of alternative methods, such as BrdU and PCNA labeling. However, for precision in cell kinetic studies, [³H]thymidine analysis is still the method of choice. In addition, for long-term birthdating studies, thymidine has a relatively low impact on normal development compared to the high teratogenicity of BrdU (see below).

B. Bromodeoxyuridine Immunohistochemistry

The introduction of monoclonal antibodies to bromodeoxyuridine (Gratzner, 1992, reviewed in Gray and Mayall, 1985) has led to considerable interest in the use of BrdU in cell proliferation studies. BrdU is phosphorylated and incorporated into DNA, where it replaces thymidine during the S phase of cell cycle. The advantages of BrdU compared with labeled thymidine are the ease of application, fast processing times, and working with radioactivity can be avoided. This has led to attempts to generalize its use. However, it soon became apparent that BrdU uptake can have dramatic long-term effects as BrdU is a potent suppressor of differentiation both *in vitro* and *in vivo* (Wilt and Anderson, 1972, Lee *et al.*, 1974, Bannigan *et al.*, 1981, Sechrist and Bronner-Fraser, 1991). The younger the chick embryo, the stronger the teratogenic effects of BrdU. For instance, treatment of a gastrulating embryo (stage 4 HH) with as low a dose as 10^{-7} *M* BrdU profoundly impairs further development (Figs. 5B and 5C). In general, BrdU labeling should not be recommended for long-term studies, such as birth-dating techniques, for which thymidine is preferable.

1. BrdU *in Vivo* Labeling

To lower the embryo in the egg shell, we first remove 1–2 ml albumen with a 5-ml syringe, 18-gauge needle introduced at the tip of the egg. The BrdU labeling protocol varies depending on the embryonic stage when the experimenter wishes to label the embryo. At very early stages (up to stage 6 HH), the embryo is very sensitive and does not respond well to rupturing the vitelline membrane. We have found that direct application of BrdU solution onto the vitelline membrane, as with thymidine, successfully labels the embryo. At later stages of development, before extraembryonic membranes surround the embryo, BrdU is directly applied on the embryo after a small opening in the vitelline membrane is made with a glass or tungsten needle. From E4, a small opening is made both in the vitelline membrane and in the amniotic sac, through which the BrdU solution is injected in the vicinity of the heart. In each case, 50 μl of a 10^{-2} *M* solution of 5-bromo-2'-deoxyuridine (Sigma) dissolved in PBS is injected with a pipette (note that lower doses of BrdU should be used when longer exposure to the base analog is desired). The egg is then resealed with tape and is incubated at 38°C for 1 to 2 hr. Embryos are then sacrificed and fixed in 4% paraformaldehyde/PBS. They are then processed for paraffin or cryostat sectioning (see below).

2. Antibody Detection

If BrdU immunohistochemistry is done in conjunction with mRNA detection, *in situ* hybridization is performed prior to incubation with the BrdU antibody. A technique for *in situ* hybridization with a cold probe on sections is described in Chapter 11. We have successfully used a technique described by Strähle *et al.* (1994). Since the diameter of a cell is approximately 10 μm, we do not recommend using thicker sections if cellular resolution of the mRNA signal and the BrdU labeling is desired. After nonisotopic *in situ* hybridization, sections are treated with 2 *N* HCl for 20 min at room temperature. HCl treatment keeps the NBT-BCIP blue precipitate and many antibody antigenic determinants intact. Sections are then washed with PBS and are incubated for 30 min with a 1:30 dilution [in PBS/1% bovine serum albumin (BSA)] of mouse anti-BrdU antibody (Becton-Dickinson). After several washes in PBS, a FITC-coupled secondary antibody (goat anti-mouse HI FITC, Antibodies Inc. Davis, CA) diluted 1:200 in PBS/1% BSA is applied to the sections for 1 hr. In other cases, the BrdU antibody is detected using diaminobenzidine and the Vectastain kit.

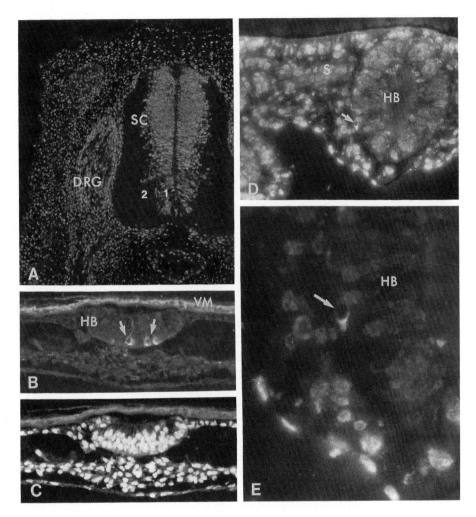

Fig. 5 Fluorescence micrographs of anti-BrdU, anti-NF-M, and combined antibody staining. (A) A 5-day (HH 26) embryo treated with BrdU (10^{-6} M) beginning at day 4 (24 hr earlier). At this rostral forelimb level the spinal cord (SC) ventricular zone (1) contains proliferating labeled nuclei whereas postmitotic motor neurons in the intermediate zone (2) are unlabeled. By this stage there are also unlabeled regions in the dorsal root ganglia (DRG) which contain postmitotic sensory neurons. (B and C) An abnormal 2-day (50 hr) embryo treated with BrdU 32 hr earlier at the late intermediate streak stage (HH 3+). At the presumptive hindbrain (HB) level, three NF-M+ neuroblasts (arrows) can be identified even though the hindbrain has not closed and contains a significantly reduced cell population (compare with D). The same section (C) secondarily stained with anti-BrdU indicates that all nuclei appear to be labeled, including the three neuroblasts. The vitelline membrane (VM) is still intact in this preparation. (D and E) A 14 somite stage embryo treated first with BrdU (10^{-3} M) 14 hr earlier at HH stage 8 (5 ss). At the level of the first somite (S), a unipolar neuroblast with a NF-M+ cytoplasm but an unstained nucleus (BrdU-, arrow) in the ventrolateral hindbrain (HB) confirms that some reticular neurons exit the cell cycle prior to neural tube closure. *Note:* These sections were cut from frozen embryos that were gelatin–sucrose embedded.

V. Selected Histological Procedures

A. Preparation of Chick Embryos for Experimental Manipulation

1. Incubate at 37–39°C until desired stage. Eggs can be removed from the incubator and allowed to cool to room temperature to slow development. They can be left out of the incubator for up to 1 day prior to use or reincubation without deleterious effects. More than this can decrease survival or increase the amount of abnormalities.

2. Opening eggs. Two methods are used to open eggs:

    a. Wash eggs with 70% EtOH. In order to sink the embryo for visualization, remove 2 ml of albumen with a 3-cc syringe with an 18-gauge needle This is usually done at the blunt end by pointing the needle to the lowest part of the egg. Place transparent Scotch magic tape on the middle of the egg. Puncture the egg with one point of the scissors and cut a circle of desired size. (For most applications, an opening of about 2.4–3 cm in diameter is best.)

    b. Puncture the egg with a small needle. Using a scalpel, cut a 1-cm² window in the shell. *Caution:* since the shell is smooth, the scalpel blade can slip easily. Using this technique, the embryo can be floated up above the egg surface by lining the square hole with vacuum grease and adding saline, drop by drop, until the embryo is floated out of the window.

3. Inking eggs: use India ink in order to improve the contrast of the embryo for manipulations. Dilute 1:10 in Howard Ringers (HR) solution and prepare a 2-cc syringe with a bent 25 ⅝-gauge needle. Puncture the vitelline membrane outside of the blastoderm. Carefully bring the needle up just beneath the embryo. Inject a small bolus of ink solution and shake the egg gently to disperse ink.

4. Removing portion of the vitelline membrane: Place a drop of HR over the embryo. Snag the membrane with a sharpened tungsten needle to tear a small window above the embryo.

5. Manipulate embryos as desired. **Always keep embryo hydrated with saline solution.** It is sometimes useful to apply dispase or saline containing 0.1% trypsin to loosen things up a bit.

6. After manipulation, the embryos are placed in the 37°C incubator. Since the embryos survival is dependent of hydration, the egg should be sealed with Scotch magic tape or electrical tape. If the embryos are to be grown for an extended period of time, add 1–2 drops of antibiotic/antimycotic solution.

B. Embryo Collection

1. Following an experiment, remove the tape covering the shell window and carefully remove the embryo with scissors. Cut a larger window if necessary.

2. Two main methods are used for removing the embryo from the yolk for fixation:

a. For older embryos: Using scissors, make four cuts in the shape of a square through the vitelline membrane and blastoderm outside the embryo. Holding one cut edge with forceps, the embryo is gently pulled from the yolk and placed into saline. Rinse embryo well.

b. For young embryos (HH stage 4–17): Place a small "lifesaver" of filter paper onto vitelline membrane such that the embryo lies beneath the hole in the paper. Using scissors, cut around the edge of the filter paper and lift off with the embryo adhering and transfer into a dish of saline as described earlier. Alternatively, a small spoon can be used to remove the embryo from the egg.

3. Trim embryos. With fine scissors, remove excess embryonic membrane while in saline and cut older embryos into smaller pieces (i.e., head removed from trunk).

4. Fix embryos. The choice of fixative and fixation time largely depend on the nature of the experiment, what antibodies are used, and the size of the embryo. For most experiments, embryos may be fixed in 4% paraformaldehyde overnight at 4°C.

5. Following fixation, rinse in saline and store or leave in paraformaldehyde. For antibody staining, overnight fixation or less (4–6 hr) is best. CAUTION: Eggs with radioactive treatment should be dispensed with according to university guidelines.

C. General Fixatives and Histological Solutions

1. 4% Paraformaldehyde in Phosphate Buffer (Used Most Often)

Add 4.0 g paraformaldehyde to 46 ml deionized water in a 100-ml Erlenmeyer flask. Heat with constant stirring until the paraformaldehyde is thoroughly mixed in the water. At this point the solution will have a milky, homogeneous appearance. Add 6 N sodium hydroxide dropwise until the solution reaches pH 7.4. The solution will become clear as the pH nears 7.4 (DO NOT use a pH meter, use pH paper). Allow the solution to cool and add 50 ml of 0.20 M phosphate buffer, pH 7.4. Mix well and dispense 10-ml aliquots into culture tubes. Store at or below 0°C.

2. 2.5% Glutaraldehyde in Phosphate Buffer

Add the contents of one ampule of 25% glutaraldehyde (Ted Pella, Inc. Redding, CA) (1 ml) to 9 ml of 0.10 M phosphate buffer. Mix well and use immediately. CAUTION: Because glutaraldehyde can give increased background fluorescence, it is not recommended for antibody staining.

3. Fixative for Plastic Sections and DiI: 4% Paraformaldehyde–0.25% Glutaraldehyde.

Mix the solution to desired concentrations; 2% paraformaldehyde and 2% glutaraldehyde (good penetration and crosslinking of proteins) is also a good combination for light and electron microscopy. Postfix with 1–2% OsO_4 in phosphate buffer.

4. Carnoy's Fix

This is good for DNA stains: glacial acetic acid (10 ml), absolute ethyl alcohol (60 ml), and chloroform (30 ml). Fix for 3–6 hr.

5. 100% Methanol or 70% Ethanol Overnight

This is good for subsequent antibody staining. CAUTION: Severe irritation can result from inhalation of vapors or contact with skin. Use gloves at all times. Prepare and use solution in fume hood. Dispose of excess and used solutions in waste containers.

6. Ink Solution

This solution is used for viewing embryos (1.5–3.5 days) after a subblastodermal injection: 1 ml Pelikan "Fount" India ink and 9 ml Howard's Ringers or PBS.

7. Howard's Ringers Solution

This solution consists of 7.20 g NaCl, 0.17 g $CaCl_2$ ($2H_2O$), 0.37 g KCl, and 1000 ml H_2O.

8. Phosphate-Buffered Saline 10× (1 M)

This solution is made up of 2.75 g $NaH_2PO_4 \cdot H_2O$, 11.25 g $NaHPO_4$, and 90 g NaCl in 1 liter H_2O. Use a stir plate to mix, adding the salt slowly to deionized water. Adjust pH to 7.4 using 1 N HCl or 1 N NaOH.

9. Phosphate Buffer

a. Monobasic Stock (0.20 M $NaH_2PO_4 \cdot H_2O$)
Molecular weight equals 137.99 g/mol. Dissolve 27.598 g of $NaH_2PO_4 \cdot H_2O$ in 1 liter of deionized water. Mix well and store at room temperature. Use a stir plate to mix, adding the salt slowly to deionized water.

b. Dibasic Stock (0.20 M Na_2HPO_4)
Molecular weight equals 141.96 g/mol. Dissolve 28.392 g of Na_2HPO_4 in 1 liter of deionized water. Mix well and store at room temperature. *Note:* The anhydrous dibasic salt dissolves very slowly so do not use the solution until the salt is completely dissolved. Use a stir plate as described with monobasic stock.

c. Ratios for Buffered Solutions

pH	Mono:Di
7.4	19:81
7.3	23:77
7.2	25.75

d. Preparation

Equimolar solutions of monobasic and dibasic salts of phosphoric acid can be mixed in various ratios to produce buffered solutions in the range of pH 6 to pH 8. Mix the stock solutions in the ratio indicated for the desired pH. This prepares a 0.20 M buffer which should be diluted to 0.1 M when used with fixations or for washing. If necessary, the pH can be adjusted with 1 N HCl or NaOH. Store at room temperature.

D. Embedding Procedures

1. Paraffin Embedding

Note: If paraffin embedding is performed for *in situ* hybridization, the following steps should be done at 4°C, up to and including the 75% ethanol dehydration solution (see below).

a. After fixation, wash embryos in PBS (1 hr for embryos up to E3, longer for older embryos—overnight at E9).

b. Dehydrate embryos in ascending ethanol series: 60, 75, 90, and 100% (2×) for 15–20 min each for embryos up to E3, longer for older embryos (1–2 hr at E9).

c. Place embryos in toluene, xylene, or Histosol (National Diagnostics, Atlanta), 2× for the same time as step b. These solvents will clear the embryo. Toluene will harden the tissue less than xylene; we routinely use Histosol in this procedure as it gives satisfactory results with a reduced toxicity.

d. Infiltrate the specimen in melted paraffin (Paraplast, VWR Scientific, Seattle, WA) poured in a mold: 2 hr for specimens up to E3 and overnight at E9. Paraffin should not be heated to more than 60°C as a higher temperature alters its sectioning properties. To remove all solvent from the previous step, one or more paraffin changes might be necessary.

e. Embed the embryo. Use warmed forceps to position the embryo. Blocks can be stored at room temperature.

f. After roughly trimming the block to the edges of the embryo, it is sectioned with a microtome. We use disposable microtome blades mounted on a blade holder (Leitz). Ribbons of 5- to 10-μm sections are floated on water dropped onto a slide which is placed on a heated plate (at 45°C). The temperature of the water will remove the wrinkles of the ribbon. If wrinkles are a problem, slightly augmenting the thickness of the section or changing the angle of the blade usually results in better quality sections. Waving a cotton swab laden with chloroform over the floating sections should also solve the problem.

2. Celloidin/Paraffin Double-Embedding Method

The celloidin/paraffin double-embedding technique is more time-consuming than the paraffin technique alone. It is best known for use in cutting large sections of whole organs or for processing hard tissue such as bone, but is excellent for the study of embryos. With a sliding microtome, wet sections (80–95% alcohol) can be cut at 3–4 μm with little shrinkage or distortion. The photographs of the Holmes silver-stained tissue (Fig. 1) are the result of this technique.

Purified celloidin (Parlodion) is shipped by dry strips. The solvent used to liquify the celloidin is equal parts of absolute alcohol/ethyl ether carried out as described below. The tissue can be processed in Stender dishes with slow rehardening of the celloidin by allowing the alcohol/ether solvent to evaporate or by use of chloroform to hasten the process. For additional details regarding embedding and sectioning, the reader is referred to Humason (1979). *Note:* This procedure is an adaptation of one utilized by Dr. Arthur LaVelle at the University of Illinois.

a. After fixation, place tissue for 30 min each in 50, 70, 95, 100, and 100% absolute alcohol/ether (1:1).

b. Place tissue in 2% celloidin (2 days), 4% celloidin (3 days), and 6% celloidin (3 days). Containers must be capped to avoid evaporation. The number of days depends on tissue size.

c. Harden celloidin overnight in a bell jar with chloroform. The next day, cut out a block including the embryo, turn it over, and leave for an extra hour.

d. Benzene (three changes for 1 hr each with agitation). Do not leave in benzene for over 6 hr even with larger embryos.

e. Paraffin infiltration. Place celloidin block in liquid paraffin for 30 min at 20 lbs. of pressure.

f. Allow paraffin in celloidin block to harden at room temperature. Mount on a chuck with paraffin and cut on a sliding microtome.

3. Embedding for Frozen Sections

Gelatin–Sucrose Embedding

a. After fixation, embryos are washed in PBS for 1 hr or more (for old embryos, see notes on lengths of washes in the paraffin-embedding section).

b. Place embryos in 5% sucrose in PBS for 4–8 hr at 4°C.

c. Place embryos in 15% sucrose/PBS for 4–8 hr at 4°C.

d. Infiltrate embryos in 15% sucrose/7.5% gelatin in PB for 2–4 hr at 37°C. To prepare this solution, heat (to 50°C) PBS into a beaker. While stirring, add 7.5% gelatin and 15% sucrose. Stir until dissolved. This solution can be kept at 4°C for up to 2 weeks. Reheat small amounts (in a microwave for a few seconds) when needed.

e. Place embryos in an embedding mold and orient. Check that orientation is kept as gelatin begins to set at room temperature. At this stage of the procedure embryos can be kept in a moist chamber at 4°C.

f. Rapidly freeze the embedded embryo in liquid nitrogen. Alternatively, a dry ice methanol bath stabilized at −70°C can be used. This will prevent the cracking of big embryos which sometimes occurs in liquid nitrogen.

g. Section on a crysotat at 10 μm.

O.C.T. Compound Embedding

We have found that gelatin–sucrose embedding is not compatible with cold probe *in situ* hybridization. For this, we have successfully used the O.C.T. compound-embedding technique. It should be noted, however, that the morphology of the embryo is not preserved as well with this embedding technique as with the gelatin–sucrose technique.

a. After fixation, embryos are washed in PBS for 1 hr at 4°C.

b. Immerse embryos in 30% sucrose in PBS at 4°C overnight.

c. Embryos are then dropped in O.C.T. compound which is poured in a mold. Let sit for 30 min at room temperature before freezing.

d. For freezing and sectioning, refer to steps f and g of the previous section.

4. Freeze-Substitution/Paraffin Embedding

Many antibodies do not work well after conventional 4% paraformaldehyde/ PBS fixation followed by paraffin embedding (Bronner-Fraser and Fraser, 1989). An alternative fixation approach which maintains better antigenic determinants is to fix embryos by methanol-freeze substitution.

a. Embryos are flash-frozen in isopentane cooled in liquid nitrogen.

b. After a few crystals form in the isopentane, the embryo (preferably held in a metal basket) should be immersed entirely for 10 sec.

c. The embryo(s) is then placed in methanol at −80°C for 3 days.

d. Transfer the specimens to fresh methanol and then to a −20°C freezer for another 3 days.

e. Transfer embryos to fresh methanol (−20°C) and then place in a 4°C freezer for another 3 days.

f. Subsequently, dehydrate and embed the embryos in Paraplast. The embryos should be serially sectioned at 5–10 μm, similar to the conventional paraffin embedding technique described earlier.

5. Plastic Embedding

Although there are many plastic resins useful for biological applications, we prefer Eponate 12 which is one of the replacements for the familiar Epon 812. The reader is encouraged to study the background information related to epoxy resins assembled by Rogers (1979). Epon is hardened uniformly by the addition of acid anhydrides (DDSA and NMA) and an amino accelerator (DMP 30).

For plastic embedding the tissue should be trimmed to small blocks before or after aldehyde fixation. This allows better penetration of OsO_4 postfixation which is recommended even for semithin sections. The following steps have worked quite satisfactorily in our laboratory (adapted from Pease, 1964).

   a. Aldehyde fix (2% paraformaldehyde, 2% glutaraldehyde in 0.1 M phosphate buffer at pH 7.4) for overnight or less.
   b. Rinse in 0.1 M PO_4 buffer (3–5 min).
   c. Postfix in 1–2% OsO_4 in 0.1 M PO_4 buffer for 1 hr.
   d. Rinse in buffer (3–5 min).
   e. Rinse once in distilled H_2O briefly.
   f. Use a platform shaker or rotator and dehydrate in ethanol:

   50%—3 to 5 min
   75%—3 to 5 min
   95%—3 to 5 min
   100%—5 to 10 min
   100%—5 to 10 min
   100%—15 to 20 min

   g. Transitional solvent, propylene oxide; two changes of 10–15 min. Drain off solvent and cover tissue with 1–2 ml of fresh solvent
   h. Resin application (mixture follows):
      1. Add resin in such an amount so that the bath will be quite fluid.
      2. Shake for 5–10 min, stir often with toothpick until bath seems homogeneous, and put on automatic shaker for 20–30 min.
      3. Double resin concentration to a point that the mixture becomes syrupy, again use toothpick to mix layers, and shake for 30–45 min.
      4. Expose blocks to the undiluted plastic mixture.
      5. Drain upside down on a paper towel.
      6. Add the undiluted mixture to a depth of 1–2 mm; stir with a toothpick.
      7. Leave blocks exposed for 1 hr with two to three stirrings.
      8. Transfer to embedding mold with fresh solution.
   i. Heat polymerization at 60°C for 2.5 days to harden. Two nights and a day seem desirable for heat polymerization. Sectioning seems to improve with standing at room temperature for days or even weeks.

Stock Resin Mixtures:

    Mixture A: 62 ml Eponate and 100 ml DDSA

    Mixture B: 100 ml Eponate and 89 ml NMA

Mixtures are stable and can be kept for many months in a refrigerator. Ordinarily they are blended and the accelerator is added just before use. We use a 1:1 mixture for soft tissue. DMP-30 is added in proportion of 1.5–2% and must be stirred in thoroughly.

E. Staining Procedures

1. Hematoxylin and Eosin Stain

This procedure is recommended as a prestain[1] for autoradiographs but can be used for routine procedures as well. Nuclei stain blue and cytoplasm stain pink. Gill's #3 ready-for-use hematoxylin can be obtained from Polysciences. Note that eosin Y is usually dissolved in a 70% ethanol solution even though it is dissolved here in water (less satisfactory).

    Histosol or xylene, 1–5 min

    Histosol or xylene, 2–3 min

    Absolute alcohol, 1–5 min

    Absolute alcohol, 2–3 min

    95% alcohol, 1–5 min

    80% alcohol, 1–5 min

    70% alcohol, 1–5 min

    Wash in distilled water (dip a few times)

    Gill's #3 hematoxylin, 3 min

    Wash in tap water, 5 min (running water)

    Wash in distilled water, two changes (dip in and out)

    Eosin–water (5 g Eosin in 1000 ml distilled water), 5 min

    Wash in distilled water, two changes for a total of 5 min

    Air dry slides completely or dehydrate and coverslip if not used for autoradiographs.

2. Toluidine Blue O Stain (for Plastic Sections)

Toluidine blue is a basic dye stain that can be applied to paraffin tissue sections but is now most widely used as a simple stain for semithin plastic sections. It

---

[1] Hematoxylin can also be used as a poststain for autoradiographs. Freshly developed slides are placed directly in the stain while still wet for 2–3 min, differentiated for 1 hr in running tap water, counterstained with eosin (if desired) for four to five dips, and then quickly dehydrated and coverslipped. The emulsion coat on the back of the slides is best removed with a razor blade during the water wash after hematoxylin staining.

provides various intensities of blue or blue-purple staining that distinguishes nuclei and cytoplasm very clearly in chick embryonic tissue. Toluidine blue is notorious for causing "fogging" in prestained autoradiographs, but this can be prevented by applying a carbon layer prior to coating with emulsion (Sechrist and Upson, 1974).

To stain, flood the sections on a warm to hot slide (on a hot plate) with 0.5% toluidine blue in 1% sodium borate (filter before use). After 15–20 sec, the stain, which may have begun to bubble or evaporate, is gently washed with a stream of distilled water and air dried. The slides can be coverslipped with an aqueous mounting medium or simply apply a drop of immersion oil to selected sections for high magnification pictures with excellent resolution (as shown in Fig. 2).

Note: Plastic sections can be deplasticized and stained with hematoxylin and eosin, but in our opinion it is not much better than toluidine blue for chick tissue. The extra effort is unnecessary.

3. Bisbenzimide

The Hoechst 33258 stain (Sigma) is DNA specific and much simpler than the classic Feulgen method. For paraffin sections, either 4% paraformaldehyde/PBS or Carnoy's solutions are good for fixation. Rehydrate sections to water and wash in PBS. The stain is 1 mg/ml in PBS and is applied for 15 min only. Following extensive rinsing in PBS, slides can be cover slipped in Gel-mount (Biomeda). A Hoechst stock solution of 10 mg/ml can be made up in distilled water and stored at 4°C for months.

A fluorescent microscope equipped with the appropriate filter (360 nm excitation, 470 nm emission) is required for viewing. Investigators without access to a fluorescent microscope may resort to the Feulgen method (as shown in Fig. 1E) to visualize DNA and to localize mitotic figures.

F. Antibody Labeling on Sectioned Material

1. Fix embryos in desired fixative and section on cryostat or microtome. If sectioned in paraffin wax, deparaffinize in two changes of histosol, followed by rehydration in 100, 100, 95, 70, and 30% ethanol for 1 min each. Wash slides in 0.1 *M* phosphate buffer.

2. Incubate with the primary antibody for 2 hr or overnight at room temperature or at 4°C, using the appropriate dilution for antibody (e.g., 1:400 for anti NF-M in 0.1% BSA in PBS; Lee *et al.,* 1987). Lay slides flat in a plastic container. In the case of hybridoma supernatants, no dilution is necessary.

3. Rinse in 0.1 *M* phosphate buffer for 10 min (two changes).

4. Incubate with a FITC- or TRITC-conjugated secondary for 1 hr at room temperature. (For HNK-1, use TRITC-goat anti-mouse IgM; for NF-M use Hi-FITC goat anti-mouse IgG.)

5. Rinse in phosphate buffer for 10 min.

6. Coverslip in an aqueous mount and view on a fluorescent microscope.

G. Preparation of Emulsion-Coated Autoradiographs

The following protocol is a modification of that formerly used in the Langman laboratory [courtesy of Dr. J. McConnell; see also Kopriwa and Leblond (1962) and Rogers (1979)].

1. Paraffin Sections

Most fixation solutions are suitable for autoradiographs except those containing salts of heavy metals. Tissue sections, cut from paraffin blocks, are floated on a standard water bath (40°F) to which 20 drops of gelatin have been added (stock solution: 5% gelatin and a crystal of thymol). Gelatin is a more reliable adhesive than albumin. The sections are then picked up from the water bath with a clean microslide and dried overnight. Slides bearing sections are routinely prestained with H&E.

2. Plastic Sections

Tissue fixed in an aldehyde (paraformaldehyde/glutaraldehyde) mixture and postfixed in osmium tetroxide is embedded in Eponate or methacrylate. Sections are cut at less than 1 μm and are mounted on previously dried gelatin-coated slides or Superfrost precoated slides (Fisher and Fedoroff, 1978). Plastic sections are routinely dipped unstained. Toluidine blue, the most common stain for plastic sections, chemically exposes the photographic emulsion. It therefore cannot be used as a prestain unless the stained sections are coated with a 1% colloidin solution or a carbon layer (Sechrist and Upson, 1974) to prevent direct contact with the emulsion.

3. Dipping Slides

The slides that are ready for autoradiography should be placed in black plastic slide boxes. Some boxes now contain a slide rack for developing which is very convenient (25 slide capacity, Clay Adams Inc., New York). The boxes should be numbered on the outside for reference. A white index card is made out on which all information regarding dipping and developing should be recorded.

The photographic emulsion, (Nuclear Track Emulsion, type NTB-2 or NTB-3, Eastman Kodak Co., Rochester, NY) is immediately placed in a refrigerator at 4°C with the date of arrival marked on the box. As soon as possible, one or two test slides are dipped to determine the amount of background fog. A blank slide is used for this and the emulsion is put back in its box and placed in the refrigerator. **Never,** at any time, should the emulsion be exposed to light. The test slides are developed the following day. The slides are allowed to dry after the rinses in distilled water. Examine the slides under the microscope (oil immersion lens) to check for background fog.

The cardboard box containing the bottle of bulk emulsion is removed from the refrigerator (4°C) and is allowed to come to room temperature. Meanwhile, plastic slide-drying racks and paper tissues are arranged within easy reach of the water bath used to melt the emulsion.

The following steps common to paraffin and plastic sections must be carried out 3 feet or more from a Wratten Safelight #2 in a completely light-tight room. The room for dipping is kept at 25°C (78°F), humidity 80%, to reduce the amount of static electricity.

The bottle with emulsion is removed from the original box and is placed in the water (40°C) for 15–30 min to melt. The water bath has a flat plastic cover in which two holes are cut to accommodate (1) the stock bottle of emulsion and (2) a Coplin jar or other special container for dipping. After the emulsion has melted, pour enough into a Coplin jar to cover three-fourths of a slide and try to maintain this level. Keep the stock bottle of emulsion in the water bath during the procedure so that it can be added to the Coplin jar to maintain the desired level of emulsion. If desired, the emulsion may be diluted 1:1 with distilled water. This does not increase the exposure time. A clean slide is dipped to determine whether the emulsion is now free of air bubbles which, if present, will produce artifacts in the emulsion coat. If air bubbles should be present, the emulsion is left at least 20 min more and is tested again in the same manner.

The slides, held at the label end, are then taken in order from the black plastic box and are dipped in the liquid emulsion for 1–2 sec. The excess is allowed to drain into the tissue paper. The slides are then placed in order on the plastic drying rack and are allowed to dry in a vertical position for 40–50 min. In the dark they are then put back in the black plastic slide box in the order described on the index card, leaving room for a small package of silica gel to absorb moisture. The box is sealed with black electrical tape (two times around) and stored in the refrigerator at 4°C for exposure. The emulsion in the stock bottle is placed back in its box and kept in the refrigerator at 4°C for future use. NOTE: Do not use emulsion for longer than 3–4 months.

4. Developing Slides

The black plastic slide box is removed from the refrigerator and is allowed to come to darkroom temperature 18°C (70°F). The developer and fixer, which are stored at room temperature in the developing room, are prepared and poured into dishes large enough to hold the metal slide baskets. Distilled water for rinses is also set out in dishes and should be at room temperature as well as the other solutions. After turning off the lights, the slides are taken from the black slide box in their own rack or are arranged in a metal slide basket. The following schedule is used for developing slides to be coverslipped:

Place the slide basket in the dish containing full-strength developer, D-19, for
   5 min with 30 sec agitation
Two rinse waters (distilled)—dip in each
Place in rapid fix for 5 min
Wash for 20–30 min
70% alcohol—5 min
80% alcohol—5 min
95% alcohol—5 min
100% alcohol—two changes (1:1)—10 min
Cedar oil—100% alcohol (1:1)—10 min
Xylene–Permount (1:1)—10 min
Permount—10–20 min

Drain and coverslip slides. Wipe off excess Permount with xylene. Dry overnight in an oven at 38°C and clean with xylene or histosol.

NOTE: Slides bearing unstained thin plastic sections should not be taken
through the alcohols, but are allowed to dry after the washes in distilled water.
These slides are then ready for poststaining with toluidine blue. If prestained,
they can be observed without a coverslip and photographed with intervening
oil immersion.

Acknowledgments

We thank Dr. Marianne Bronner-Fraser for her encouragement and helpful comments on the
manuscript. Drs. Kristin Artinger and Mark Selleck helped assemble several of the methods presented
in Section V. Their contributions are appreciated. We also thank Cell Press for granting permission
to use Fig. 2B-D, F; 3I; and 5D,E which were first published in *Neuron* **7**, 947–963 (1991).

References

Alberts, B., Bray, D., Lewis, J., Raff, M., Roberts, K., and Watson, J. D. (1994). "Molecular Biology
   of the Cell," 3rd Ed. Garland Publishing, New York.
Balls, M., and Billet, F. (1973). "The Cell Cycle in Development and Differentiation." Cambridge
   University Press, London.
Bannigan, J., Langman, J., and van Breda, A. (1981). The uptake of 5-bromodeoxyuridine by the
   chicken embryo and its effects upon growth. *Anat. Embryol.* **162**, 425–434.
Bennett, G., and DiLullo, C. (1985). Transient expression of a neurofilament protein by replicating
   neuroepithelial cells of the embryonic chick brain. *Dev. Biol.* **107**, 107–127.
Boswald, M., Harasim, S., and Mauer-Schultze, B. (1990). Tracer dose and availability time of
   thymidine and bromodeoxyuridine: Application of bromodeoxyuridine in cell kinetic studies. *Cell
   Tissue Kinet.* **23**, 169–181.
Boulder Committee (1970). Embryonic vertebrate central nervous system: Revised terminology.
   Anat. Rec. **166**, 257–262.
Bronner-Fraser, M., and Fraser, S. (1989). Developmental potential of avian trunk neural crest cells
   in situ. *Neuron* **3**, 755–766.

Cajal, S., and Ramon, y. (1960). "Studies on Vertebrate Neurogenesis." Charles C. Thomas, Springfield. [English translation by L. Guth]

Christ, B., and Ordahl, C. (1995). Early stages of chick somite development. *Anat. Embryol.* **191**, 381–396.

Cowdry, E. (1914). The development of the cytoplasmic constituents of the nerve cells of the chick. *Am. J. Anat.* **15**, 389–429.

Dupin, E. (1984). Cell division in the ciliary ganglion of quail embryos *in situ* and after back-transplantation into the neural crest migration pathways of chick embryos. *Dev. Biol.* **105**, 288–289.

Fisher, K., and Fedoroff, S. (1978). The development of chick spinal cord in tissue culture. II. Cultures of whole chick embryos. *In Vitro* **14**, 878–886.

Fujita, S. (1962). Kinetics of cellular proliferation. *Exp. Cell Res.* **28**, 52–60.

Fujita, S. (1963). The matrix cell and cytogenesis in the developing central nervous system. *J. Comp. Neurol.* **120**, 37–42.

Gratzner, H. (1982). Monoclonal antibody to 5-bromo- and 5-iododeoxyuridine: A new reagent for detection of DNA replication. *Science* **218**, 474–475.

Gray, J., and Mayall, B. (1985). "Monoclonal Antibodies against Bromodeoxyuridine." A. R. Liss, New York.

Hamburger, V., and Hamilton, H. (1951). A series of normal stages in the development of the chick embryo. *J. Morphol.* **88**, 49–92.

Hayat, M. A. (1989). "Principles and Techniques of Electron Microscopy: Biological Applications," 3rd Ed. CRC Press, Boca Raton, FL.

Henrique, D., Adam, J., Myat, M., Chitnis, A., Lewis, J., and Ish-Horowicz, D. (1995). Expression of a *Delta* homologue in prospective neurons in the chick. *Nature* **375**, 787–790.

Holmes, W. (1943). Silver staining of nerve axons in paraffin sections. *Anat. Rec.* **86**, 157–187.

Holtzer, H., Rubinstein, N., Fellini, S., Yeoh, G., Chi, J., Birnbaum, J., and Okayama, M. (1975). Lineages, quantal cell cycles and the generation of cell density. *Quart. Rev. Biophys.* **8**, 523–557.

Humason, G. L. (1979). "Animal Tissue Techniques," 4th Ed. Freeman, San Francisco.

Kaehn, K., Jacob, H., Christ, B., Hinrichsen, K., and Poelmann, R. (1988). The onset of myotome formation in the chick. *Anat. Embryol.* **177**, 191–201.

Kopriwa, B., and LeBlond, C. (1962). Improvements in the coating technique of radioautography. *J. Histochem. Cytochem.* **10**, 269–284.

Langman, J., Guerrant, R., and Freeman, B. (1966). Behavior of neuro-epithelial cells during closure of the neural tube. *J. Comp. Neurol.* **127**, 399–412.

Langman, J., and Haden, C. (1970). Formation and migration of neuroblasts in the spinal cord of the chick embryo. *J. Comp. Neurol.* **138**, 419–432.

Langman, J., and Nelson, G. (1968). A radioautographic study of the development of the somite in the chick embryo. *J. Embryol. Exp. Morph.* **19**, 217–226.

Layer, P. G., and Sporns, O. (1987). Spatiotemporal relationship of embryonic cholinesterases with cell proliferation in chicken brain and eye. *Proc. Natl. Acad. Sci. USA* **84**, 284–288.

Lee, H., Deshpande, A., and Kalmus, G. (1974). Studies on effects of 5-bromodeoxyuridine on the development of explanted early chick embryos. *J. Embryol. Exp. Morph.* **32**, 835–848.

Lee, V., Carden, M., Schlaepfer, W., and Trojanowski, J. (1987). Monoclonal antibodies distinguish several differentially phophorylated states of the two largest rat neurofilament subunits (NF-H and NF-M) and demonstrate their existence in the normal nervous system of adult rats. *J. Neurosci.* **7**, 3474–3489.

Marcelle, C., Eichmann, A., Halevy, O., Bréant, C., and Le Douarin N. (1994). Distinct developmental expression of a new avian fibroblast growth factor receptor. *Development* **120**, 683–694.

Marcelle, C., Wolf, J., and Bronner-Fraser, M. (1995). The *in vivo* expression of the FGF receptor FREK mRNA in avian myoblasts suggests a role in muscle growth and differentiation. *Dev. Biol.* **172**, 100–114.

Martin, A., and Langman, J. (1965). The development of the spinal cord examined by autoradiography. *J. Embryol. Exp. Morphol.* **14**, 25–35.

McConnell, J., and Sechrist, J. (1980). Identification of early neurons in the brainstem and spinal cord. I. An autoradiographic study in the chick. *J. Comp. Neurol.* **192,** 769–783.

Okazaki, K., and Holtzer, H. (1966). Myogenesis: Fusion, myosin synthesis, and the mitotic cycle. *Proc. Natl. Acad. Sci. USA* **56,** 1484–1490.

Pease, D. C. (1964). "Histological Techniques for Electron Microscopy," Academic Press, N.Y.

Pownall, M., and Emerson, C. (1992). Molecular and embryological studies of avian embryogenesis. *Sem. Dev. Biol.* **3,** 229–241.

Rogers, A. (1979). "Techniques of Autoradiography." Elsevier/North-Holland Biomedical Press, Amsterdam.

Rohrer, H., and Thoenen, H. (1987). Relationship between differentiation and terminal mitosis: Chick sensory and ciliary neurons differentiate after terminal mitosis of precursor cells, whereas sympathetic neurons continue to divide after differentiation. *J. Neurosci.* **7,** 3739–3748.

Rothman, T., Gershon, M., and Holzter, H. (1978). The relationship of cell division to the acquisition of adrenergic characteristics by developing sympathetic ganglion cell precursors. *Dev. Biol.* **65,** 322–341.

Sauer, M. E., and Walker, B. E. (1959). Radioautographic studies of interkinetic nuclear migration in the nedural tube. *Proc. Soc. Exp. Biol. Med.* **101,** 557–560.

Sechrist, J. (1968). "Initial Cytodifferentiation of Neuroblasts." Doctoral Thesis, University of Illinois at the Medical Center, Chicago, IL.

Sechrist, J. (1969). Neurocytogenesis. I. Neurofibrils, neurofilaments, and the terminal mitotic cycle. *Am. J. Anat.* **124,** 117–134.

Sechrist, J., and Bronner-Fraser, M. (1991). Birth and differentiation of reticular neurons in the chick hindbrain: Ontogeny of the first neuronal population. *Neuron* **7,** 947–963.

Sechrist, J., and Upson, R. (1974). Prevention of chemography in prestained epoxy autoradiographs by an intervening carbon film. *Stain Technol.* **49,** 297–300.

Sidman, R. (1970). Autoradiographic methods and principles for study of the nervous system with thymidine-H^3. *In* "Contemporary Research Methods in Neuroanatomy" (W. Nauta and S. Ebbesson, eds.), pp. 252–274. Springer-Verlag, New York.

Stern, C. (1993). Transplantation in avian embryos. *In* "Essential Developmental Biology: A Practical Approach" (C. D. Stern and P. W. H. Holland, eds.), pp. 111–117. Oxford University Press, London.

Strähle, U., Blader, P., Adam, J., and Ingham, P. (1994). A simple and efficient procedure for nonisotopic in situ hybridization to sectioned material. *TIG* **10,** 74–75.

Tapscott, S. J., Bennett, G. S., and Holtzer, R. (1981). Neuronal precursor cells in the chick neural tube express neurofilament proteins. *Nature* **292,** 836–838.

Tapscott, S., Davis, R., Thayer, M., Cheng, P., Weintraub, H., and Lassar, A. (1988). MyoD1: A nuclear phosphoprotein requiring a Myc homology region to convert fibroblasts to myoblasts. *Science* **242,** 405–411.

Tapscott, S., Lassar, A., Davis, R., and Weintraub, H. (1989). 5-Bromo-2'-deoxyuridine blocks myogenesis by extinguishing expression of MyoD1. *Science* **245,** 532–536.

Wachtler, F., and Christ, B. (1992). The basic embryology of skeletal formation in vertebrates: The avian model. *Sem. Dev. Biol.* **3,** 217–227.

Watson, M. (1958). Staining of tissue sections for electron microscopy with heavy metals. *J. Biophys. Biochem. Cytol.* **4,** 475–478.

Weintraub, H., Davis, R., Tapscott, S., Thayer, M., Krause, M., Benezra, R., Blackwell, T., Turner, D., Rupp, R., Hollenberg, S., *et al.* (1991). The myoD gene family: Nodal point during specification of the muscle cell lineage. *Science* **251,** 761–766.

Wilt, F., and Anderson, M. (1972). The action of 5-bromodeoxyuridine on differentiation. *Dev. Biol.* **28,** 443–447.

Wright, W. (1992). Muscle basic helix-loop-helix proteins and the regulation of myogenesis. *Curr. Opin. Genet. Dev.* **2,** 243–248.

Yablonka-Reuveni, Z., and Rivera, A. (1994). Temporal expression of regulatory and structural muscle proteins during myogenesis of satellite cells on isolated adult rat fibers. *Dev. Biol.* **164,** 588–603.

CHAPTER 17

Time-Lapse Cinephotomicrography, Videography, and Videomicrography of the Avian Blastoderm

H. Bortier,★ M. Callebaut,★ and L. C. A. Vakaet†

★ Laboratory of Human Anatomy and Embryology
University Centre Antwerpen (RUCA)
2020 Antwerpen, Belgium

† Laboratory of Experimental Cancerology
University Hospital
9000 Gent, Belgium

  I. Introduction
 II. General Methods
       A. Material
       B. Instruments
       C. Procedures
III. Time-Lapse Cinephotomicrography, Videography, and Videomicrography Installation
       A. Time-Lapse Cinephotomicrography Installation
       B. Time-Lapse Videography Installation
       C. Time-Lapse Videomicrography Installation
 IV. Critical Aspects of Time-Lapse Video Registration
  V. Results and Discussion
       A. Normal Developments
       B. Experiments
 VI. Conclusions and Perspectives
     References

I. Introduction

Because development occurs slowly, developmental movements cannot be observed directly. Morphogenetic movements can be revealed by time-lapse cinephotomicrography or videography. Time-lapse cinephotomicrography or videography is now in widespread use in research and is an essential tool in the modern teaching of developmental biology (Bortier, 1991). That this technique is essential can be learned from the history of avian research. Prior to the advent of time-lapse cinephotomicrography, it was believed that no morphogenetic movements in the avian blastoderm occur before the appearance of the primitive streak. Gräper (1929) was the first to use stereocinematography in the chick blastoderm *in ovo*. This technique, combined with vital staining, allowed observation of ingression at the primitive streak. Later, De Haan (1963) described the migration of clusters of precardiac mesoderm with cinematography.

Vakaet (1967) combined the *in vitro* technique of New (1955) with time-lapse cinephotomicrography and carbon marks to study early chick morphogenetic movements. He recorded and published photographs of film sequences of normal developments, the regression of Hensen's node and shortening of the primitive streak. In addition, he observed the final placement of the definitive endoblast, and the induction of secondary neurulation and secondary primitive streaks. With time-lapse cinephotomicrography, Vakaet (1970) developed a staging from oviposition to the appearance of the headfold.

The goal of our research is to understand the mechanisms and dynamics of morphogenetic movements during gastrulation and neurulation. To this end, we have developed setups for time-lapse videography and videomicrography. Videography has superseded cinematography because sequences are copied faster, tape does not break as easy as film and does not scratch, videosequences can be observed forward and backward and as still images, and editing video sequences is less time-consuming.

II. General Methods

A. Material

For our research we used chick eggs (White Rock, from the Rijksstation voor Pluimveeteelt, Merelbeke, B-9820) and quail eggs (*Coturnix coturnix japonica*, from laboratory stock).

The shell of the egg covers the egg white and the yolk ball. The shell is composed of a calcified layer and the outer and the inner shell membranes. At the blunt edge of the egg, the outer and the inner shell membranes are split by the air chamber (Fig. 1). The inner shell membrane surrounds the thin and thick egg white. At the periphery, the thin egg white is in contact with the inner shell membrane; centrally, it contacts the outer yolk membrane, with both membranes being egg white derived. The thick egg white is a more or less closed capsule. It is transpeared at the poles of the egg by the chalazae that extend from the inner shell membrane to the outer yolk membrane. These chalazae are spun out from the egg white during the descent and rotation of the yolk ball in the uterus. The inner part of the yolk membrane corresponds to the zona pellucida in

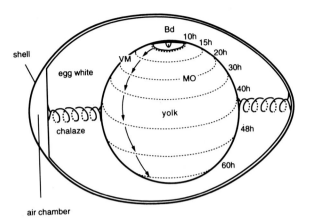

Fig. 1 Chick egg. Bd, blastoderm; MO, margin of overgrowth; VM, vitelline membrane; arrows, direction of epiboly; h, hours of incubation.

mammalian eggs. Inside it is tapered by the plasma membrane of the yolk. After oviposition the plasma membrane of the yolk extends as the subgerminal membrane under the blastoderm, separating it from the yolk ball (Fig. 2). An unincubated chick blastoderm does not adhere to the vitelline membrane or to the plasma membrane. After 5 to 10 hr of incubation the margin of overgrowth forms at the edge of the blastoderm (Fig. 3) as a ring that is six to seven cells thick that adheres to the vitelline membrane after about 10 hr of incubation. The margin of overgrowth migrates over the yolk ball during epiboly (Fig. 1). The chick margin of overgrowth also adheres to the vitelline membrane of other avian species, but it adheres only to the inner side of the vitelline membrane.

When other avian strains are used, it is necessary to check the correspondence of their development to the stages of Vakaet (1970) (V) and to the stages of Hamburger and Hamilton (1951) (HH), as development may slightly differ among species.

A chick blastoderm at stage 5V of Vakaet (1970) has an area pellucida about 2 mm long and 1.5 mm wide. The overall thickness of the area pellucida is about 0.1 mm. The vitelline membrane, the area opaca, the area pellucida, and the primitive streak are recognized by differences in translucency (see Fig. 7).

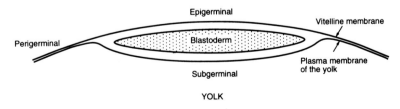

Fig. 2 Position of the avian blastoderm on the yolk.

B. Instruments

Ringer's solution: 9 g NaCl, 0.42 g Kcl, 0.24 g CaCl$_2$, aqd. 1000 ml; other saline solutions also can be used.

Culture dish; glass or plastic

Culture medium

In the original description of New (1955) the culture medium is thin egg white. For microsurgery, a semisolid medium that allows microsurgery as well as normal culturing *in vitro* up to 48 hr of incubation is preferable. We use a mixture of 25 ml thin egg white and a gel made of 150 mg Bacto-agar (Difco, Detroit, MI) in 25 ml Ringer's solution. It is possible to use more or less Bacto-agar, depending on the thickness of the egg white of the avian strain used.

Bowl (see Fig. 6)

Micosurgical instruments

For microsurgery, several instruments can be used. Some use cactus needles, others glass needles. We prefer watchmaker's tungsten needles and a Pasteur pipette with a tip bent in an angle of 135° to the shaft and with a diameter of 0.20 to 0.25 mm (Bortier and Vakaet, 1987a) (Fig. 4). It is essential that the edge of the tip be even.

Glass rings

Spoon; plastic or metal

Scissors; straight, curved, or Wecker scissors (see Fig. 6)

Sterilization

Bacterial infections are rare because of the lysozyme content of the egg white. Normal sterility precautions, cleaning of the metal instruments with ethanol, and autoclaving the glassware can be utilized to completely eliminate contamination.

Incubator for the observation of multiple cultures

In order to observe multiple experiments one after the other without having to open the incubator and thus varying the temperature, an incubator with moveable trays (Fig. 5) can be used; other incubators at 37.5–38°C are also acceptable.

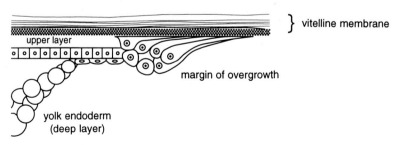

Fig. 3 Margin of overgrowth.

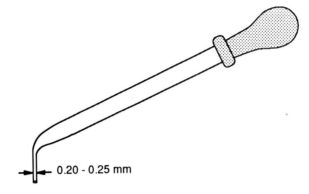

Fig. 4 Pasteur pipette with a tip diameter of 0.20–0.25 mm and a rubber bulb.

C. Procedures

1. New Culture

Open the blunt end of the egg shell with a forceps to expose the egg white and yolk ball. Discard the thick egg white and place the egg ball in a bowl with Ringer's solution. The membrane that surrounds the yolk is the vitelline membrane. In fertilized eggs the blastoderm lies directly below it as the white circular area floating on the egg yolk. The germ disk of unfertilized eggs can be recognized as a small mass of irregular whitish dots containing large oil drops visible under the stereomicroscope. Using a blunt forceps, clean the yolk ball thoroughly from the adhering thin egg white. Cleaning the egg from the egg white can be tedious depending on the avian strain. This cleaning step is critical in the New culture procedure. Avian blastoderms can easily be cultured *in vitro* because the blastoderm adheres to the vitelline membrane by the margin of overgrowth. The vitelline membrane can be incised at the equator and lifted from the yolk together with the blastoderm (Fig. 6).

After a complete circular incision of the vitelline membrane, gently peel the vitelline membrane away from the yolk with a forceps in a slow but continuous movement parallel to the yolk surface. Be careful not to interrupt the movement when the margin of overgrowth of the blastoderm is reached. When the vitelline membrane with the blastoderm is isolated, transfer the vitelline membrane to a culture dish in a spoon with saline.

The ventral side of the blastoderm should be toward the observer. If there is doubt about the side, try to remove some yolk droplets from the blastoderm with a forceps. As the ventral side of the blastoderm is the side closest to the yolk, yolk droplets adhere to this side. If the dorsal side is up, turn the vitelline membrane upside down with a forceps.

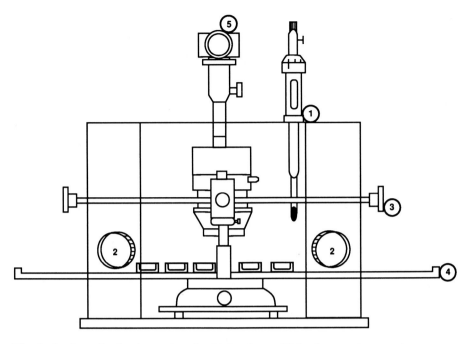

Fig. 5 Incubator for the observation of multiple cultures. (1) Incubator and contact thermometer, (2) entrances, (3) focus screw, (4) moveable Plexiglas tray with culture dishes, and (5) stereomicroscope M5 (Wild, Heerbrugg, CH-9435) with an ocular piece.

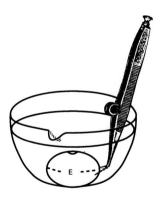

Fig. 6 Incision in the vitelline membrane. E, equator.

1. Suck away the Ringer's solution in the culture dish.
2. Place a glass ring on the vitelline membrane and center it on the blastoderm.
3. Curl the edges of the vitelline membrane until they reach over the inside of the glass ring.
4. Take the glass ring with a forceps to transfer the vitelline membrane and the blastoderm into a culture dish with culture medium. The result should be as shown in Fig. 7.

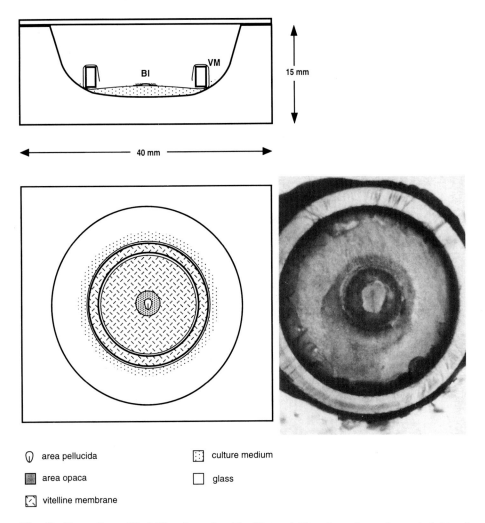

area pellucida   culture medium

area opaca   glass

vitelline membrane

Fig. 7 New culture. (Top) View from the side. (Bottom) View from above; the ventral side of the blastoderm is up, toward the observer. (Right) A chick blastoderm in New culture. Bl, blastoderm; VM, vitelline membrane.

338   H. Bortier *et al.*

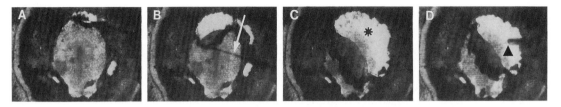

Fig. 8 The aspiration-punching procedure. The ventral side of the blastoderm faces the observer, the cranial is up. (A) Loosening of the deep layer at the endophyll wall with a tungsten needle. (B) Reclining the deep layer with a tungsten needle (arrow). (C) Bare upper layer in the proamnion (asterisk). (D) Aspiration punching of a wound in the bare upper layer with a Pasteur pipette (arrowhead).

2. Microsurgery

We developed a technique for experimental excision wounding, and xenografting in the upper layer of the chick blastoderm (Bortier and Vakaet, 1987a,b) using the Pasteur pipette described in Fig. 4. It should be closed with a soft rubber bulb. To reach the upper layer directly, incise the yolk

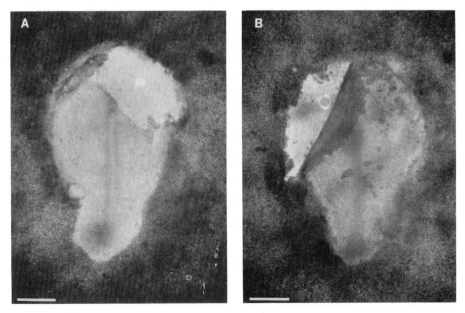

Fig. 9 Results of the aspiration-punching procedure. (A) Excision wound in the bare chick upper layer (indicated by arrow). (B) Isochronic, isotopic, and isotropic quail xenograft in the chick upper layer. Bar: 500 μm.

endoderm at the cranial periphery of the area pellucida and recline the deep layer with a microsurgical needle (Fig. 8). Partially fill a Pasteur pipette with Ringer's solution. Approach the bare upper layer with the pipette while gently squeezing the rubber bulb to release one drop of Ringer's solution. Simultaneously, press the pipette against the upper layer and gently release the rubber bulb and suck out a fragment of the upper layer. The result should be as illustrated in Fig. 9A.

For xenografting, recline the deep layer of a quail blastoderm with a microsurgical needle and repeat the aspiration punch procedure on the upper layer described earlier. Then, gently release the quail graft from the pipette over the wound in the host upper layer (Fig. 9B). To prevent the graft from floating away, suck dry with a filter paper and reposition the deep layer. In xenografting experiments the grafts can be isochronically (at a similar stage), isotopically (in a similar region), and isotropically (in the same dorsoventral polarity) or heterochronically, heterotopically, and heterotropically, in any combination.

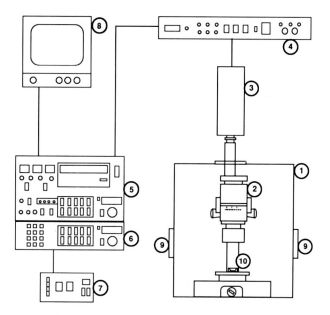

Fig. 10 Time-lapse videography installation. (1) Incubator, (2) Wild M8 stereomicroscope, (3) WV-1850 camera (Panasonic, Osaka, Japan), (4) time–date generator WJ-810 (Panasonic, Osaka, Japan), (5) U-matic video recorder VO-5850P (Sony, Tokyo, Japan), (6) animation control unit EOS AC580 (Electronics, Barry, South Glamorgan), (7) interval timer (Vel, Leuven, B-3030), (8) WV-5340 monitor (Panasonic, Osaka, Japan), (9) entrances, and (10) culture dish.

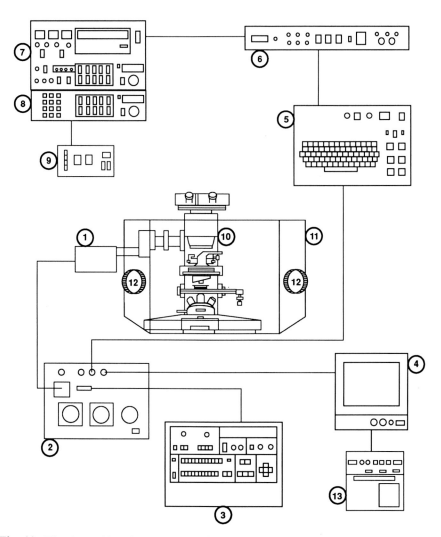

Fig. 11 Time-lapse videomicrography installation. (1) Camera C-1966-01 (Hamamatsu, Phototonics, Hamamatsu-City, Japan), (2) image processor (Hamamatsu, Phototonics, Hamamatsu-City, Ja-
pan), (3) contrast adjustment (Hamamatsu, Phototonics, Hamamatsu-City, Japan), (4) TV monitor
(Hamamatsu, Phototonics, Hamamatsu-City, Japan), (5) video typewriter VTW-210 FOR.A (Japan),
(6) time–date generator WJ-810 (Panasonic, Osaka, Japan), (7) U-matic video recorder VO-5850P
(Sony, Tokyo, Japan), (8) animation control unit EOS AC580 (EOS Electronics A.V., Barry, South
Glamorgan), (9) interval timer (VEL, Leuven, B-3030), (10) inverted microscope (Fluovert, Leitz,
Wetzlar, BRD), (11) incubator, (12) entrances, and (13) video graphic printer UP-811 (Sony,
Tokyo, Japan).

III. Time–Lapse Cinephotomicrography, Videography, and Videomicrography Installation

A. Time–Lapse Cinephotomicrography Installation

Refer to the description and illustrations of Vakaet (1970).

B. Time–Lapse Videography Installation

For time-lapse videomicrography (Bortier and Vakaet, 1987b, 1992b; Bortier, 1991). (Fig. 10), we used M8 stereomicroscope (Wild, Heerbrugg, CH-9435), on top of which a WV-1850 camera (Panasonic, Osaka, Japan) was mounted in a Plexiglas incubator at $38 \pm 1°C$. The camera was linked to a U-matic video recorder VO-5850P (Sony, Tokyo, Japan) through an animation control unit EOS AC580 (EOS Electronics A. V., Barry, South Glamorgan). A time–date generator WJ-810 (Panasonic, Osaka Japan) displays the chronological information on a WV-5340 monitor (Panasonic, Osaka, Japan). One video image was recorded every 30 sec, yielding an acceleration of $750\times$ at normal projection speed (25 images/sec). Other types of microscopes, cameras, monitors, video recorders, and time date generators can be used.

C. Time–Lapse Videomicrography Installation

For time-lapse videomicrography (Bortier and Vakaet, 1989; Bortier *et al.*, 1993), we used an inverted microscope (Fluovert, Leitz, Wetzler, BRD) with Nomarski optics (obj. NPL Fluotar L 40/0.60) (Fig. 11). An AVEC (Allen's video enhanced contrast)/VIM (video intensified microscope) system C-1966-01 (Hamamatsu Phototonics, Hamamatsu-City, Japan) was linked to a U-matic video recorder VO-5850P (Sony, Tokyo, Japan) in an incubator at $38 \pm 1°C$. One video image was recorded every 18 sec, yielding an acceleration of $325\times$ in projection. Other types of microscopes, cameras, video recorders, and monitors can also be used.

Data from the time-lapse recording experiments were registered on the video-cassette using a video typewriter VTW-210 (FOR. A, Japan). Still images were

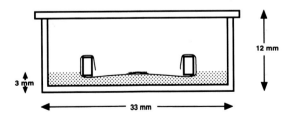

Fig. 12 Culture dish for time-lapse videomicrography.

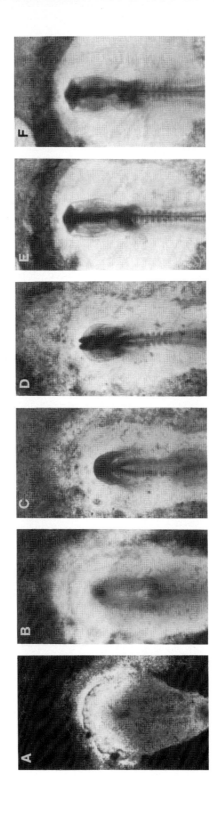

photographed from the video screen with a Leicaflex SL (Leitz, Wetzler, BRD) (obj. Makro-Elmarit 1:2.8/50) on Technical Pan film 15 din (Kodak). Exposure was at least 1 sec. After video recording, the images can be transferred to a computer with image processing capabilities.

IV. Critical Aspects of Time-Lapse Video Registration

The heat transmitted by the lamp of the microscope can cause two unwanted effects: (a) drying of the blastoderm and (b) damping of the glass or plastic lid of the culture dish. To prevent the first effect from occurring:

1. Be sure there is enough saline solution in the glass ring around the blastoderm, without drowning it.
2. Close the culture dish completely with hot paraffin if the culture dish is a glass dish that is reusable. Use silicone glue when disposable plastic dishes are used.

To prevent the second effect from occurring:

1. Use a heat filter to reduce the temperature gradient or place an open, transparent well filled with distilled water, close to the culture.
2. If reducing the temperature gradient does not prevent dampness, apply a thin layer of glycerin on the inside of the lid.

The culture dish used for time-lapse videography has a thick and irregular bottom (Fig. 7). For time-lapse videomicrography, the height of the culture dish will probably have to be adapted. Use a culture dish with a thin flat bottom and a thin layer of culture medium to reduce the distance from the blastoderm to the front lens of the objective (Fig. 12).

V. Results and Discussion

A. Normal Developments

In the following description of normal avian development *in vitro,* the stages are according to Vakaet (1970) (V) and Vakaet and Bortier (1995). The staging

---

Fig. 13 Development of a chick blastoderm in New culture with time-lapse videography. (A) Stage 7V, the cranial half of the primitive streak starts to regress toward the caudal part of the area pellucida. (B) Stage 8/9V, the head process is visible and the progression of the middle layer is apparent. Neurulation becomes visible with the formation of the neural plate; the neural plate can be recognized as the dark areas cranial to the primitive streak. (C) Stage 6 HH, closure of the neural lips at the mesencephalic region, first somites. (D) Stage 7 HH, closure of the neuroporus anterior, six somites. (E) Stage 9 HH, optic cups, heart formation, progression of the anterior intestinal portal. (F) Stage 10 HH, the neural crest is visible through the skin of the head.

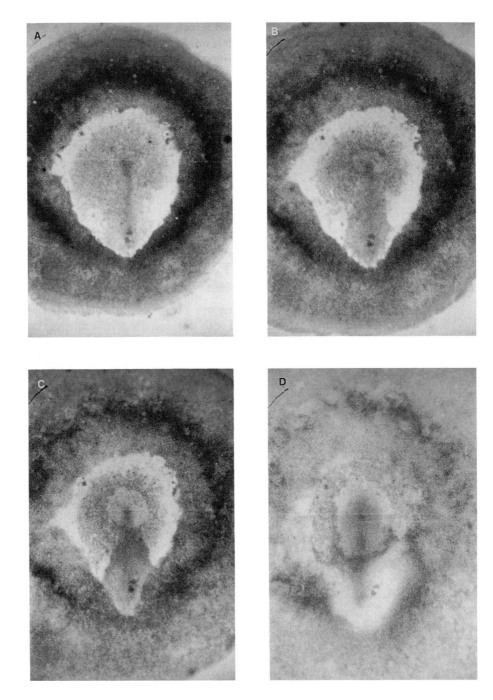

system of Hamburger and Hamilton (1951) is adequate for older stages, but there is a gap of about 12 hr between stages 3HH and 4HH. In that period, Vakaet distinguishes stages 4V, 5V, and 6V; stage 7V corresponds to stage 4HH.

In unincubated freshly laid blastoderms the difference between the darker area opaca and the more transparent area pellucida is obvious. During development, most extraembryonic structures are derived from the area opaca. All intraembryonic structures are derived from the area pellucida. Between stages 0V and 1V, the diameter of the blastoderm shrinks about 10% (personal video observations). At stage 1V polonaise movements (Gräper, 1929) occur, marking the area where the primitive streak will develop. The primitive streak at stage 2V appears as a slender dark rod at the future caudal part of the area pellucida. After an hour or two it extends cranially as a pyramid-shaped structure and is called stage 3V. At the end of stage 4V the primitive streak first becomes grooved at the tip of the primitive streak. Whereas the grooving proceeds caudally, the primitive streak grows cranially. At the end of stage 5V the primitive streak is fully grooved. From stage 6V onward, the most cranial part of the primitive streak is called Hensen's node. At stage 7V the cranial half of the primitive streak starts to regress toward the caudal part of the area pellucida (Fig. 13A). At stage 8V the head process is visible and the progression of the middle layer is apparent (Fig. 13B). The headfold appears at stage 9V as a crescent-shaped fold at the cranial end of the area pellucida. The headfold contributes to the anterior intestinal portal.

Neurulation becomes apparent with the formation of the neural plate, which can be recognized as the darker areas cranial to the primitive streak (Fig. 13B). The edges of the neural plate fold to form the neural lips that fuse to form the neural tube. Fusion of the neural lips is first observed at the future mesencephalic region (Fig. 13C). The fusion extends cranially and caudally. At the cranial end of the neural tube, closure of the anterior neuropore is evident (Fig. 13D). Whereas neurulation progresses at the cranial part of the embryo, the caudal part of the embryo is still gastrulating. The development of the somites, the optic cups, and the formation of the heart can be visualized (Figs. 13D and 13E).

B. Experiments

Time-lapse cinephotomicrography, videography, and videomicrography make it possible to visualize phenomena that cannot be made by classic microscopic observations and histology.

Fig. 14 Final placement of the definitive endoblast recorded with time-lapse cinephotomicrography (Vakaet, 1967). (A) The ventral side of a stage 5V blastoderm is toward the observer, the cranial is up, and the deep layer is removed. Time intervals after reincubation are (B) 1 hr 40 min, (C) 3 hr 20 min, and (D) 6 hr 40 min. (B and C) The definitive endoblast area is seen as more translucent around Hensen's node; a small layer of yolk is pushed away by the definitive endoblast during its final placement.

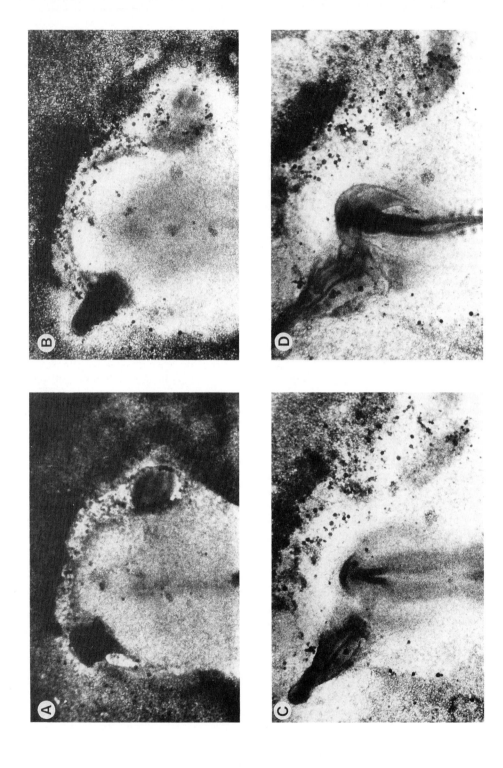

1. Formation of the Definitive Endoblast

In a stage 5V blastoderm the deep layer was totally discarded. Time-lapse cinephotomicrography demonstrates the final placement of the definitive endoblast by ingression through the primitive streak (Fig. 14).

2. Experimental Inductions

Induction means the development of a structure in an area where it normally would not develop. Time-lapse cinephotomicrography and videography visualize the induction of secondary neural plates and the induction of secondary primitive streaks in the upper layer of the proamnion (Vakaet, 1981; Bortier and Vakaet, 1991, 1995). Both types of experiments demonstrate that the upper layer of the proamnion can form either a neural plate or a primitive streak, while it normally forms skin of the head or neck. Induction thus appears to be a choice among morphogenetic potencies.

Insertion of a stage 6V quail Hensen's node in the endophyllic crescent of a stage 6V chick blastoderm induces secondary neurulation in the upper layer of the host. With time-lapse cinephotomicrography (Fig. 15), the autonomous regression of Hensen's node is seen after 5 hr and neurulation is obvious after 8 hr.

The insertion of a stage 4V quail posterior node in the endophyllic crescent of a stage 5V chick blastoderm induces a secondary primitive streak in the upper layer of the hsot. With time-lapse cinephotomicrography the graft is initially seen to disappear. Without time-lapse cinematography this experiment might have been discarded after 24 hr for absence of a reaction. Indeed, after 5 hr of incubation a more transparent area around the site of the graft is seen (Fig. 16B). After 8 hr a secondary primitive streak appears in the area (Fig. 16C). The secondary primitive streak appears to recruit presumptive neural plate cells from the neural lip of the host to become cells that ingress through the secondary primitive streak.

3. Movements of Xenografts

Time-lapse videography was used to follow the movements of quail xenografts in the chick upper layer (Bortier and Vakaet, 1987b, 1992a,b). The quail grafts

---

Fig. 15 Experimental induction of a secondary neurulation (stage 6V quail Hensen's node in the endophyllic crescent of a chick host stage 6V) recorded with time-lapse cinephotomicrography (Vakaet, 1967). A stage 6V quail Hensen's node inserted in the endophyllic crescent of a stage 6V chick host (left). A stage 6V quail midpiece primitive streak inserted in the endophyllic crescent has not developed (right). (A) At the start of the culture, the ventral side of the stage 6V blastoderm is toward the observer and the cranial is up. Time intervals after reincubation are (B) 5 hr, (C) 8 hr 20 min, and (D) 11 hr 40 min. (B) Autonomous regression of Hensen's node. (C) Neurulation is obvious. (D) The secondary neural tissue influences the neural tissue of the host.

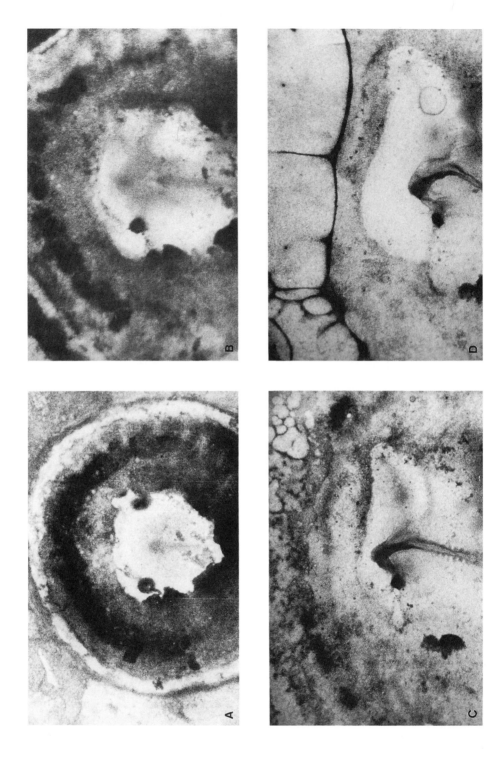

are visible because the quail cells contain less yolk than the chick cells and stay together so that they appear as a more transparent patch in the chick upper layer. The movements of the quail grafts can be followed as long as they move in the upper layer. After ingression, grafts can be followed only vaguely for an hour or two.

The advantages of using time-lapse videography to follow the morhogenetic movements of the xenografts are gain of time and precision. Time-lapse videography indeed allows one to observe movements directly. Moreover, one single xenograft experiment followed with time-lapse videography represents innumerable xenografting experiments on every point of the track of the graft. Without time-lapse videography, only the histological result of a single xenograft experiment in one particular area of the upper layer at a certain time can be demonstrated. With time-lapse videography, all the areas and stages of the blastoderm are covered in one experiment. It is possible to see quail grafts becoming part of the neural tube of the host, extending into the epiblast or ingressing through the primitive streak. Some grafts appear to be incorporated in two areas: becoming part neural tissue or ingressing through the primitive streak. Such observations are crucial for reconstructing early fate maps.

The grafts in the neural plate narrow laterolaterally during gastrulation and extend craniocaudally during neurulation. This convergence–extension is visible directly within one graft with time-lapse videography (Fig. 17). The movements within the epiblast areas are expansion movements of the quail graft that are seen directly.

The presumptive notochord, somites, and lateral plate areas in the upper layer converge from cranial to caudal toward the anterior half of the primitive streak. These movements of the more transparent quail grafts from cranial-lateral to caudal-media are seen directly (Bortier and Vakaet, 1992a,b).

4. Wound Closure of Experimental Excision Wounds in the Bare Upper Layer

From the observed morphogenetic movements, questions arise about the mechanism and dynamics that guide cells during these movements: what is the driving force for these movements, what guides the movements, and how do the cells

---

Fig. 16 Experimental induction of a secondary primitive streak (stage 4V midpiece primitive streak in the endophyllic crescent of a chick host stage 5V) recorded with time-lapse cinephotomicrography (Vakaet, 1967). A stage 4V quail midpiece primitive streak is inserted in the endophyllic crescent of the chick host (right). A stage 4V Hensen's node inserted in the endophyllic crescent of the chick host has not developed (left). (A) At the start of the culture, the ventral side of a stage 5V chick blastoderm is toward the observer and the cranial is up. Time intervals after reincubation are (B) 5 hr, (C) 11 hr 40 min, and (D) 16 hr 40 min. (B) A more translucent area at the site of the quail midpiece. (C and D) A secondary primitive streak; presumptive neural plate cells of the chick host are recruited to become cells that ingress through the secondary primitive streak.

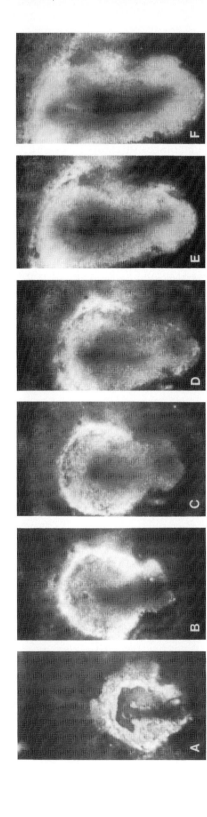

move? These questions prompted the study of the closure of experimental wounds in the bare upper layer of the proamnion in the chick blastoderm (Bortier and Vakaet, 1987b; Bortier *et al.*, 1993). We observed that experimental excision wounds in the upper layer closed, even when the deep layer was not repositioned. Time-lapse videography (Fig. 18) and videomicrography demonstrate a global movement of the upper layer toward the wound and movements of individual cells of the wound submarginal region. The wound submarginal regions change shape during closure while the upper layer cells move in respect to one another.

With histological techniques we demonstrated that these wounds do not close by classic mechanisms such as an increase in mitotic figures, contraction of the wound rim, and migration on a substrate. Counts of metaphases plus anaphases around wound submarginal zones and mirror image areas at the opposite side of the primitive streak of the blastoderm are indeed not significantly different. S-phases counted after autoradiography with tritiated thymidine also showed no significant difference between the wound submarginal zones and their mirror image area. These findings demonstrate that wounds do not close by increased cell division.

A second classic mechanism could be a contraction of the wound rim. One then would expect an even wound rim during closure. This was not seen with time-lapse videography. To the contary, the wound rims are irregular during closure, with their shape changing from circular to split like and again to circular. A continuous ring of microfilament bundles has not been found around the wounds. Even if microfilament bundles were present, this would not prove that there is contraction, as microfilament bundles can be propulsive (Theriot and Mitchison, 1992).

A third classic mechanism could be migration on a substrate. There are, however, no other cell layers at the wound submarginal zones. The only candidate as a substrate is the basal lamina. With transmission electron microscopy and scanning electron microscopy, no basal lamina was found within the wounds. With immunohistochemistry for laminin, no laminin was found inside the wounds. The structure of the cells of the wound submarginal region remains unchanged throughout closure: the cells do not acquire a flattened shape as do cells migrating on a substrate.

Fig. 17 Morphogenetic movements of a stage 5V quail isochronic, isotopic, and isotropic xenograft in a stage 5V chick host recorded with time-lapse videography. (A) At the start of the culture, the ventral side of a stage 5V chick blastoderm is toward the observer, the cranial is up, and the quail xenograft is cranial to the cranial tip of the primitive streak. Time intervals after reincubation are (B) 3 hr 10 min, (C) 6 hr 39 min, (D) 9 hr 37 min, (E) 12 hr 34 min, and (F) 15 hr 10 min. (A–C) The edges of the quail graft and the wound in the upper layer are seen. (D–F) The healed xenograft is seen as a more translucent area in the chick upper layer. After 24 hr of incubation, fixation, paraffin embedding, and staining, the quail cells were found in the brain extending from the prosencephalon through the mesencephalon.

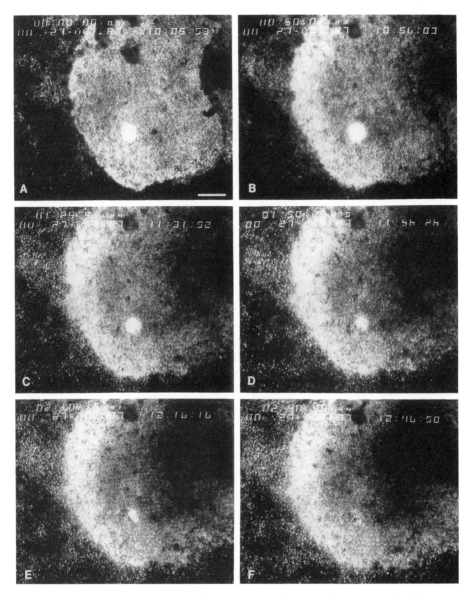

Fig. 18 Closure of an experimental excision wound in the bare upper layer of the chick blastoderm recorded with time-lapse videography. (A) At the start of the culture, the ventral side of a stage 4V blastoderm is toward the observer, the cranial is to the left, the more translucent area is the bare upper layer, and the whitish area is the experimental excision wound. Time intervals after reincubation are (B) 50 min, (C) 1 hr 25 min, (D) 1 hr 50 min, (E) 2 hr 5 min, and (F) 2 hr 40 min. The wound submarginal region changes shape during closure. Bar: 250 μm.

If none of these three classic mechanisms explains wound closure, how do these wounds close? The observations with time-lapse videography and videomicrography allowed us to look for other possible mechanisms. We propose a new paradigm to explain the global movement of the upper layer toward the wound and the movements of individual wound submarginal region cells. During wound closure the movements of the cells are driven by "mitotic pressure" (Bortier *et al.*, 1993); the horizontal pressure exerted by the addition of daughter cells and by the parting of the anaphase nuclei and telophase cells. This moving apart brings about changes in the relative positioning of neighboring cells. Connecting processes bridging one or more apical cell surfaces are observed during these movements; in chick blastoderms, most of the mitotic figures are lying at the dorsal side of the upper layer and parallel to it. The individual movements of cells result in a global movement of the upper layer toward the wound, where there is no mitotic pressure because there are no cells within the wound.

For mitotic pressure to initiate movements, the cells of the upper layer need to be able to move freely on their basal lamina. We have demosntrated that the upper layer cells do indeed move on their basal lamina during morphogenetic movements (unpublished observations). The direction of the movements may therefore be toward areas where there is a sink in mitotic pressure. In experimental wound closure, this is in the direction of the wound whereas in gastrulation it is in the direction of the primitive streak. This is clearly illustrated by the attraction of cells of a presumptive neural lip by an actively ingressing primitive streak (Fig. 16).

VI. Conclusions and Perspectives

Time-lapse cinephotomicrography, videography, and videomicrography have been essential in the studies of normal development, formation of the definitive endoblast, induction experiments, movements of xenografts in the upper layer, and wound closure. Video registrations have led to the new concept of "mitotic pressure" as a major mechanism of morphogenetic movements during gastrulation and neurulation.

Video registration is a basic technique in the study of developmental biology as "life" is movement and only video registration allows morphogenetic movements to be observed directly. It allows access to the fourth dimension: the evolution of shape in time, as morphogenesis may be called.

References

Bortier, H. (1991). Chicken organogenesis. *In* "A Dozen Eggs: Time-Lapse Microscopy of Normal Development" (R. Fink, ed.), pp. 28–29. Sinauer Associates, Sunderland, MA.
Bortier, H., and Vakaet, L. (1987a). Wound healing in the upper layer of the chicken blastoderm. *Cell Diff.* **20** (Suppl.), 114S.

Bortier, H., and Vakaet, L. (1987b). Videomicrography in the study of morphogenetic movements in the early chicken blastoderm. *Cell Diff.* **20** (Suppl.), 114S.

Bortier, H., and Vakaet, L. (1989). Videomicrography with Nomarski optics and AVEC-system of wound closure in the upper layer of the chicken blastoderm. *Cell Diff. Dev.* **27** (Suppl.), 101.

Bortier, H., and Vakaet, L. (1991). Videography of experimental teratology in the chicken embryo. *Teratology* **44,** 13A–14A.

Bortier, H., and Vakaet, L. C. A. (1992a). Mesoblast anlage fields in the upper layer of the chicken blastoderm at stage 5V. *In* "Formation and Differentiation of Early Embryonic Mesoderm" (R. Bellairs, E. J. Sanders, and J. W. Lash, eds.), pp. 1–7. Plenum press, New York.

Bortier, H., and Vakaet, L. C. A. (1992b). Fate mapping the neural plate and the intraembryonic mesoblast in the upper layer of the chicken blastoderm with xenografting and time-lapse videography. *Development* (Suppl.), 93–97.

Bortier, H., and Vakaet, L. C. A. (1995). Morphogenetic movements in the avian blastoderm: Mechanism and dynamics. *In* "Organization of the Early Vertebrate Embryo" (N. Zagris *et al.,* eds.), pp. 131–137. Plenum Press, New York.

Bortier, H., Vandevelde, S., and Vakaet, L. (1993). Mechanism of closure of experimental excision-wounds in the bare upper layer of the chick blastoderm. *Int. J. Dev. Biol.* **37,** 459–466.

De Haan, L. (1963). Migration patterns of the precardiac mesoderm in the early chick embryo. *Exp. Cell Res.* **29,** 544–560.

Gräper, L. (1929). Die Primitiventwicklung des Huhnchens nach stereokinematographischen Untersuchungen, kontrolliert durch vitale Farbmarkierung und verglichen mit der Entwicklung anderer Wirbeltier. *Roux' Arch.* **116,** 382–429.

Hamburger, V., and Hamilton, H. L. (1951). A series of normal stages in the development of the chick embryo. *J. Morphol.* **88,** 49–92.

New, D. A. T. (1951). A new technique for the cultivation of the chick embryo in vitro. *J. Embryol. Exp. Morphol.* **3,** 326–331.

Theriot, J. A., and Mitchison, T. J. (1992). Actin microfilament dynamics in locomoting cells. *Nature* **352,** 126–131.

Vakaet, L. (1967). Contribution à l'étude de la prégastrulation et de la gastrulation de l'embryon de poulet en culture in vitro. *Mém. Acad. Ro. Med. Belgique* **3,** 231–257.

Vakaet, L. (1970). Cinephotomicrographic investigations of gastrulation in the chick blastoderm. *Arch. Biol.* **81/3,** 387–426.

Vakaet, L. (1981). Neurale inductie bij vogels. *Verhandelingen van de koninklijke academie voor geneeskunde van België* **XLIII nr2,** 78–102.

Vakaet, L. C. A., and Bortier, H. (1995). Mapping of gastrulation movements in birds. *In* "Organization of the Early Vertebrate Embryo" (N. Zagris *et al.,* eds.), pp. 123–129. Plenum Press, New York.

INDEX

A

Adenoviral vectors, gene transfer technique, 168–172
  life cycle, 168–169
  recombinant vector generation, 169–170
  stock preparation, 170–171
  stock titer, 171–172
Adhesion assays
  cell–extracellular matrix interactions, 285–299
    materials, 285–287
    methods, 287–299
      cell migration assay, 292–295
      protocol, 287–292
      substrata preference assay, 295–299
  retinal cell–substratum interactions, 279–280
Antibodies
  cell division detection, bromodeoxyuridine antibodies, 313–315
  in situ hybridization, 232–233
  labeling methods, 324–325
  microinjection methods, neural crest cells, 70–72
  quail–chick transplantation, differential embryo diagnosis, 29
Apical ectodermal ridge
  manipulation techniques, 139–141
  retrovirus-mediated gene expression manipulation, 206–211
Autoradiography
  cell division detection
    emulsion-coated autoradiographs, 325–327
    [^{3}H]thymidine method, 309–313
      embryo staging, 309–310
      grain count interpretation, 313
      [^{3}H]thymidine application, 310–311
      protocol, 311–313
    staining methods, 323
Avian embryo, *see also specific manipulation*
  culture technique, 1–14
    agar method, 13
    in ovo approach, 3–7
    New culture method, 7–12
    overview, 1–2
    plasma clot method, 13

embryo slices, 109–123
  applications, 117–123
    neurite guidance mechanisms assay, 118–120
    in situ studies, 120–122
  characteristics, 116–117
  culture, 110–116
    adherent culture, 112–113
    cutting, 112
    embryo preparation, 111–112
    floating culture, 113–114
    media, 115–116
    mounting procedure, 114
    peanut agglutinin lectin labeling, 114–115
  overview, 109–110
gene transfer technique, viral vector injection, 173–174
limb bud operations, 125–144
  apical ectodermal ridge manipulations, 139–141
  enzymatic dissociation, 142–144
  extraembryonic membranes, 131–133
  grafting techniques
    chorioallantoic grafts, 133–135
    flank grafts, 135–136
    intracoelomic grafts, 136
    limb-to-limb grafts, 137–139
    polarizing activity test, 141–142
    somite grafts, 136–137
  overview, 125–126
  preparation, 126–130
    egg incubation, 126
    fenestration, 127–130
    solutions, 127
    tools, 127
  tissue recombination, 142–144
microsurgery, 13–18
  dissection enzymes, 17–18
  donor embryo explantation, 14–17
  instruments, 13–14
  methods, 18
segmental plate manipulation, *in vivo,* 81–92
  applications, 91–92
  critical procedural aspects, 90–91

materials, 82–84
methods, 84–90
donor embryo preparation, 84
donor segmental plate implantation,
88–90
donor segmental plate removal, 84–86
experimental embryo harvesting, 90
host embryo preparation, 86–88
host segmental plate removal, 88
overview, 81–82
transplantation methods, 23–54
applications, 51–54
blastodisc transplantations, 40–44
blastodermal chimeras, 40
epiblasts, 43–44
germ layer combinations, 40–43
streak fragments, 43–44
differential diagnosis, 27–29
antibodies, 29
nucleic probes, 29
nucleolar marker, 27–28
egg preparation, 35
hemopoietic organ rudiment
transplantations, 44–51
bursa of fabricius rudiments, 48–49
chorioallantoic membrane grafts, 44–45
dorsal mesentery grafts, 45
parabiosis, 45–46
somatopleure grafts, 45
thymus rudiments, 46–48
yolk sac chimeras, 49–51
materials and equipment, 29–35
egg holders, 31
Feulgen–Rossenbeck stain, 35
incubators, 31
microsurgery instruments, 32
optical equipment, 31
transplant equipment, 32–35
neural tissue transplantations, 35–40
brain vesicles, 39–40
folds, 38–39
plate tissue, 38–39
tubes, 36–38
overview, 24–27

B

Bisbenzimide, cell stain, 324
Blastoderm
blastodisc transplantation methods,
quail–chick embryos, 40–44
blastodermal chimeras, 40
epiblasts, 43–44

germ layer combinations, 40–43
streak fragments, 43–44
development, time-lapse videography,
331–353
critical registration aspects, 343
equipment installation, 341–343
experimental applications, 343–353
definitive endoblast formation, 347
induction, 347
normal development, 343–345
wound closure, 349–353
xenograft movement, 347–349
overview, 331–335
instruments, 334–335
material choice, 332–333
procedures, 335–340
microsurgery, 338–340
New culture, 335–338
Brain vesicles, quail–chick embryo
transplantation, 39–40
Bromodeoxyuridine immunohistochemistry,
cell division detection, 313–315
Buds, see Limb buds
Bursa of fabricius, quail–chick transplantation
methods, 48–49

C

Carbocyanine dyes, see Iontophoretic dye
labeling
Cell culture
avian embryo, 1–14
agar method, 13
in ovo approach, 3–7
New culture method, 7–12
overview, 1–2
plasma clot method, 13
blastoderm cells, time-lapse videography,
335–338
embryo slices, 110–116
adherent culture, 112–113
cutting, 112
embryo preparation, 111–112
floating culture, 113–114
media, 115–116
mounting procedure, 114
peanut agglutinin lectin labeling, 114–115
limb bud micromass culture, 237–246
methods, 238–245
critical aspects, 241
isolation, 239–240
materials, 238–239

mesenchyme–ectoderm coculture,
241–242
microtiter technique, 241
nucleopore filtration, 243–244
solutions, 238–239
overview, 237–238
teratology applications, 245–246
neural crest cells, 62–70
cranial region primary culture, 68
medium preparation, 62–64
secondary cultures, 68–69
three-dimensional substrate preparation,
64–65
trunk region primary culture, 65–68
two-dimensional substrate preparation, 64
whole trunk explants, 69–70
neurons, 249–262
critical aspects, 259–261
culturing, 260–261
dissection, 259
dissociation, 259–260
materials, 251–252
methods, 252–259
ganglia dissection, 252–255
ganglia dissociation, 255–256
protocol, 256–259
overview, 249–250
retinal cells, 265–282
methods, 275–278
β-galactosidase expression detection,
277–278
protocol, 276
transfection, 276–277
neuronal cell assays, 278–282
cell–substratum adhesion assay, 279–280
crystal violet stain, 280–281
neurite outgrowth assay, 281–282
substrate preparation, 278–279
overview, 265–266
primary cell acquisition, 266–275
explant mounts, 272–275
ganglion cell isolation, 270
percoll gradient, 271–272
retinal dissection, 268–269
retinal strips, 272–275
suspension preparation, 270–271
trypsinization, 269–270
somite strips, 99
Cell differentiation, 301–327
cell cycle, 301–302
detection methods, 309–315
bromodeoxyuridine
immunohistochemistry, 313–315

[^{3}H]thymidine autoradiography, 309–313
histological procedures, 316–327
antibody labeling, 324–325
collection methods, 316–317
embedding procedures, 319–323
embryo preparation, 316
emulsion-coated autoradiographs, 325–327
solutions, 317–319
staining procedures, 323–324
neural differentiation, 303–306
somite differentiation, 307–309
specialization, 301–302
Cell division, 301–327
cell cycle, 301–302
detection methods, 309–315
bromodeoxyuridine
immunohistochemistry, 313–315
[^{3}H]thymidine autoradiography, 309–313
histological procedures, 316–327
antibody labeling, 324–325
collection methods, 316–317
embedding procedures, 319–323
embryo preparation, 316
emulsion-coated autoradiographs, 325–327
solutions, 317–319
staining procedures, 323–324
neural differentiation, 303–306
somite differentiation, 307–309
specialization, 301–302
Cell grafting, see Grafting techniques
Cell lineage
iontophoretic tracers, microinjection
technique, 149–158
injection apparatus, 150–152
protocol, 154–158
tools, 152–154
retroviral vector elucidation method,
179–180
Chick cells, see Avian embryo
Chorioallantoic membrane
limb bud grafting techniques, 133–135
quail–chick transplantation methods, 44–45
Cinephotomicrography, see Time-lapse
videography
Coelom, limb bud grafting techniques, 136
Crystal violet stain, retinal assay, 280–281
Culture technique, see Cell culture

D

Dextran, see Iontophoretic dye labeling
Differentiation, see Cell differentiation

Dye labeling, *see* Iontophoretic dye labeling;
  Vital dyes

E

Ectoderm
  apical ectodermal ridge
    manipulation techniques, 139–141
    retrovirus-mediated gene expression
      manipulation, 206–211
  limb bud micromass culture,
    mesenchyme–ectoderm coculture,
    241–242
Embedding procedures, 319–323
  celloidin-paraffin double-embedding method,
    320
  freeze-substitution–paraffin method, 321
  gelatin-sucrose method, 320–321
  O.C.T. compound method, 321
  paraffin method, 319–320
  plastic method, 322
Embryo culture, *see* Avian embryo; Cell
  culture
Embryo slices, 109–123
  applications, 117–123
    in situ studies, 120–122
    neurite guidance mechanisms assay,
      118–120
  characteristics, 116–117
  culture, 110–116
    adherent culture, 112–113
    cutting, 112
    embryo preparation, 111–112
    floating culture, 113–114
    media, 115–116
    mounting procedure, 114
    peanut agglutinin lectin labeling,
      114–115
  overview, 109–110
Enzymes
  limb bud dissociation, 142–144
  microsurgery dissection technique,
    17–18
Eosin stain, autoradiography, 323
Extracellular matrix, interaction assays,
  285–299
  materials, 285–287
  methods, 287–299
    cell adhesion assay, 287–292
    cell migration assay, 292–295
    substrata preference assay, 295–299

F

Feulgen–Rossenbeck staining method,
  quail–chick transplantation, 35
Fluorescent labeling, *see* Iontophoretic dye
  labeling

G

β-Galactosidase, expression detection, 277–278
Gene expression, retrovirus-mediated
  manipulation, 185–217
  infection–phenotype correlation, 214–215
  materials, 195–196
  methods, 196–214
    lumenal space injection protocols, 211–213
    novel infection protocol development,
      213–214
    preparation, 205–206
    solid tissue injection protocols, 206–211
    virus construction, 196–200
    virus production, 200–205
  overview, 186–195
    advantages, 186
    optimization, 193–195
    vector choice, 186–189
    virology, 189–193
  viral spread restriction, 215–216
Gene transfer technique, 161–181
  adenoviral vectors, 168–172
    expression patterns, 172
    life cycle, 168–169
    recombinant vector generation, 169–170
    safety issues, 172
    stock preparation, 170–171
    stock titer, 171–172
  applications, 177–181
    bioactive gene insertion, 180–181
    cell migration, 180
    lineage studies, 179–180
    methods comparison, 177–179
  chick embryo injection, 173–174
  histology, 174–177
    fixation, 174
    lacZ activity stain, 174–175
    microscopy, 177
    tissue sectioning, 175–177
  retroviral vectors, 162–168
    life cycle, 162–164
    replication-competent virus testing, 167
    replication-defective vector generation,
      164–165
    safety issues, 167–168

stock preparation, 165–166
stock titer, 166–167
Grafting techniques, *see also* Transplantation
hemopoietic organ
chorioallantoic membrane grafts, 44–45
dorsal mesentery grafts, 45
somatopleure grafts, 45
limb bud operations
chorioallantoic grafts, 133–135
flank grafts, 135–136
intracoelomic grafts, 136
limb-to-limb grafts, 137–139
polarizing activity test, 141–142
somite grafts, 136–137
neural crest cells, 74–78
fold ablations, 75
notochord ablations, 77–78
notochord implants, 76–77
tube rotations, 74–75

H

Hematoxylin stain, autoradiography, 323
Hemopoietic organ, quail–chick
transplantation methods, 44–51
bursa of fabricius rudiments, 48–49
chorioallantoic membrane grafts, 44–45
dorsal mesentery grafts, 45
parabiosis, 45–46
somatopleure grafts, 45
thymus rudiments, 46–48
yolk sac chimeras, 49–51
Horseradish peroxidase, *see* Iontophoretic dye
labeling

I

Immunochemistry, *see also* Antibodies
cell division detection, 313–315
in situ hybridization, 232–233
In situ hybridization, avian embryo analysis
embryo slices, 120–122
fluorescence labeling, 230
overview, 220–221
protein detection, 229–230
rational, 221
RNA detection, 228–230
solution preparation, 221–222
tissue sections, 230–233
immunocytochemical detection, 232–233
posthybridization washing, 232–233
precautions, 231

prehybridization treatments, 232
subbed slide preparation, 231–232
troubleshooting, 233–234
whole mount procedure, 222–228
embryo pretreatment, 224–225
labeled RNA probe preparation, 222–224
photography, 227–228
posthybridization washing, 225–227
probe detection, 225–227
sectioning, 227–228
Iontophoretic dye labeling
applications, 158–160
in situ hybridization combined, 230
lineage tracer microinjection, 149–158
injection apparatus, 150–152
protocol, 154–158
tools, 152–154
overview, 147–149

L

Labeling methods, *see specific method*
LacZ, activity detection, histochemical staining,
174–175
Lectin, peanut agglutinin, embryo slice
labeling, 114–115
Limb buds
micromass cultures, 237–246
methods, 238–245
critical aspects, 241
isolation, 239–240
materials, 238–239
mesenchyme–ectoderm coculture,
241–242
microtiter technique, 241
nucleopore filtration, 243–244
solutions, 238–239
overview, 237–238
teratology applications, 245–246
operation techniques, 125–144
apical ectodermal ridge manipulations,
139–141
enzymatic dissociation, 142–144
extraembryonic membranes, 131–133
grafting techniques
chorioallantoic grafts, 133–135
flank grafts, 135–136
intracoelomic grafts, 136
limb-to-limb grafts, 137–139
polarizing activity test, 141–142
somite grafts, 136–137
overview, 125–126
preparation, 126–130

egg incubation, 126
 fenestration, 127–130
 solutions, 127
 tools, 127
 tissue recombination, 142–144
 retrovirus-mediated gene expression
  manipulation, injection protocols,
  206–211
Lineage, *see* Cell lineage
Lipid-soluble carbocyanine dyes, *see*
 Iontophoretic dye labeling

M

Markers, quail–chick transplantation,
 27–28
Mesenchyme cells, *see* Limb buds
Microinjection
 iontophoretic lineage tracers, 149–158
  injection apparatus, 150–152
  protocol, 154–158
  tools, 152–154
 neural crest cells, 70–72
Micromass culture, limb buds, 237–246
 methods, 238–245
  critical aspects, 241
  isolation, 239–240
  materials, 238–239
  mesenchyme–ectoderm coculture,
   241–242
  microtiter technique, 241
  nucleopore filtration, 243–244
  solutions, 238–239
 overview, 237–238
 teratology applications, 245–246
Microsurgery
 avian embryo dissection, 13–18
  dissection enzymes, 17–18
  donor embryo explantation, 14–17
  instruments, 13–14
  methods, 18
 blastoderm development, time-lapse
  videography, 338–340
 transplantation methods, 32
Migration assays
 materials, 285–287
 methods, 287–299
  cell adhesion assay, 287–292
  gene transfer detection, 180
  protocol, 292–295
  substrata preference assay,
   295–299

N

Neural crest cells, *see also* Somites
 culture, 62–70
  cranial region primary culture, 68
  medium preparation, 62–64
  secondary cultures, 68–69
  three-dimensional substrate preparation,
   64–65
  trunk region primary culture, 65–68
  two-dimensional substrate preparation, 64
  whole trunk explants, 69–70
 grafting techniques, 74–78
  fold ablations, 75
  notochord ablations, 77–78
  notochord implants, 76–77
  tube rotations, 74–75
 labeling, *in vivo,* 72–74
 microinjection methods, 70–72
 quail–chick embryo transplantation, 35–40
  brain vesicles, 39–40
  folds, 38–39
  plate tissue, 38–39
  tubes, 36–38
Neurites
 guidance determination
  embryo slice assay, 118–120
  somite strip assay, 104–105
 outgrowth assay, 281–282
Neurons
 autonomic and sensory neuron cultures,
  249–262
  critical aspects, 259–261
   culturing, 260–261
   dissection, 259
   dissociation, 259–260
  materials, 251–252
  methods, 252–259
   ganglia dissection, 252–255
   ganglia dissociation, 255–256
   protocol, 256–259
  overview, 249–250
 differentiation, 303–306
 retinal culture, 265–282
  methods, 275–278
   β-galactosidase expression detection,
    277–278
   protocol, 276
   transfection, 276–277
  neuronal cell assays, 278–282
   cell–substratum adhesion assay, 279–280
   crystal violet stain, 280–281
   neurite outgrowth assay, 281–282

substrate preparation, 278–279
overview, 265–266
primary cell acquisition, 266–275
    explant mounts, 272–275
    ganglion cell isolation, 270
    percoll gradient, 271–272
    retinal dissection, 268–269
    retinal strips, 272–275
    suspension preparation, 270–271
    trypsinization, 269–270
New culture
    avian embryo culture, 7–12
    blastoderm development, time-lapse
        videography, 335–338
Notochord, grafting techniques
    ablations, 77–78
    implants, 76–77
Nucleic probes, quail–chick transplantation,
    differential embryo diagnosis, 29
Nucleolar markers, quail–chick
    transplantation, 27–28
Nucleopore filtration technique, limb bud
    micromass cultures, 243–244

P

Peanut agglutinin lectin, embryo slice labeling,
    114–115
Percoll gradient, retinal primary cell
    acquisition, 271–272
Plasma clot culture method, avian embryo
    culture, 13
Polarizing activity zone, graft assay, 141–142

Q

Quail cells, *see* Avian embryo

R

Retina, cell culture, 265–282
    methods, 275–278
        β-galactosidase expression detection,
            277–278
        protocol, 276
        transfection, 276–277
    neuronal cell assays, 278–282
        cell–substratum adhesion assay, 279–280
        crystal violet stain, 280–281
        neurite outgrowth assay, 281–282
        substrate preparation, 278–279
    overview, 265–266

primary cell acquisition, 266–275
    explant mounts, 272–275
    ganglion cell isolation, 270
    percoll gradient, 271–272
    retinal dissection, 268–269
    retinal strips, 272–275
    suspension preparation, 270–271
    trypsinization, 269–270
Retroviral vectors
    cell lineage elucidation, 179–180
    gene expression manipulation, 185–217
        infection–phenotype correlation, 214–215
        materials, 195–196
        methods, 196–214
            lumenal space injection protocols,
                211–213
            novel infection protocol development,
                213–214
            preparation, 205–206
            solid tissue injection protocols, 206–211
            virus construction, 196–200
            virus production, 200–205
        overview, 186–195
            advantages, 186
            optimization, 193–195
            vector choice, 186–189
            virology, 189–193
        viral spread restriction, 215–216
    gene transfer technique, 162–168
        life cycle, 162–164
        replication-competent virus testing, 167
        replication-defective vector generation,
            164–165
        safety issues, 167–168
        stock preparation, 165–166
        stock titer, 166–167
RNA, *in situ* hybridization
    double detection method, 228–230
    labeled probe preparation, 222–224

S

Segmental plate, manipulation, *in vivo,*
    81–92
    applications, 91–92
    critical procedural aspects, 90–91
    materials, 82–84
    methods, 84–90
        donor embryo preparation, 84
        donor segmental plate implantation,
            88–90
        donor segmental plate removal, 84–86
        experimental embryo harvesting, 90

host embryo preparation, 86–88
host segmental plate removal, 88
overview, 81–82
Somatopleure, quail–chick transplantation
    methods, 45
Somites, *see also* Neural crest cells
differentiation, 307–309
embryo fillet preparation, 93–107
    critical aspects, 101–104
        border visibility, 103
        neuron sprouting efficiency, 104
        population contamination, 103
        temporal–spatial concerns, 102–103
        tissue architecture, 101–102
    future research directions, 105–107
    guidance interactions, 104–105
    methods, 94–101
        culture, 99
        dissection, 95–99
        neuron labeling, 100
        strip fixation, 101
        substrata preparation, 95
    neurite analysis, 104–105
    overview, 94
limb bud grafting techniques, 136–137
Staining methods, *see specific method*

T

Teratology, limb bud micromass culture,
    245–246
[^{3}H]Thymidine autoradiography, cell division
    detection, 309–313
embryo staging, 309–310
grain count interpretation, 313
[^{3}H]thymidine application, 310–311
protocol, 311–313
Thymus, quail–chick transplantation methods,
    46–48
Time-lapse videography, blastoderm
    development, 331–353
critical registration aspects, 343
equipment installation, 341–343
experimental applications, 343–353
    definitive endoblast formation, 347
    induction, 347
    normal development, 343–345
    wound closure, 349–353
    xenograft movement, 347–349
overview, 331–335
    instruments, 334–335
    material choice, 332–333
procedures, 335–340

microsurgery, 338–340
New culture, 335–338
Toluidine blue O stain, plastic sections,
    323–324
Transplantation, *see also* Grafting techniques
quail–chick embryos, 23–54
    applications, 51–54
    blastodisc early transplantations, 40–44
        blastodermal chimeras, 40
        epiblasts, 43–44
        germ layer combinations, 40–43
        streak fragments, 43–44
    differential diagnosis, 27–29
        antibodies, 29
        nucleic probes, 29
        nucleolar marker, 27–28
    egg preparation, 35
    hemopoietic organ rudiment
        transplantations, 44–51
        bursa of fabricius rudiments, 48–49
        chorioallantoic membrane grafts, 44–45
        dorsal mesentery grafts, 45
        parabiosis, 45–46
        somatopleure grafts, 45
        thymus rudiments, 46–48
        yolk sac chimeras, 49–51
    materials and equipment, 29–35
        egg holders, 31
        Feulgen–Rossenbeck stain, 35
        incubators, 31
        microsurgery instruments, 32
        optical equipment, 31
        transplant equipment, 32–35
    neural tissue transplantations, 35–40
        brain vesicles, 39–40
        folds, 38–39
        plate tissue, 38–39
        tubes, 36–38
    overview, 24–27
Trypsinization, retinal primary cell acquisition,
    269–270

V

Videomicrography, *see* Time-lapse videography
Viral vectors
gene transfer technique, 161–181
    adenoviral vectors, 168–172
        expression patterns, 172
        life cycle, 168–169
        recombinant vector generation, 169–170
        safety issues, 172
        stock preparation, 170–171

stock titer, 171–172
applications, 177–181
    bioactive gene insertion, 180–181
    cell migration, 180
    lineage studies, 179–180
    methods comparison, 177–179
chick embryo injection, 173–174
histology, 174–177
    fixation, 174
    lacZ activity stain, 174–175
    microscopy, 177
    tissue sectioning, 175–177
retroviral vectors, 162–168
    life cycle, 162–164
    replication-competent virus testing, 167
    replication-defective vector generation, 164–165
    safety issues, 167–168
    stock preparation, 165–166
    stock titer, 166–167
retrovirus-mediated gene expression manipulation, 185–217
    infection–phenotype correlation, 214–215
    materials, 195–196
    methods, 196–214

lumenal space injection protocols, 211–213
    novel infection protocol development, 213–214
    preparation, 205–206
    solid tissue injection protocols, 206–211
    virus construction, 196–200
    virus production, 200–205
overview, 186–195
    advantages, 186
    optimization, 193–195
    vector choice, 186–189
    virology, 189–193
viral spread restriction, 215–216
Vital dyes, neural crest cell labeling, *in vivo*, 72–74

X

Xenograft movement, time-lapse videography, 347–349

Z

Zone of polarizing activity, graft assay, 141–142

VOLUMES IN SERIES

Founding Series Editor
DAVID M. PRESCOTT

Volume 1 (1964)
Methods in Cell Physiology
Edited by David M. Prescott

Volume 2 (1966)
Methods in Cell Physiology
Edited by David M. Prescott

Volume 3 (1968)
Methods in Cell Physiology
Edited by David M. Prescott

Volume 4 (1970)
Methods in Cell Physiology
Edited by David M. Prescott

Volume 5 (1972)
Methods in Cell Physiology
Edited by David M. Prescott

Volume 6 (1973)
Methods in Cell Physiology
Edited by David M. Prescott

Volume 7 (1973)
Methods in Cell Biology
Edited by David M. Prescott

Volume 8 (1974)
Methods in Cell Biology
Edited by David M. Prescott

Volume 9 (1975)
Methods in Cell Biology
Edited by David M. Prescott

Volume 10 (1975)
Methods in Cell Biology
Edited by David M. Prescott

Volume 11 (1975)
Yeast Cells
Edited by David M. Prescott

Volume 12 (1975)
Yeast Cells
Edited by David M. Prescott

Volume 13 (1976)
Methods in Cell Biology
Edited by David M. Prescott

Volume 14 (1976)
Methods in Cell Biology
Edited by David M. Prescott

Volume 15 (1977)
Methods in Cell Biology
Edited by David M. Prescott

Volume 16 (1977)
Chromatin and Chromosomal Protein Research I
Edited by Gary Stein, Janet Stein, and Lewis J. Kleinsmith

Volume 17 (1978)
Chromatin and Chromosomal Protein Research II
Edited by Gary Stein, Janet Stein, and Lewis J. Kleinsmith

Volume 18 (1978)
Chromatin and Chromosomal Protein Research III
Edited by Gary Stein, Janet Stein, and Lewis J. Kleinsmith

Volume 19 (1978)
Chromatin and Chromosomal Protein Research IV
Edited by Gary Stein, Janet Stein, and Lewis J. Kleinsmith

Volume 20 (1978)
Methods in Cell Biology
Edited by David M. Prescott

Advisory Board Chairman
KEITH R. PORTER

Volume 21A (1980)
**Normal Human Tissue and Cell Culture, Part A: Respiratory, Cardiovascular,
    and Integumentary Systems**
Edited by Curtis C. Harris, Benjamin F. Trump, and Gary D. Stoner

Volume 21B (1980)
Normal Human Tissue and Cell Culture, Part B: Endocrine, Urogenital, and Gastrointestinal Systems
Edited by Curtis C. Harris, Benjamin F. Trump, and Gary D. Stoner

Volume 22 (1981)
Three-Dimensional Ultrastructure in Biology
Edited by James N. Turner

Volume 23 (1981)
Basic Mechanisms of Cellular Secretion
Edited by Arthur R. Hand and Constance Oliver

Volume 24 (1982)
The Cytoskeleton, Part A: Cytoskeletal Proteins, Isolation and Characterization
Edited by Leslie Wilson

Volume 25 (1982)
The Cytoskeleton, Part B: Biological Systems and *in Vitro* Models
Edited by Leslie Wilson

Volume 26 (1982)
Prenatal Diagnosis: Cell Biological Approaches
Edited by Samuel A. Latt and Gretchen J. Darlington

Series Editor
LESLIE WILSON

Volume 27 (1986)
Echinoderm Gametes and Embryos
Edited by Thomas E. Schroeder

Volume 28 (1987)
***Dictyostelium discoideum:* Molecular Approaches to Cell Biology**
Edited by James A. Spudich

Volume 29 (1989)
Fluorescence Microscopy of Living Cells in Culture, Part A: Fluorescent Analogs, Labeling Cells, and Basic Microscopy
Edited by Yu-Li Wang and D. Lansing Taylor

Volume 30 (1989)
Fluorescence Microscopy of Living Cells in Culture, Part B: Quantitative Fluorescence Microscopy—Imaging and Spectroscopy
Edited by D. Lansing Taylor and Yu-Li Wang

Volume 31 (1989)
Vesicular Transport, Part A
Edited by Alan M. Tartakoff

Volume 32 (1989)
Vesicular Transport, Part B
Edited by Alan M. Tartakoff

Volume 33 (1990)
Flow Cytometry
Edited by Zbigniew Darzynkiewicz and Harry A. Crissman

Volume 34 (1991)
Vectorial Transport of Proteins into and across Membranes
Edited by Alan M. Tartakoff

Selected from Volumes 31, 32, and 34 (1991)
Laboratory Methods for Vesicular and Vectorial Transport
Edited by Alan M. Tartakoff

Volume 35 (1991)
Functional Organization of the Nucleus: A Laboratory Guide
Edited by Barbara A. Hamkalo and Sarah C. R. Elgin

Volume 36 (1991)
***Xenopus laevis:* Practical Uses in Cell and Molecular Biology**
Edited by Brian K. Kay and H. Benjamin Peng

Series Editors
LESLIE WILSON AND PAUL MATSUDAIRA

Volume 37 (1993)
Antibodies in Cell Biology
Edited by David J. Asai

Volume 38 (1993)
Cell Biological Applications of Confocal Microscopy
Edited by Brian Matsumoto

Volume 39 (1993)
Motility Assays for Motor Proteins
Edited by Jonathan M. Scholey

Volume 40 (1994)
A Practical Guide to the Study of Calcium in Living Cells
Edited by Richard Nuccitelli

Volume 41 (1994)
Flow Cytometry, Second Edition, Part A
*Edited by Zbigniew Darzynkiewicz, J. Paul Robinson,
  and Harry A. Crissman*

Volume 42 (1994)
Flow Cytometry, Second Edition, Part B
*Edited by Zbigniew Darzynkiewicz, J. Paul Robinson,
  and Harry A. Crissman*

Volume 43 (1994)
Protein Expression in Animal Cells
Edited by Michael G. Roth

Volume 44 (1994)
***Drosophila melanogaster:* Practical Uses in Cell and Molecular Biology**
Edited by Lawrence S. B. Goldstein and Eric A. Fyrberg

Volume 45 (1994)
Microbes as Tools for Cell Biology
Edited by David G. Russell

Volume 46 (1995)
Cell Death
Edited by Lawrence M. Schwartz and Barbara A. Osborne

Volume 47 (1995)
Cilia and Flagella
Edited by William Dentler and George Witman

Volume 48 (1995)
***Caenorhabditis elegans:* Modern Biological Analysis of an Organism**
Edited by Henry F. Epstein and Diane C. Shakes

Volume 49 (1995)
Methods in Plant Cell Biology, Part A
Edited by David W. Galbraith, Hans J. Bohnert, and Don P. Bourque

Volume 50 (1995)
Methods in Plant Cell Biology, Part B
Edited by David W. Galbraith, Don P. Bourque, and Hans J. Bohnert

Volume 51 (1996)
Methods in Avian Embryology
Edited by Marianne Bronner-Fraser

ISBN 0-12-564153-2

90018